AI for Medical Image Analysis

Najib Ben Aoun • Sadique Ahmad •
Mohamed Hammad
Editors

AI for Medical Image Analysis

Reconciling Innovation and Ethical Considerations

Springer

Editors
Najib Ben Aoun
Al-Baha University
Al Aqiq, Saudi Arabia

Sadique Ahmad
Prince Sultan University
Riyadh, Saudi Arabia

Mohamed Hammad
Prince Sultan University
Riyadh, Saudi Arabia

ISBN 978-3-032-02962-1 ISBN 978-3-032-02963-8 (eBook)
https://doi.org/10.1007/978-3-032-02963-8

This Springer imprint is published by the registered company Springer Nature Switzerland AG
The registered company address is: Gewerbestrasse 11, 6330 Cham, Switzerland

Preface

The way doctors identify, treat, and manage illnesses has been completely transformed by the introduction of artificial intelligence (AI) into healthcare. The application of image processing and computer vision technologies is one of the most impactful advancements, which has boosted the accuracy and effectiveness of medical image analysis, enhanced treatment planning, and enabled more personalized care. With the use of these technologies, healthcare professionals may now "see beyond" the limits of conventional imaging techniques, gaining deeper understanding and more thorough analyses—both essential for efficient patient care.

However, applying AI techniques for medical image analysis has to be conducted while upholding the ethical considerations to ensure the technology benefits patients and healthcare providers while minimizing potential risks. In fact, it is essential to establish a thorough framework that incorporates stringent validation on diverse and representative datasets to mitigate bias and guarantee accuracy across different populations.

AI systems must exhibit transparency and explainability, enabling healthcare professionals to comprehend and trust their outputs, while accountability measures distinctly delineate responsibility for AI-generated judgments. In addition, AI systems have to support, not replace, the clinicians, guaranteeing that they continue to play a crucial role in decision-making. The development and deployment of AI-based medical image analysis systems have to be guided by ethical oversight committees to address any emerging issues.

This book, *AI for Medical Image Analysis: Reconciling Innovation and Ethical Considerations*, delves into the use of AI in medical image analysis while adhering to ethical considerations. It will cover the technological advancements, applications, strategies, and ethical considerations around the use of AI in healthcare imaging. It presents a holistic perspective on how AI-driven computer vision and image processing are reshaping the healthcare landscape and expanding the realm of what is conceivable for medical diagnostics and treatment.

We believe that as the area develops, this book will stimulate more investigation and creativity, which will eventually result in discoveries and uses. We are grateful to the contributors and reviewers who have helped make this work possible, and we are eager to see how it will affect the community.

Have fun reading the articles!

Al-Baha, Saudi Arabia Najib Ben Aoun

Acknowledgment First and foremost, we thank God for our excellent health and well-being, which allowed us to finish this book.

In addition, we would like to dedicate this book to our families.

Contents

Introduction to AI in Medical Image Analysis

Muhammad Umraiz, Asim Niaz, and Kwang Nam Choi

1 Introduction to Artificial Intelligence in Medical Imaging

Artificial Intelligence (AI) has emerged as a transformative force in healthcare, particularly in the field of medical imaging [45]. AI refers to a broad spectrum of computer techniques that enable machines to perform tasks requiring cognitive functions such as learning and decision-making. In healthcare, AI technologies can assist in diagnosing diseases, interpreting complex medical data, and even suggesting treatment options. Within medical imaging, AI algorithms—especially those based on machine learning—are capable of analyzing radiological images (such as X-rays [2], CT scans, MRIs, etc.) with high speed and accuracy, often matching or exceeding human expert performance in specific tasks. This potential to achieve radiologist-level accuracy has positioned AI as a pivotal innovation poised to revolutionize diagnostic imaging and improve patient care.

1.1 Overview of AI in Healthcare

In the broader healthcare landscape, AI techniques have been applied to diverse problems ranging from predictive analytics in electronic health records to personalized medicine [24]. Radiology and medical imaging have become leading domains for healthcare AI applications, in part due to the digital and visual nature of imaging data. Early applications of AI in medicine date back to expert systems in the 1970s and 1980s that attempted to assist in diagnosis using rule-based logic. However, it

M. Umraiz · A. Niaz (✉) · K. N. Choi
Department of Computer Science and Engineering, Chung-Ang University, Seoul, South Korea
e-mail: umraiz@vim.cau.ac.kr; asim@vim.cau.ac.kr

N. Ben Aoun et al. (eds.), *AI for Medical Image Analysis*,
https://doi.org/10.1007/978-3-032-02963-8_1

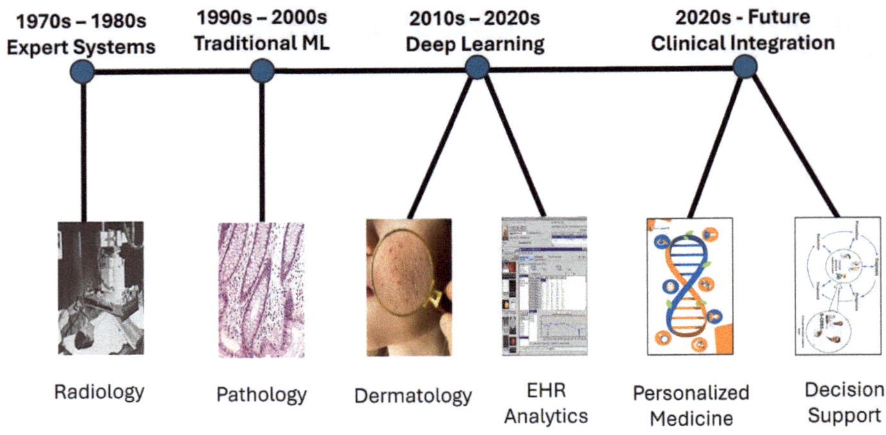

Fig. 1 Evolution of AI in healthcare and its key application areas across time

wasn't until the 2010s—with advances in machine learning (ML) and deep neural networks—that AI demonstrated dramatic improvements in performance and began to see serious adoption in clinical imaging. For example, modern deep learning models can detect pathologies in images such as tumors or lesions at times with performance comparable to human specialists. AI's presence in healthcare is rapidly growing: hospitals and clinics are beginning to integrate AI-based decision support tools for radiology, pathology, dermatology, and more [26]. The appeal lies in AI's ability to process large volumes of data efficiently and consistently, assisting doctors in making more accurate diagnoses and reducing human error. This is particularly important given the rising demand for medical imaging and the burden on radiologists to interpret an ever-increasing number of scans, as illustrated in Fig. 1.

1.2 Evolution of AI in Medical Imaging

The journey of AI in medical imaging has been a decades-long evolution [47]. Initial forays into computerized image analysis began with basic pattern recognition techniques in the late twentieth century. One historical milestone was in 1992, when a computer system was first utilized for detecting microcalcifications in mammography. These early Computer-Aided Detection (CAD) systems were fairly limited and rule-based, but they demonstrated that automated image analysis was possible. Through the 1990s and early 2000s, machine learning methods like decision trees, support vector machines, and Bayesian classifiers were explored for tasks such as lung nodule detection on chest X-rays and tumor classification. However, results were modest due to limitations in algorithms and computing power. The late 2000s to 2010s saw a paradigm shift with the rise of deep learning. In 2012, a deep convolutional neural network won the ImageNet competition in computer vision, heralding a new era for image analysis algorithms. This breakthrough quickly translated into medical imaging: researchers started applying deep convolutional neural networks (CNNs) to medical images with impressive results. By the mid-2010s, deep learning-based AI systems could outperform classical approaches and even match expert radiologists in certain tasks. For instance, a deep learning algorithm developed at Stanford called CheXNet was shown to detect pneumonia in chest X-rays at a level exceeding individual radiologists, while also highlighting on the image where the pneumonia is likely located.

Likewise, in breast cancer screening, a prospective study demonstrated that an AI system reading mammograms was non-inferior to a double-reading by two radiologists—essentially performing as well as experienced doctors in detecting cancers. These milestones mark how far AI in imaging has progressed: from simple experiments to robust models capable of near-human diagnostic performance. The evolution has been fueled by several factors: the availability of big data (large annotated medical image datasets), improvements in hardware (GPUs enabling faster training of deep networks), and algorithmic innovations. Today's AI in medical imaging builds upon decades of research and is characterized by sophisticated models that can learn complex patterns directly from image pixels.

1.3 Importance and Scope

The importance of AI in medical imaging cannot be overstated. Medical images are central to clinical decision-making—radiologists interpret scans to detect diseases, plan treatments, and monitor progress. AI has the potential to enhance this process in multiple ways [13, 39]. Firstly, AI can increase diagnostic accuracy: by catching subtle patterns or early signs of disease that might be missed by the human eye, thereby improving early detection. For example, AI algorithms have identified early signs of diabetic retinopathy in retinal images and early lung cancers in CT scans that are challenging for humans to discern.

Secondly, AI offers efficiency gains—an algorithm can analyze an image in seconds, which may help triage urgent cases (like flagging a brain hemorrhage on a scan for immediate attention) and reduce backlogs. This is crucial given that in many regions the number of images to be read far exceeds the capacity of available specialists. Thirdly, AI provides consistency; unlike humans, an algorithm's performance does not vary with fatigue or time of day—this consistency can reduce variability in interpretations. The scope of AI in imaging spans all medical imaging modalities and specialties: from radiology (X-rays, CT, MRI, ultrasound) to pathology (microscopic slides), cardiology (echocardiograms, angiography), ophthalmology (retinal scans), and beyond

Virtually any scenario where images are used for diagnosis or guidance, AI can play a supportive role. Furthermore, AI is extending imaging capabilities—for instance, helping generate quantitative measurements (like organ volumes, tumor diameters) automatically, which can support treatment planning. The impact also extends to healthcare accessibility: AI tools can assist less experienced practitioners or serve regions with a shortage of specialists. One notable statistic highlighting AI's growth is the market projection for AI in healthcare. The global market for AI in medical imaging is expected to grow roughly ten-fold over a decade—from about 21 billion in 2018 to an estimated 265 billion in 2028.

This reflects the enormous expectations and investment in this technology. In summary, AI's importance lies in its promise to augment human expertise, improve diagnostic accuracy and efficiency, and ultimately enhance patient outcomes. The scope continues to expand as new algorithms and applications are developed, making AI an integral part of the future of medical imaging.

2 Fundamental Concepts of AI in Medical Imaging

To appreciate the applications of AI in medical image analysis, it is essential to understand the fundamental concepts of how AI works in this context. The term AI encompasses a variety of approaches, but most current successes in image analysis are achieved through machine learning techniques, particularly deep learning [41]. This section will outline the basics of machine learning and deep learning as applied to medical imaging, and highlight key algorithms and architectures commonly used in this domain.

2.1 Basics of Machine Learning

Machine learning (ML) is a branch of AI focused on developing algorithms that can learn patterns from data and make predictions or decisions. In the context of medical imaging, an ML system might learn to distinguish between normal and abnormal scans by training on a collection of labeled examples [38, 43]. The two primary learning paradigms in ML are supervised learning and unsupervised learning.

In supervised learning, the algorithm is trained on input images paired with known output labels (for example, MRI scans with labels indicating the presence or absence of a tumor). Through this training process, the model "learns" a mapping from image to label, enabling it to predict labels for new, unseen images. Supervised learning can address tasks like classification (e.g., classify an X-ray as showing pneumonia or not) or regression (e.g., predict the volume of an organ from a scan).

Unsupervised learning, on the other hand, involves learning from images without explicit labels. The goal in unsupervised learning may be to discover inherent structures or patterns in the data—for instance, clustering images into groups that share similar features, or detecting anomalies that deviate from normal patterns. An example in imaging would be training a model on a large number of normal images so that it can later identify an outlier image that looks abnormal (useful for

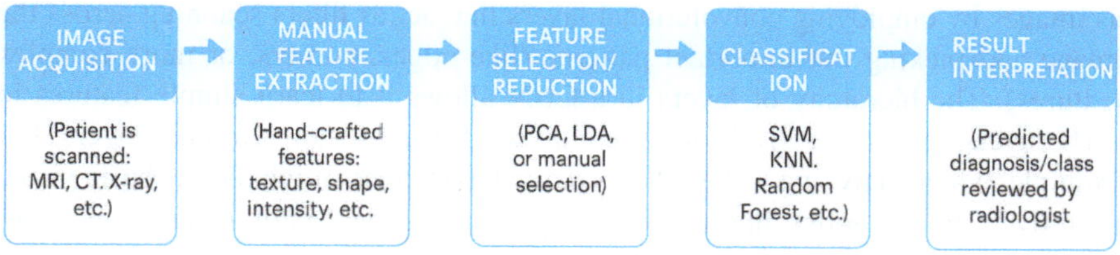

Fig. 2 Traditional machine learning workflow for medical imaging, involving manual feature extraction and classification using algorithms like SVM or KNN

anomaly detection). Another unsupervised approach is dimensionality reduction, where complex image data is distilled into a simpler representation (e.g., using algorithms like PCA—Principal Component Analysis). In practice, supervised learning has been the dominant approach in medical image analysis, because many tasks (diagnosis, segmentation) have clear definitions of desired output that can be used to train models. However, obtaining labeled medical images can be labor-intensive (requiring expert annotation), so unsupervised and semi-supervised techniques are also explored to leverage large amounts of unlabeled data. In addition to these learning modes, reinforcement learning is a third paradigm where an agent learns by interacting with an environment and receiving feedback. While less common in image interpretation, reinforcement learning has niche uses in medical imaging such as optimizing imaging device parameters or navigating robotic surgery tools under imaging guidance.

A traditional machine learning workflow for medical imaging, as shown in Fig. 2, typically involved first extracting hand-crafted features from images and then training a classifier on those features. Early systems relied on features like edges, textures, or shapes identified by algorithms (for example, using edge detectors or Haralick texture features) and then used classifiers such as support vector machines (SVMs), k-nearest neighbors (KNN), or random forests to classify images based on those features. These classical methods had some success—indeed, SVMs were long popular for medical image classification—but they often plateaued because designing effective features by hand is challenging. This is where deep learning changed the game: deep learning algorithms automatically learn the features from the raw images, eliminating the need for manual feature engineering and often achieving far superior performance.

2.2 *Deep Learning Techniques and Architectures*

Deep learning refers to neural network algorithms with multiple layers ("deep" refers to having many layers of neurons) that can learn rich representations of data. In image analysis, the most prevalent deep learning architecture is the Convolutional Neural Network (CNN). CNNs are specially designed to process grid-like data such as images by employing convolutional layers that act as filters scanning across the image and picking out important patterns (like edges, corners, or more complex textures). The hierarchy of layers in a CNN allows it to learn simple features in early layers and progressively more complex, abstract features in later layers. For example, when analyzing a chest X-ray, early CNN layers might detect basic visual primitives (lines, blobs), intermediate layers might detect parts of anatomy (ribs, lung fields), and deeper layers might recognize high-level indicators of disease (an opacity in the lung that suggests pneumonia). This automatic feature learning is a key advantage of deep learning over earlier approaches [42].

Several deep network architectures have been influential in medical imaging. LeNet-5 was one of the first CNNs (developed for digit recognition) [52], but modern CNNs are far deeper. AlexNet (2012) demonstrated the power of deep CNNs on general images and spurred adoption in other domains. Later architectures like VGG (which showed the effect of depth with many convolution layers), ResNet (which introduced skip connections to allow very deep networks of 50+ layers without training degradation) and DenseNet (which connects each layer to subsequent layers to encourage feature reuse) have all been applied successfully to medical image tasks. In fact, many medical AI models use these architectures (or their variants) as backbones. For instance, a deep network for classifying brain tumors might use a ResNet or DenseNet architecture as its core for feature extraction [14]. Researchers also commonly use transfer learning: taking a CNN model pre-trained on a large general image dataset (like ImageNet) and fine-tuning it on medical images. This leverages learned feature representations and is very useful when medical data is limited.

Beyond classification, deep learning architectures have been devised for other tasks like segmentation and detection. A notable architecture for image segmentation is the U-Net, which was originally developed for biomedical image segmentation [40]. U-Net has an encoder-decoder structure: the encoder path is like a regular CNN that downsamples the image (capturing context and features), and the decoder path upsamples to produce a pixel-wise prediction map, with skip connections linking corresponding levels of the encoder and decoder. This design allows U-Net to precisely localize structures in images. U-Nets and their variants are now standard for segmentation problems (for example, delineating tumor boundaries on MRI or segmenting organs on CT scans). For object detection in images (identifying and localizing findings, e.g., detecting and bounding a lung nodule in a CT slice), there are deep learning models like R-CNN and YOLO that are used in general computer vision and have been adapted to medical images to pinpoint lesions with bounding boxes or contours.

Another important set of deep learning models are Generative Adversarial Networks (GANs). GANs consist of two networks (a generator and a discriminator) that compete, leading the generator to learn how to create synthetic data that mimics real data. In medical imaging, GANs have been used for data augmentation (generating realistic synthetic medical images to expand training datasets), for image improvement (e.g., converting low-resolution or low-dose images into higher quality images), and even for modality translation (such as generating a pseudo-MRI from a CT scan). For example, GAN-based models can produce enhanced images from noisy low-dose CT scans, potentially enabling lower radiation doses while maintaining image quality [44].

Beyond classification, segmentation is a major AI application of Vision Transformers and large vision-language models applied to imaging. Transformers, which have revolutionized NLP, are now being explored for medical images as well, sometimes in combination with CNNs or as part of multi-modal models that can handle images and text (such as radiology reports). These are cutting-edge research areas aiming to create "foundation models" that could understand a variety of medical images with minimal task-specific training.

In summary, deep learning techniques—especially CNN-based architectures—form the backbone of modern AI in medical image analysis. Key architectures include CNNs for classification and detection, encoder-decoder networks like U-Net for segmentation, and GANs for generative tasks and enhancement. The algorithmic toolkit in medical imaging also still includes some classic ML algorithms (like random forests or SVMs) in applications where deep learning might not be feasible or necessary, but the trend overwhelmingly favors deep learning due to its superior performance on image recognition tasks.

2.3 Key Algorithms Used in Medical Imaging

To highlight specific algorithms commonly encountered in this field: Convolutional Neural Networks (CNNs): As discussed, CNNs (and their many variants) are the primary algorithm for image classification, lesion detection, and even patch-based analysis in pathology slides. Networks such as ResNet (with skip connections) have been used to classify diseases on X-rays, while DenseNet was employed in a well-known chest X-ray study (CheXNet) to detect multiple pathologies [37]. These deep CNNs have millions of parameters and require large datasets and computational power to train, but they excel at learning image features.

Segmentation Networks: The U-Net and derived architectures (V-Net for 3D data, etc.) are standard for segmentation. They allow pixel-level labeling, for example segmenting a brain tumor on MRI or outlining the heart muscle on an ultrasound. There are also fully convolutional networks (FCNs) and more recent transformer-based segmenters, but U-Net remains highly popular in medical challenges due to its effectiveness on biomedical images.

Ensembles and Hybrid Models: In some cases, combining models can yield better results. Ensembles of CNNs (multiple networks voting or averaged) are used to improve robustness. There are also hybrid approaches that integrate deep learning with classical techniques—for instance, using CNNs to generate features which are then fed into a traditional classifier, or combining multiple algorithms (one to detect a region of interest, another to classify it).

Support Vector Machines (SVM) and Other ML: Before deep learning dominance, SVMs were a go-to algorithm for many medical imaging tasks, such as classifying tissue samples or breast cancer lesions using pre-extracted features [17].

Decision trees and ensembles like random forests have been used for tasks like identifying disease patterns in scans (they are still occasionally used in radiomics pipelines where engineered features are extracted from images). While these algorithms may not reach the accuracy of CNNs on large image datasets, they can perform well on smaller problems or when paired with good feature extraction. They also tend to be more interpretable, which is why some radiology researchers still explore these simpler models for certain problems where interpretability is crucial.

Clustering and Anomaly Detection Algorithms: Unsupervised algorithms like k-means clustering, autoencoders, and One-Class SVMs find use in anomaly detection—for example, learning what healthy anatomy looks like and then flagging an outlier image that might contain a pathology. Variational autoencoders (VAEs) and other deep generative models can detect anomalies by reconstructing an image and highlighting differences.

Reinforcement Learning: A niche but interesting use is in optimizing imaging procedures. For example, reinforcement learning algorithms have been investigated to plan MRI sequences or to control the movement of an ultrasound probe to get the best image. They are also used in treatment settings like radiation therapy planning, where an AI agent learns to modify beam settings based on feedback (though this crosses into treatment rather than pure imaging analysis).

It is also worth noting that data preprocessing and augmentation algorithms are key parts of applying AI to medical images. Techniques to normalize image intensity, crop or resize images, and augment data (rotations, flips, adding noise, etc.) are routinely used to make the algorithms more robust. These are not "AI algorithms" per se, but they are an important aspect of the pipeline that improves model performance.In summary, the fundamental concepts of AI in medical imaging revolve around teaching machines to recognize patterns in images. Traditional ML provided the foundation, but deep learning has vastly expanded the capabilities. Understanding these basics—how supervised learning works, what a CNN does, how a U-Net segments an image—is crucial for researchers and practitioners who aim to develop or utilize AI tools in medical imaging. With these concepts in hand, we can explore the myriad applications of AI across different imaging modalities. Table 1 provides an overview of key AI algorithms used in medical imaging, highlighting their types, examples, and primary applications.

3 Applications of AI in Imaging Modalities

AI techniques have now been applied across all major medical imaging modalities, enhancing image interpretation and clinical decision support in each domain. In this section, we examine how AI is used in Magnetic Resonance Imaging (MRI), Computed Tomography (CT), Ultrasound, and other imaging modalities such as X-rays and nuclear imaging [46]. For each modality, we will discuss representative applications and highlight case studies or practical examples that demonstrate AI's capabilities in real clinical scenarios, as summarized in Fig. 3.

Table 1 Key AI algorithms in medical imaging

Algorithm category	Examples	Medical image analysis applications
Machine learning algorithms	SVM, KNN, k-Means, Random Forest, XGBoost	Classification, segmentation, radiomics analysis, outlier/anomaly detection, feature selection, and small dataset analysis
Deep learning algorithms	CNN, ResNet, DenseNet, U-Net, FCN, V-Net, GAN, Autoencoder	Image classification, lesion/tumor detection, organ and tissue segmentation, pathology analysis, image synthesis, reconstruction, and denoising
Ensemble learning	Random Forest, XGBoost, CNN Ensembles, Hybrid Models	Robust prediction, multi-stage analysis, region classification, improved generalization and robustness
Reinforcement learning	Q-Learning, Deep Q-Network (DQN), Policy Gradient, Actor-Critic	Imaging parameter optimization, robotic navigation, ultrasound probe control, automated view planning

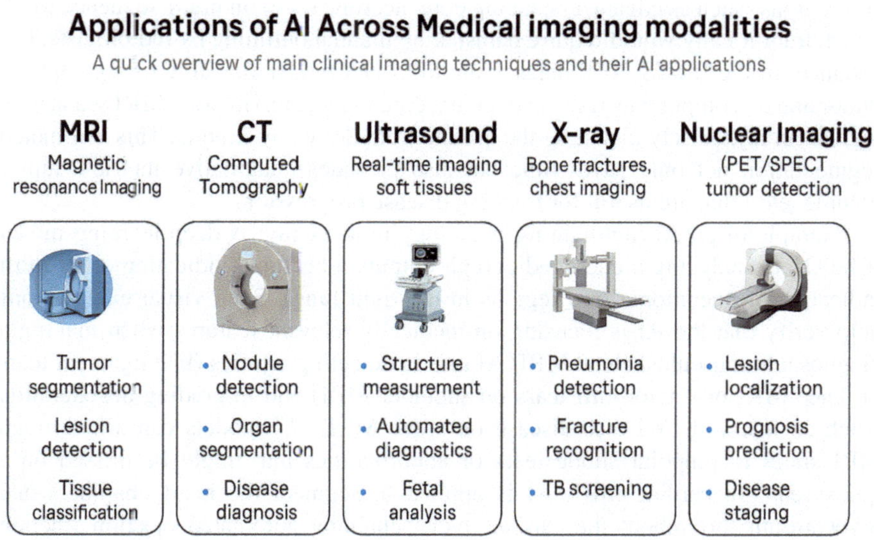

Fig. 3 Applications of AI across major medical imaging modalities, highlighting key clinical use cases in MRI, CT, ultrasound, X-ray, and nuclear imaging

3.1 Magnetic Resonance Imaging (MRI)

MRI is a powerful imaging modality that provides detailed images of soft tissues, making it invaluable for neurological, musculoskeletal, abdominal, and cardiovascular imaging, among others [19]. AI has been leveraged extensively in MRI for tasks ranging from detection of abnormalities to image enhancement [6]. One of the prominent applications is in neuroimaging. For example, AI algorithms can assist in identifying neurological disorders: deep learning models have been trained on brain MRIs to detect conditions like Alzheimer's disease, multiple sclerosis lesions, or brain tumors. In one study, researchers at Mount Sinai used deep learning on brain MR images to successfully identify features associated with Alzheimer's disease. Similarly, for brain tumors, AI can both detect and classify tumor types. A deep CNN applied to MRI scans achieved an impressive 98.5% accuracy in classifying types of brain tumors in one experiment, distinguishing, for instance, between gliomas of different grades. This level of accuracy approaches that of expert neuroradiologists, showing AI's potential in supporting brain tumor diagnosis.

Beyond classification, segmentation is a major AI application in MRI. Segmenting tumors, organs, or other structures in MRI images is vital for surgical planning and treatment. AI models like U-Net have been widely used to automatically segment brain tumors in MRI (as part of challenges like the Brain Tumor Segmentation BraTS challenge). These models can delineate the tumor's boundaries and even its sub-regions (such as edema, enhancing core, necrotic core) on multi-sequence MRI, which traditionally would require painstaking manual outlining by radiologists. For instance, in the BraTS 2019 dataset, an AI U-Net model was able to segment the tumor and its components (edema in green, core in red, etc.) in brain MRI scans with high accuracy, closely matching the ground truth drawn by experts. This automated segmentation not only saves time but also provides quantitative metrics (tumor volume, etc.) that are useful for tracking disease progression.

Example of an AI highlighting pathology in an X-ray: A deep learning model (CheXNet) analyzing a chest radiograph outputs a heatmap indicating areas most indicative of pneumonia (red regions in the right lung). Such visual explanations help verify that the AI is focusing on medically relevant features when making a diagnosis.In musculoskeletal MRI, AI aids in detecting injuries (like ligament tears on knee MRI or rotator cuff tears on shoulder MRI) and in grading degeneration (such as intervertebral disc disease on spine MRI). AI models can sift through MRI slices to pinpoint subtle tears or abnormalities that might be missed on a quick read. In cardiac MRI, AI is applied to segment the heart chambers and myocardium throughout the cardiac cycle, enabling automated ejection fraction calculations and detection of wall-motion abnormalities. This has significant implications for diagnosing cardiomyopathies or ischemic heart disease faster and more consistently.Another exciting area is MRI image reconstruction and enhancement. Deep learning is being used to reconstruct MRI images from undersampled data, effectively accelerating MRI scans. By allowing fewer measurements and then using AI to fill in the missing information, one can obtain good quality images much faster—a technique known as AI-assisted accelerated MRI. This is transformative because MRI scans are often lengthy; reducing scan time improves patient comfort and increases scanner throughput. AI-driven reconstruction has shown that even when an MRI is done at a lower resolution or with faster (but noisier) sequences, a neural network can upscale or denoise the image to high quality. This concept is akin to having a smart "photoshop" for MRI that makes a fast, low-detail scan look like a slower, high-detail one, and it's enabled by training on lots of image data.

3.2 Computed Tomography (CT)

CT scans provide cross-sectional images using X-rays and are widely used for imaging the chest, abdomen, head, and vascular structures [3, 50]. AI applications in CT imaging are prolific, especially in the areas of detection and quantification [51]. One of the earliest successes of medical imaging AI was in lung CT: for screening and diagnosing lung cancer. AI algorithms can automatically detect pulmonary nodules (small potential tumors) on CT scans of the lungs. These nodules can be very tiny and easily overlooked, but AI CAD (computer-aided detection) systems highlight them for the radiologist. Modern deep learning detectors go further, characterizing nodules to suggest which are likely benign and which suspicious for cancer, thus aiding in lung cancer screening programs. The FDA has approved multiple AI tools for this purpose, given lung cancer's high mortality if not caught early.

AI has also been instrumental during the COVID-19 pandemic by analyzing chest CT scans. Early in the pandemic, AI models were developed to detect COVID-19 pneumonia patterns on lung CT and even quantify the extent of infection (percentage of lung involvement) to help assess severity. This quantitative analysis by AI could track patient progress (e.g., how lung opacities clear or worsen over time). Beyond COVID-19, for typical pneumonias or other lung diseases, AI can flag areas of consolidation or fibrosis on CT.

In neuroimaging with CT, one critical application is detecting strokes and intracranial hemorrhages on head CT scans [8]. Time is absolutely critical in stroke—faster diagnosis can enable quicker treatment (like thrombolytic therapy for ischemic stroke). AI-powered triage software is now in use in some hospitals: the moment a head CT is done, the AI algorithm analyzes it within seconds and if it detects a hemorrhage or large vessel occlusion, it sends an urgent alert to the radiologist and stroke team. This can cut down the notification time for critical findings dramatically. Studies have shown these AI tools achieve high sensitivity in detecting intracerebral hemorrhages, sometimes finding tiny hemorrhages that might be subtle for human readers. The result is that patient outcomes can improve because treatment is administered sooner for conditions like stroke or head trauma bleeding.

In abdominal CT, AI assists in tasks such as identifying liver lesions, classifying kidney tumors, or detecting colon polyps on CT colonography. For example, AI can help differentiate a small benign cyst in the liver from a small metastasis, based on learned texture and contrast patterns. In oncology, whole-body CT scans can be laboriously assessed by AI to find enlarged lymph nodes or new lesions, which is valuable in cancer staging and follow-up.

Another important contribution of AI in CT is quantification and risk prediction. CT scans can be quantitatively analyzed for markers that predict disease. For instance, calcium scoring on cardiac CT (for coronary artery disease risk) can be automated by AI—the algorithm identifies calcifications in coronary arteries and measures their volume and density to produce a calcium score. This was traditionally done manually, but AI can do it in a fraction of the time. Similarly, bone mineral density can be opportunistically measured by AI from routine CT scans to flag patients at risk of osteoporosis, even if the scan was done for another reason. In lung CT, AI can quantify emphysema, air trapping, or fibrosis patterns, giving doctors objective metrics of disease burden.

It's also worth noting that like MRI, CT benefits from AI in image enhancement. Low-dose CT is desirable to reduce radiation exposure, but it results in noisier images. AI algorithms (often using deep learning noise reduction or even GANs) can clean up low-dose CT images to make them nearly as good as standard dose, enabling safer imaging practices.

3.3 *Ultrasound and Other Modalities*

Ultrasound imaging is a real-time, operator-dependent modality used widely in obstetrics, cardiology (echocardiography), and point-of-care examinations (like FAST scans in trauma) [5, 25]. Ultrasound images can be harder for AI because they are noisy and vary with the operator's skill and angle of acquisition. Nonetheless, AI is making inroads in ultrasound as well. One area is in automated interpretation of obstetric ultrasound [21]. For example, determining fetal gestational age and position is crucial during pregnancy. Google Health recently demonstrated an AI approach where even non-expert operators could perform an ultrasound sweep of a pregnant abdomen, and an AI model would interpret it to determine things like the baby's gestational age and orientation with accuracy comparable to experienced sonographers. This has huge potential for increasing access to prenatal ultrasound in low-resource settings, where trained sonographers are scarce. By following a simple protocol and letting AI analyze the images, mid-level health providers could screen pregnant patients effectively.

In cardiology, echocardiograms (heart ultrasounds) are being analyzed by AI to measure heart function automatically [35]. An AI tool can, for instance, identify the chamber borders in each frame of an echo and compute ejection fraction (how much blood the heart pumps out), detect valve malfunctions, or see if the heart muscle motion is abnormal in any region (suggesting an infarct). Some deep learning models have shown ability to interpret echocardiograms at a level approaching cardiologists—even identifying subtle hypertrophy or early heart failure signs.

Automating these measurements can save clinicians a lot of time and ensure consistency in results.

In general ultrasound (e.g., abdominal ultrasound), AI can help in recognizing organs and lesions. An AI system can guide a less experienced user by recognizing that, say, the current view is a transverse section of the liver and highlighting if any lesion is present. Efforts are also underway to use AI for standardizing image acquisition—for instance, prompting the user to adjust probe position if the AI sees that an optimal view is not yet obtained (like telling the user to rotate slightly to see the whole kidney).

X-rays (Radiography) imaging is one of the "other modalities" where AI has had a huge impact. Chest X-rays, being the most common imaging exam globally, have been a major focus [15]. AI models (like the aforementioned CheXNet) can detect a variety of findings on chest X-rays—from pneumonia, pleural effusions, and pneumothorax to nodules and signs of heart failure. These algorithms often output both a probability of a condition and a heatmap localizing the regions of the image associated with that condition (providing some explainability, as shown in the example figure above with pneumonia). In clinical use, such AI tools can serve as a second reader, assisting radiologists by ensuring no important finding is missed (for example, if the radiologist overlook a small pneumothorax on a busy day, the AI might flag it). There are case studies of AI detecting tuberculosis on chest X-rays in screening programs with accuracy high enough that it's being deployed in areas with limited radiologist availability—the AI screens out normal X-rays and refers only suspicious ones for further review, greatly improving efficiency of TB screening.

Mammography (a specialized X-ray for breast cancer screening) is another area with extensive AI application [48, 49]. Mammograms are challenging to interpret and historically had computer-aided detection systems since the 1990s. Modern AI has revitalized mammography CAD. Deep learning algorithms can identify calcifications, masses, and architectural distortions with high sensitivity. More interestingly, AI is used to assess the risk from a mammogram: research has shown that patterns in a mammogram (even if no overt tumor is visible) can predict a woman's future risk of developing breast cancer. AI models have been trained to analyze a mammogram and output a risk score for developing cancer in the next 5 years. In one study, an AI system assigned the highest risk scores to 87.6% of cases that were screen-detected cancers, indicating that AI can stratify which patients might need more vigilant surveillance. These risk models could personalize screening intervals in the future.

Nuclear Medicine (PET/SPECT) AI is also being applied to modalities like PET (Positron Emission Tomography) and SPECT, often in combination with CT or MRI (as in PET/CT or PET/MR) [28, 33]. For instance, in oncology, a PET scan highlights metabolic activity (like uptake of a glucose analog in FDG-PET). AI can automatically delineate areas of abnormal uptake (identifying tumors or metastases) and even quantify it (standardized uptake values) to help in treatment response assessment. Additionally, there are efforts to use AI to improve image quality in nuclear medicine; similar to low-dose CT, PET scans with lower dose or shorter acquisition time (hence noisier images) can be cleaned up by AI to look like full-dose scans, potentially reducing radiation or speeding up scans.

Pathology and Ophthalmology (Other Imaging Domains) Expanding "other modalities" to include pathology slides and retinal images (which are types of medical images too), AI has made remarkable achievements [16, 23]. In digital pathology, whole-slide images are extremely large (gigapixel images of tissue biopsies). AI can scan through a pathology slide to find regions that contain cancer cells (for example, identifying metastatic tumor in a lymph node biopsy slide) and even grade tumors or detect subtle features (like perineural invasion or lymphovascular invasion) that are important for prognosis. These tasks are like finding needles in haystacks due to slide size, and AI's exhaustive and tireless analysis is well-suited to assist pathologists. In ophthalmology, AI applied to retinal fundus photographs can detect diabetic retinopathy, glaucoma, and age-related macular degeneration signs with very high accuracy. One of the first instances of FDA approval for an autonomous AI system was an AI for diabetic retinopathy screening that can be used in a primary care setting without a specialist: it takes a retinal photo and immediately tells if more evaluation is needed, allowing earlier intervention and treatment to prevent vision loss.

3.4 *Case Studies and Practical Examples*

To ground these applications in concrete examples, let's briefly survey a few:

- Neurological MRI Case: An AI model for anomaly detection in brain MRIs was deployed to screen for any unusual findings in scans taken for various reasons. In a reported case, the AI flagged a subtle abnormal signal in the hippocampus region of a patient's brain MRI that the radiologist had initially not commented on. On closer inspection, it turned out to be an early sign of sclerosis that correlated with the patient's history of seizures, thus aiding in an earlier diagnosis of epilepsy. This kind of anomaly detection (where the AI knows what "normal" looks like and alerts when something deviates) can be a safety net in busy clinical workflows.
- Brain Tumor Classification: Researchers trained a CNN on hundreds of brain MRI scans labeled with the type of tumor determined by biopsy. The AI learned to differentiate glioblastomas from lower-grade gliomas and metastases, achieving over 95% accuracy. In practice, this could support radiologists by providing a second opinion on the likely tumor type before surgery, potentially guiding how aggressive a surgery or therapy to plan. Moreover, another team in the UK developed a non-invasive AI technique using diffusion-weighted MRI to classify pediatric brain tumors, avoiding the need for immediate biopsy in some cases. By analyzing water molecule diffusion patterns in the MRI, their AI could distinguish tumor types with high accuracy, illustrating how AI might reduce invasive procedures.

- Chest X-Ray TB Screening: In a public health project, an AI system was used to screen chest X-ray images for tuberculosis (TB) in rural clinics. The system processed each X-ray in seconds and gave a score of how likely TB was present. Patients above a certain score were flagged for further testing (sputum tests or expert review). This deployment found numerous TB cases that would have otherwise been missed due to lack of radiologists, demonstrating AI's value in resource-limited settings. The sensitivity of the AI was comparable to experienced radiologists, and it significantly reduced the burden on the few specialists available by filtering out normals.
- Mammography AI in Practice: A recent study in Sweden integrated an AI tool to read screening mammograms alongside radiologists. The AI would mark suspicious areas and provide a cancer risk score for each mammogram. They found that using the AI as an aid increased cancer detection slightly and could potentially allow for single-radiologist reading (with AI as the second reader) instead of the traditional two radiologist review, with no loss in accuracy. This could make screening programs more efficient. However, the study also noted that the AI might not catch every cancer the humans do (and vice versa), underscoring that collaboration between AI and human readers is likely the optimal approach.
- Automated Ultrasound for Fetal Health: A practical example comes from rural healthcare where midwives used a handheld ultrasound device. Guided by an AI (which told them if the angle was correct and when to capture an image), they performed "blind sweeps" over the abdomen. The AI later interpreted these sweeps to determine fetal presentation (whether the baby is head-down or breech) and estimate gestational age by analyzing anatomical landmarks. In trials, this AI's assessments matched those of expert sonographers in a majority of cases. This suggests that in areas with no sonographers, AI could help fill the gap by enabling basic ultrasound exams for pregnant women, improving prenatal care.

These examples illustrate not only the breadth of AI applications across modalities but also how AI is being practically used to solve real clinical problems—from speeding up image analysis and reducing errors to expanding access to diagnostic imaging in underserved areas. Each imaging modality presents unique challenges (for instance, MRI's varied sequences, CT's radiation and resolution issues, ultrasound's operator dependence), yet AI techniques have shown adaptability in tackling each of these and enhancing what clinicians can do with the modality.

4 AI for Automated Image Analysis

A core promise of AI in medical imaging is automation—the ability for machines to perform image analysis tasks automatically that would otherwise require extensive human time and effort. In this section, we delve into specific automated image analysis tasks powered by AI, including anomaly detection and diagnosis, image

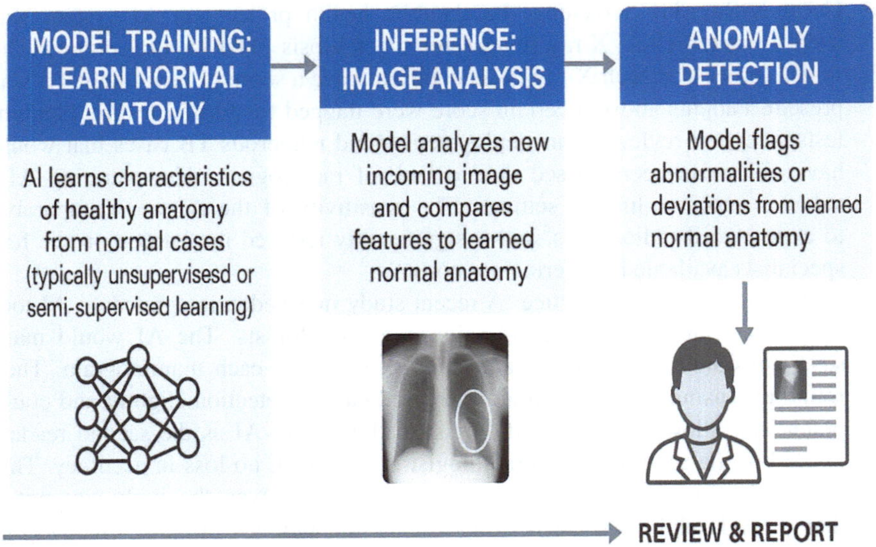

Fig. 4 Concise workflow illustrating the progression of AI applications in medical imaging for anomaly detection, highlighting learning from normal anatomy and flagging abnormalities

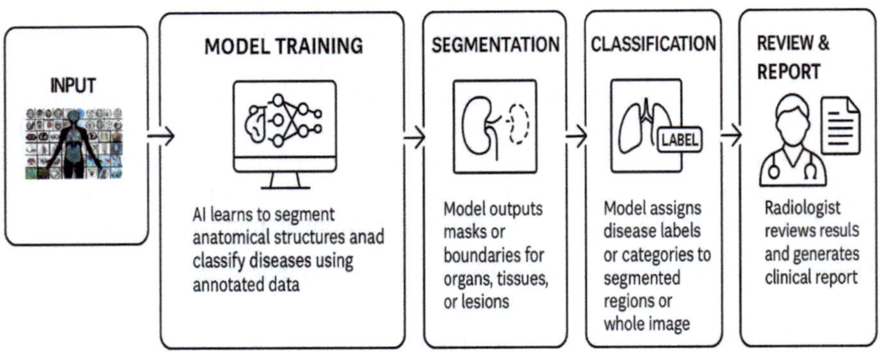

Fig. 5 Concise workflow illustrating the progression of AI applications in medical imaging for image segmentation and classification, outlining structure delineation and disease labeling

segmentation and classification, and predictive modeling in clinical contexts. These tasks form the crux of how AI systems assist clinicians: by sifting through images to find abnormalities, categorizing findings, quantifying structures, and even predicting patient outcomes or disease trajectories based on imaging data. AI systems streamline critical imaging tasks such as detecting abnormalities, segmenting structures, classifying findings, and predicting clinical outcomes, as illustrated in the workflows shown in Figs. 4, 5 and 6.

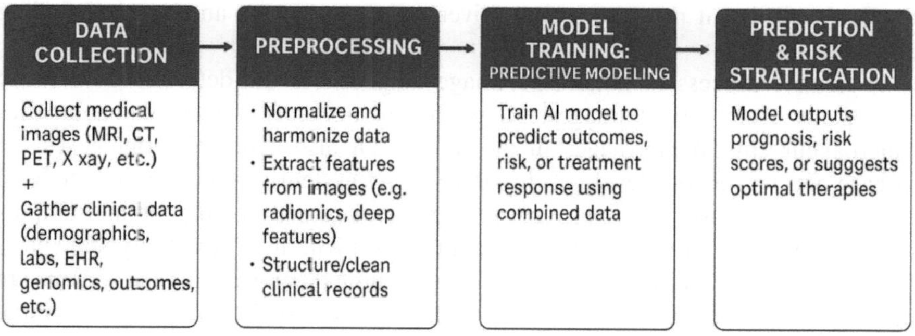

Fig. 6 Concise workflow depicting the progression of AI applications in medical imaging for predictive modeling. The process integrates medical image features and clinical data to enable prognosis, risk stratification, and personalized treatment planning, supporting clinical decision-making at every stage

4.1 Anomaly Detection and Diagnosis

Anomaly detection refers to identifying unusual or abnormal findings in data [32]. Traditional diagnostic processes rely on clinicians to notice anything out of the ordinary in an image. AI anomaly detection systems aim to replicate this ability by learning what normal anatomy looks like and then flagging regions in an image that deviate from the norm [53]. For example, an AI model might be trained on thousands of normal chest X-rays. When it encounters a new X-ray, it compares it to the learned profile of normal and if there's something like an unexpected shadow or nodule, it highlights it as a potential anomaly. This is particularly useful in scenarios like screening, where the prevalence of abnormality is low—the AI can quickly dismiss normal studies and draw attention to the few that need detailed review. Some AI systems use deep generative models (like variational autoencoders) for this: they reconstruct an input image in their learned normal way, and any significant difference between the reconstructed (normal) image and the actual image can indicate an abnormal region.

Once an anomaly is detected, the next step is diagnosis, i.e., determining what that anomaly represents. AI algorithms are increasingly capable of providing differential diagnoses for image findings. For instance, if a lung nodule is detected on CT, an AI could analyze its shape, margins, density, and behavior across phases to suggest whether it's likely a benign granuloma, a malignant tumor, or an infectious lesion. In brain MRI, an anomaly in white matter might be classified by AI as more consistent with multiple sclerosis plaques versus small vessel ischemic changes, based on characteristics like location and appearance on different sequences. These diagnostic suggestions are typically arrived at through classification algorithms trained on datasets where the ground truth diagnosis is known (often confirmed by biopsy, surgery, or follow-up). AI thus acts as a diagnostic assistant: it doesn't make the final call, but it provides a data-driven opinion on what an abnormal finding could be.

A notable success in automated image diagnosis is the detection of diabetic retinopathy from retinal images. Here, the AI not only detects the anomalies (microaneurysms, hemorrhages in the retina) but also essentially diagnoses the disease and its severity level [1]. In 2018, an AI system for autonomous diabetic retinopathy detection was approved: it examines a retinal photograph and outputs if referable diabetic retinopathy is present (yes/no) with high sensitivity and specificity, effectively performing an automated screening diagnosis. Similar systems are being developed for skin lesions—an AI can look at a dermoscopic image of a mole and decide if it's suspicious for melanoma (the anomaly being irregular structure) or likely benign.

An important aspect of AI-driven anomaly detection is minimizing false negatives (missed abnormalities). The systems are often tuned to be very sensitive so as to catch anything potentially important. This sometimes comes at the cost of more false positives (flagging things that turn out normal), but as a second reader or screening tool, high sensitivity is usually desired. Over time, as these systems incorporate more data, including negative feedback when radiologists disagree with AI, the goal is to improve specificity as well, so that the AI alerts become increasingly reliable.

4.2 Image Segmentation and Classification

Image segmentation is the process of dividing an image into meaningful regions or objects to facilitate analysis, often used in medical imaging for tasks like tumor detection and organ delineation [29–31]. Image segmentation and classification are two cornerstone tasks in medical image analysis that AI automates. Image segmentation involves partitioning an image into meaningful regions—essentially drawing boundaries around structures of interest (organs, lesions, etc.) or labeling each pixel/voxel with a class (tumor, normal tissue, blood vessel, background, etc.) [4]. Manual segmentation by experts is extremely time-consuming. For example, delineating a brain tumor on dozens of MRI slices can take a radiologist or technician a couple of hours. AI can perform the same segmentation in seconds once trained. Segmentation is crucial for quantifying volumes (like tumor size), for surgical and radiation therapy planning (knowing exact extents), and for tracking changes over time.

Deep learning has greatly advanced segmentation quality. Models like U-Net can often achieve segmentations that closely match an expert's manual contour. Automated segmentation has been applied to numerous problems: demarcating the heart chambers in cardiac MRI, segmenting the liver and any lesions in abdominal CT, outlining cartilage on knee MRI, segmenting neonatal brain structures on ultrasound, and more. In radiotherapy, AI-generated segmentations of tumors and organs-at-risk from planning CT scans can dramatically speed up the treatment planning process, which traditionally required manual contouring of each slice by an oncologist. With AI doing the initial contour, the physician only needs to fine-tune it, saving valuable time.

Segmentation is not just binary (object vs background); it can be multi-class. For instance, in pathology, an AI might segment a slide into regions of tumor, stroma, necrosis, etc. Or in ophthalmology OCT scans, segment the different layers of the retina and any abnormal fluid regions. Meanwhile, image classification is about assigning a label to an entire image or an identified region. In medical imaging, classification tasks include things like classifying an image as normal vs abnormal, classifying the disease present (pneumonia vs heart failure markings on a chest X-ray), or determining the grade of a finding (e.g., mild, moderate, severe osteoarthritis on a knee X-ray). Classification often goes hand-in-hand with detection: first detect a lesion, then classify what type of lesion it is. For example, an AI system could detect multiple lung nodules on a CT scan and then classify each one as likely benign or suspicious. Similarly, an algorithm could detect that there is a fracture on a limb X-ray and classify the fracture type (transverse, oblique, comminuted, etc.).

One successful example of classification is in breast imaging: AI algorithms can classify mammogram findings or whole mammograms on a BI-RADS scale (the standardized category for suspicion of malignancy). They analyze the shapes and patterns of calcifications and masses and assign a category that correlates with cancer likelihood. Another example is liver lesions on MRI: AI can look at dynamic contrast-enhanced MRI sequences and classify a lesion as a hemangioma vs cyst vs hepatocellular carcinoma vs metastasis by recognizing their characteristic enhancement patterns. Such classification aids radiologists in making the correct diagnosis without always needing an invasive biopsy.

It's worth highlighting AI's role in multi-label classification on images. Medical images can have multiple findings. A chest X-ray might show cardiomegaly, nodules, and a pleural effusion all at once. AI models (often deep CNNs) have been trained to output probabilities for a range of possible findings on a single image. For instance, one deep learning model given a chest X-ray might output: 90% probability of cardiomegaly, 70% probability of pleural effusion, 5% probability of pneumonia, etc., effectively classifying the presence or absence of dozens of pathologies simultaneously. This comprehensive classification capability is something that can greatly assist radiologists by ensuring all aspects of an image are considered.

4.3 Predictive Modeling in Clinical Contexts

Beyond interpreting what is in an image, AI is increasingly used to correlate imaging findings with broader clinical predictions—essentially using images (sometimes in combination with other data) to predict future outcomes or guide clinical management [12]. This is where predictive modeling comes in. In a clinical context, we may ask questions like: Given this patient's scans (and possibly other info), what is the likelihood of a certain outcome? AI models can analyze imaging features (some visible, some subtle or abstract) to predict things like disease progression, treatment response, or even survival.

One example of this is in oncology prognosis. After a cancer is diagnosed and imaged (say a CT scan of lung cancer), an AI model could be used to extract a large number of features from the tumor's image (size, shape, texture heterogeneity, etc.—a field often called radiomics) and then predict the likelihood that the cancer will respond to chemotherapy, or the risk of recurrence after surgery [11]. These predictive models can help in tailoring treatments—for instance, if the AI predicts a poor response to standard therapy, perhaps the patient should be considered for a clinical trial or a more aggressive treatment upfront.

Another burgeoning area is using imaging to predict genetic information—sometimes called imaging genomics or radiogenomics. For certain tumors, AI has been able to predict the presence of specific gene mutations just from MRI or CT scans. For example, in glioblastomas, AI models analyzing MRI have predicted IDH mutation status or MGMT promoter methylation status with decent accuracy. These are important genetic markers that traditionally required tissue sampling; if AI can non-invasively predict them, it can guide treatment decisions (since some therapies work better with certain mutations).

In cardiovascular imaging, predictive modeling can mean using imaging findings to predict the risk of future cardiac events. A coronary CT angiography may show plaques in the arteries. AI could quantify the characteristics of these plaques (volume, composition, etc.) and predict the 5-year risk of a heart attack. Similarly, in echocardiography, subtle patterns of heart motion detected by AI might predict which patients are at risk of developing heart failure even before overt symptoms or ejection fraction drop.

AI is also used to predict treatment outcomes—for example, in patients with liver tumors [36], analyze the pre-treatment CT and predict who will respond to radioembolization; or in patients with rectal cancer, analyze MRI to predict who might achieve a complete response to neoadjuvant chemo-radiation (potentially avoiding surgery if the prediction is of complete tumor eradication). These are very valuable because they allow more personalized and optimized patient care.

Integrating clinical data with images enhances these predictive models. Modern approaches sometimes feed not only the images into a deep network but also patient metadata (age, lab results, genomics). For instance, a model might take a lung CT and the patient's pulmonary function test results and output a prediction of risk for postoperative complications if lung surgery is done. The combination helps capture factors that imaging alone might miss.

One more example: in neuroimaging, AI models are being researched that look at brain PET or MRI scans and predict the likelihood of conversion from mild cognitive impairment to Alzheimer's dementia in the next few years [9]. This can help in selecting patients for early intervention trials.

In all these predictive tasks, validation is key. Such models require large studies to ensure the predictions are reliable and add value over existing clinical scoring systems. But the potential is that AI could reveal subtle imaging biomarkers—

patterns not obvious to human observers—that correlate strongly with outcomes. This is essentially precision medicine: using rich data like images in algorithms to stratify patients by risk or likely benefit, leading to more individualized care.

In conclusion, AI-driven automated image analysis covers a spectrum from finding what is in the image (anomalies, segments, classes) to inferring what that means for the patient. The ability to automatically mark up images with regions and labels simplifies many workflows and frees up expert time for more complex decision-making. Meanwhile, predictive modeling opens the door to using imaging not just for diagnosis but for prognostication and treatment planning, moving imaging into a central role in guiding patient management strategies. As these AI tools become more refined and integrated with hospital systems, we can expect faster diagnoses, more consistent quantifications, and data-informed predictions that improve patient care on an individualized level.

5 Challenges and Limitations

While the promise of AI in medical imaging is great, there are significant challenges and limitations that must be acknowledged and addressed. These challenges span technical issues, data concerns, ethical and legal implications, and practical deployment hurdles. This section examines some of the key challenges: data privacy and security, ethical considerations in AI deployment, and bias and fairness in AI models. Understanding these limitations is crucial, as it tempers the hype and guides researchers and clinicians to implement AI in a responsible and effective manner [18].

Medical images are considered sensitive health data, often containing both anatomical information and metadata like patient names or IDs. Large-scale AI development requires access to vast imaging datasets, raising concerns about privacy—especially across institutions and jurisdictions with regulations like HIPAA or GDPR. De-identification is a basic requirement, but risks remain that models may inadvertently memorize or expose identifiable features.

Security is another concern, particularly when AI systems operate in cloud environments or are integrated with hospital infrastructure. Cyberattacks or malicious tampering could lead to incorrect diagnoses or data breaches. Ensuring encryption, access control, and software validation is essential.

To address privacy, federated learning allows model training across multiple institutions without transferring raw data. Instead, model weights are shared and updated locally, reducing the risk of central data exposure. Combined with differential privacy and anonymization techniques (e.g., facial blurring, cropping), such approaches offer promising directions for secure and privacy-preserving AI in healthcare.

5.1 Ethical Considerations in AI Deployment

Deploying AI in healthcare raises important ethical questions, particularly around accountability. If an AI system misdiagnoses a condition, responsibility still typically lies with the human clinician. However, as AI becomes more autonomous, the line of accountability may blur. Ethically, AI should support—not replace—clinical judgment unless rigorously validated and regulated for independent use [20].

Transparency and explainability are also critical. Many AI models function as "black boxes," offering little insight into their decision-making. In medicine, both clinicians and patients need understandable justifications for AI-driven recommendations. Techniques like heatmaps or textual explanations are steps toward explainable AI, but achieving interpretability without compromising accuracy remains a challenge. Clinicians must be able to trust and understand AI outputs, and patients should be informed when AI is part of their care.

Trust and validation go hand in hand. Even high-performing models must undergo thorough testing—ideally in prospective clinical trials—to ensure they improve patient outcomes. Without such validation, using AI tools risks patient safety and undermines ethical standards. Ongoing trials, such as those in breast cancer screening, are examples of efforts to establish clinical trust and efficacy.

Another concern is over-reliance. There is a risk that heavy dependence on AI may erode clinicians' skills over time. For instance, trainees exposed to AI-generated interpretations might not develop the depth of diagnostic reasoning needed when AI is unavailable. To prevent de-skilling, AI should remain a support tool, and clinical training must continue to emphasize foundational expertise.

5.2 Bias and Fairness in AI Models

Bias in AI poses a serious risk in healthcare, where unfair predictions can harm underrepresented patient groups [7]. A primary source of bias is non-representative training data. For example, models trained predominantly on adult or Caucasian patient data may underperform on children or racially diverse populations. Studies have shown that dermatology AIs often struggle with darker skin tones due to biased datasets. In radiology, models have even been shown to predict patient race from images—despite it being imperceptible to human experts—suggesting the risk of models learning spurious correlations tied to demographics.

Bias can also arise from spectrum bias or domain shift. A model trained in tertiary hospitals may overfit to severe cases and miss mild ones in community settings. Similarly, models trained on data from a specific scanner or imaging protocol may not generalize to different devices.

Addressing fairness requires diverse, representative datasets and subgroup-level performance evaluation. If disparities are found, techniques like stratified retraining or augmenting underrepresented data can help. Regulatory agencies increasingly expect bias audits and documentation. Initiatives like "bias bounties" have been proposed to crowdsource identification of hidden biases.

Finally, generalization remains a challenge. AI models often perform worse when tested outside their development environment. External validation across institutions is essential before clinical deployment. Transparency is also crucial—proprietary models can obscure data sources and training methods, making it difficult to detect bias. Standards are emerging to require clear reporting on dataset composition and subgroup analysis in published studies.

5.3 *Ethical and Technical Limitations*

Bias in AI decisions can reinforce health disparities. If an AI performs poorly on certain groups, those patients may receive substandard care. Thus, fairness is not just a technical issue but a moral imperative in medical AI. Researchers are developing mitigation strategies such as re-sampling, re-weighting, adversarial training, and algorithmic debiasing to ensure predictions are not influenced by sensitive attributes like race or gender.

Several technical limitations also challenge the effective use of AI in healthcare:

- **Data Requirements:** Deep learning models require large, labeled datasets. This creates a gap in performance between common and rare diseases, where annotated data is scarce but clinical need is often high.
- **Model Updating:** Current regulatory frameworks often approve "locked" AI models that cannot learn from new data without re-approval. As medical practices and disease patterns evolve, the inability to update models limits their long-term utility. Adaptive AI and safe continuous learning are active areas of research and regulation.
- **Adversarial Vulnerability:** AI models can be sensitive to imperceptible perturbations in input data. Slight modifications, intentional or not, can cause incorrect predictions—highlighting the need for robust model design.

While these challenges remain, they are the focus of ongoing research. The successful integration of AI in healthcare depends on protecting patient privacy, securing systems, ensuring fairness, and maintaining clinician oversight. AI should support, not replace, medical judgment. Recognizing and addressing these limitations is crucial for safe, equitable, and effective deployment.

6 Standardization and Protocols for AI in Medical Imaging

As AI systems transition from research to clinical practice, there is a pressing need for standardization, protocols, and regulatory frameworks to ensure these tools are safe, effective, and interoperable with existing healthcare systems. This section covers key aspects of this integration: regulatory frameworks, quality assurance and validation, and interoperability in AI-driven systems. Establishing standards and protocols is essential to move AI in medical imaging from promising prototypes to trustworthy, routine tools in hospitals [10].

6.1 Regulatory Frameworks

Medical AI tools, especially those involved in diagnosis or treatment guidance, are regulated as medical devices [22]. In the United States, the Food and Drug Administration (FDA) oversees such software under its medical device framework. As of early 2024, the FDA has authorized over 600 AI/ML-enabled medical devices—most in radiology—for tasks like stroke detection, chest X-ray interpretation, and MRI analysis. These are primarily cleared via the 510(k) pathway for moderate-risk devices, the De Novo pathway for novel but moderate-risk tools, or the more rigorous PMA route for high-risk applications.

A key challenge with AI is its adaptability. Traditional devices remain static post-approval, whereas AI can evolve through retraining. Currently, the FDA only approves "locked" algorithms, requiring a new submission for performance-impacting updates. To address this, the FDA has proposed a framework allowing limited pre-approved changes under its "Software as a Medical Device (SaMD) Pre-Specifications and Algorithm Change Protocol." In collaboration with other regulators, the FDA also released principles for Good Machine Learning Practice (GMLP), emphasizing data quality, transparency, and ongoing monitoring.

In the European Union, AI tools are regulated under the Medical Device Regulation (MDR), which classifies many imaging AIs as class IIa or IIb devices. These require certification via Notified Bodies, clinical evaluation, and post-market surveillance. Software updates may trigger re-certification, making regulatory planning essential during development.

While regulatory requirements vary by region, the overall trend is toward cautious acceptance with a focus on patient safety. Developers must incorporate regulatory readiness early—tracking performance, maintaining data traceability, and ensuring mechanisms for reporting malfunctions. Table 2 summarizes key approval pathways, update policies, and monitoring standards in the USA and EU.

6.2 Quality Assurance and Validation

Any AI tool influencing patient care must undergo rigorous validation—both technical (e.g., accuracy, sensitivity, specificity) and clinical (e.g., impact on diagnosis, workflow, or outcomes) [27]. Validation begins during development using cross-validation and independent test sets, but performance in real-world clinical settings may differ due to varying disease prevalence, image quality, or workflow integration.

Table 2 Regulatory frameworks for AI in medical imaging

Aspect	USA (FDA)	European Union (MDR)
Regulation type	Medical device regulations (AI = Software as a Medical Device, SaMD)	AI falls under EU MDR, replacing MDD
Approval pathways	510(k) (equivalence), De Novo (moderate risk), PMA (high risk)	Class IIa/IIb: Certification via Notified Bodies
AI-specific challenges	AI must be "locked" at approval; updates require re-approval	AI updates may trigger re-certification
Adaptive AI	FDA exploring SaMD Pre-Specifications for updates	Post-market surveillance ensures updates comply
Key guidelines	FDA + MHRA + Health Canada: Good Machine Learning Practice (GMLP)	"State of the art" compliance, clinical evaluation required
Monitoring	Performance tracking, error reporting mandatory	Ongoing safety/performance monitoring required

Hospitals often perform local validation before deploying AI tools. This may include retrospective testing on archived data or prospective "shadow mode" evaluations where AI runs in parallel without influencing decisions. Clinical protocols are then adapted based on observed performance.

Professional bodies such as the ACR and RSNA have established initiatives like ACR's Data Science Institute to promote continuous monitoring. Institutions are encouraged to maintain QA logs—tracking AI agreement with radiologists, critical errors, or false positives—to ensure ongoing reliability, similar to equipment calibration.

Clinical trials are also emerging to assess patient outcomes. For example, studies have shown AI can triage mammograms, reducing radiologist workload without compromising detection rates.

From a regulatory perspective, agencies like the FDA require evidence from reader studies or multi-center testing. Post-market surveillance includes collecting user feedback and monitoring performance. If issues arise—such as consistent errors on a new scanner—updates or corrective actions may be required.

Calibration of AI outputs is another QA component. A probability score (e.g., 90%) should reflect actual risk. Poor calibration can mislead clinicians, so local calibration and interpretability are key.

Finally, interoperability is essential for real-world adoption. AI tools must integrate with healthcare IT systems using standards like DICOM for imaging and HL7/FHIR for clinical data. Seamless communication and standardized outputs ensure that AI systems function reliably within clinical workflows.

6.3 Interoperability and Standardization

For AI to function effectively in radiology, it must integrate with existing systems like the PACS (Picture Archiving and Communication System). AI algorithms typically receive imaging data, process it, and return outputs—such as annotations, heatmaps, or structured reports—back into the PACS or reporting system. The DICOM standard has been extended to support AI-generated outputs, including Secondary Capture images and Structured Reports (SR) for results like lung nodule detection. The DICOM Standards Committee emphasizes the use of standard formats to ensure compatibility across systems.

Initiatives like Integrating the Healthcare Enterprise (IHE) further support workflow integration by defining how AI results should be encoded and attached to studies. For instance, AI-generated overlays or structured findings can be auto-attached to CT scans, making them immediately accessible to radiologists within their existing workflow.

Interoperability also includes managing multiple AI systems within a single environment. A radiology department may use numerous specialized AI tools, and platforms are emerging to unify their outputs through standard APIs (e.g., RESTful interfaces, FHIR), reducing the need for clinicians to interact with separate user interfaces.

Model interoperability—sharing and deploying AI models across institutions—is another focus. Formats like ONNX (Open Neural Network Exchange) enable models to be transferred across frameworks, facilitating customization, retraining, or federated development.

Standardization efforts are supported by collaboration among regulatory bodies and professional organizations such as the FDA, RSNA, and ACR. These groups work on defining performance metrics, establishing documentation standards, and developing fair comparison protocols—such as RSNA's structured-format AI challenges.

Deployment protocols also include user guidance. Institutions should provide clear usage policies—for example, stating that an AI tool is validated only for adult chest X-rays, not pediatric cases. Proper training ensures users understand the tool's capabilities and limitations.

Finally, the concept of a "continuous learning system with a Predetermined Change Control Plan (PCCP)" is under discussion. Such frameworks would allow approved models to be updated in the field within predefined limits, avoiding the need for re-approval. These updates would follow internal validation procedures and monitoring protocols to ensure

6.4 Quality Assurance Standards

Organizations might also adopt QA standards like ISO 13485 (for medical device quality management) when developing AI, and hospitals might use something akin to IEC 62304 (medical device software lifecycle processes) to manage the integration [34]. These ensure that the software development and maintenance follow high quality standards (though these are more manufacturer-side). Finally, documentation protocols are important. Every time an AI provides a result that is used clinically, it should be documented (for medico-legal reasons, traceability). If a radiologist overrules an AI, that's fine, but some system might log that interaction for improvement purposes or auditing. Hospitals will likely keep logs of AI suggestions vs final decisions both to improve the AI (if it's being retrained) and to review if any incident occurs. In summary, the move from innovation to implementation for AI in medical imaging depends on robust standardization and protocols. Regulatory frameworks are coming into place to ensure safety and efficacy, requiring evidence and providing oversight for AI tools. Quality assurance processes, both pre- and post-deployment, are essential to maintain trust in these tools—AI in medicine must be continuously monitored just like any critical equipment. And for AI to truly augment clinical practice, it must speak the same language as existing systems (DICOM, HL7, etc.) and fit into workflows seamlessly. Significant progress is being made on all these fronts, with multi-stakeholder collaborations. The goal is that a radiologist or clinician shouldn't have to worry about the technicalities of AI integration—if standards are followed, the AI results will appear where they should, in a form they expect, and with known reliability—allowing the focus to remain on patient care.

7 Future Directions and Opportunities

Looking ahead, the field of AI in medical image analysis is poised for even greater advancements. As both imaging technologies and AI algorithms evolve, their synergy will open up new frontiers. In this section, we discuss several future directions and opportunities: innovations in AI and imaging technologies, the potential for enhanced clinical workflows, and the expanding role of AI in personalized medicine. These areas highlight how AI's integration with medical imaging could further revolutionize diagnosis, treatment, and healthcare delivery in the coming years.

7.1 Innovations in AI and Imaging Technologies

AI itself is a fast-moving target, with novel algorithms and paradigms emerging that could benefit medical imaging. One major trend is the development of foundation models and large-scale multi-modal AI systems. These are models trained on extremely large datasets (sometimes across image and text domains) that can be adapted to various tasks. In radiology, researchers are exploring whether a single large model can be trained to handle many types of images and tasks—for instance, a model that could analyze not just one kind of scan but X-rays, CTs, and MRIs, and not just detect one condition but many. Early work, for example, is looking at applying vision-language models like GPT-4 Vision to radiology. The idea is a model that could take an imaging study and even output a textual report (effectively mimicking what a radiologist would dictate) by combining image analysis with language generation. While still in nascent stages (and requiring careful safety checks), this approach might eventually produce AI that can draft full radiology reports which radiologists then edit—significantly speeding up reporting.

Transformers and attention-based architectures, which have dominated natural language processing, are also making inroads into imaging. Vision Transformers (ViTs) have shown performance comparable to CNNs on some imaging tasks and could potentially capture global image context even better in certain cases. We might see hybrid models that use both convolutional layers and transformers to leverage the strengths of each (convolutions for local detail, transformers for long-range dependency). These could further improve accuracy or allow AI to handle more complex images (like whole 3D volumes at once, rather than slice by slice).

On the imaging technology side, modalities themselves are advancing—higher resolution imaging, new contrast mechanisms (like photoacoustic imaging), etc. AI will be critical in extracting information from these richer images. For example, as 7-Tesla MRI becomes more common (with finer detail of brain structures), AI could help navigate the more complex images to identify micro-lesions or subtle anomalies that even expert eyes might struggle with due to detail overload. In pathology, whole slide scanners now produce multi-gigapixel images; future high-throughput microscopy might integrate AI directly at the point of image capture to zero in on regions of interest in real-time. Another area of innovation is real-time AI integration in image acquisition. We touched on this with ultrasound guiding operators. This can expand to MRI/CT—e.g., "smart" MRI sequences that decide on the fly (via AI) whether a particular sequence is needed or if the images acquired so far are sufficient because AI is confident about a diagnosis. There's research on adaptive imaging: an AI monitors the MRI acquisition and can say "stop, we already see the tumor clearly" or "we need an extra sequence with contrast because something looks off." This could optimize scanning time per patient.

AI-driven image reconstruction will continue to advance. Deep learning reconstruction techniques may become standard in MRI and CT, making scans faster and lower dose. We might see AI reconstructors that are vendor-neutral and become part of the DICOM standard image formation pipeline. With better reconstruction, we could also see new types of imaging that were not previously clinically viable become feasible. For example, in MRI, sequences that were too slow or images that were too noisy might now be usable thanks to AI cleaning them up.

7.2 *Enhanced Clinical Workflows*

The future radiology workflow could be dramatically different with AI deeply embedded. Envision a scenario in a radiology department in a few years: As images are acquired, a suite of AI algorithms in the background triages studies (urgent findings like acute brain bleed on CT head are immediately flagged and pushed to the top of the worklist for radiologists with an alert; normal screening mammograms might be preliminarily read by AI and queued separately for later double-checking). By the time a radiologist opens a study, AI might have already segmented any lesions, measured them, compared to prior scans, retrieved relevant prior cases from the archives for reference, and even drafted key images and preliminary impressions. The radiologist then acts more as a conductor—verifying and finalizing the compilation of AI outputs into a coherent report.

Such an AI-augmented workflow could greatly reduce mundane tasks: for example, automated report drafting where AI fills in normal findings sections so radiologists just confirm them, and highlights only areas that need attention. Natural language processing (NLP) integrated with the AI vision could also help ensure that measurements in the image (like the diameter of a tumor) are automatically inserted into the text report accurately, eliminating human transcription errors. AI can also help in workflow orchestration beyond image analysis. For example, scheduling and protocoling: AI might predict that a certain MRI exam is likely to need contrast based on the clinical question and initial sequences, and recommend it, saving time. Or in managing radiology workflow: predicting no-shows, optimizing scanner utilization by analyzing past data, etc., which some institutions are already exploring.

Another future aspect is continuous education and feedback. Workflow integrated AI could gather interesting cases or ones where it was less confident and flag them for teaching files. Radiologists can benefit from AI as a second reader that not only helps in real-time but also helps them learn. If an AI consistently spots something a radiologist missed, that feedback can be looped to the radiologist (gently, in a QA meeting for instance) to help improve human performance—a reversal of roles where AI helps train humans, after humans have trained AI. In interventional radiology and surgery, augmented reality (AR) with AI is a exciting area. Future operating rooms might use AI to overlay CT or MRI data onto the patient in real time with AR glasses, guiding surgeons to the exact location of a tumor beneath the surface. The AI would do the registration and tracking, essentially fusing imaging with the patient in front of the surgeon. Already, prototypes exist for spinal surgery where AI helps identify the correct vertebrae levels on fluoroscopy images. We can expect more of this cross-over, where imaging AI helps during procedures (like highlighting blood vessels to avoid, or estimating margins to cut).

7.3 Personalized Medicine and Integration with Other Data

Perhaps the most profound long-term direction is using imaging AI as part of a broader personalized medicine approach. Medical images provide phenotypic information about a disease; when combined with genomic data, lab results, and patient history (all fodder for AI as well), we can create comprehensive models of a patient's health. AI could discover patterns linking imaging findings with gene expression profiles or proteomics. For example, in oncology, a future AI system might take a patient's MRI, plus their genomic sequencing of the tumor, plus clinical data, and predict which therapy that specific patient will respond best to. There is a concept of developing a "virtual patient" or digital twin—a computational model of a patient that can be used to simulate disease progression or treatment response. Imaging is vital for that because it provides spatial and functional context about the disease in the body. AI can help build and update these digital twins with each new scan.

Personalized medicine also includes using AI to tailor follow-up and screening. AI risk models might determine that one patient's scans show they are at high risk for rapid disease progression, so they need more frequent imaging follow-ups; whereas another patient is low risk and can avoid unnecessary scans (reducing radiation exposure and cost). This dynamic adjustment of care based on continuously learning AI models will push medicine from guideline-based (one size fits all) to truly individualized.

Multi-modal AI is a key enabler for personalization. We will see more AI that simultaneously processes images and other data. For instance, an AI for dementia might take MRI brain scans, FDG-PET images, and neurocognitive test results together to diagnose and predict progression, rather than treating them separately. Such holistic AI models will align more with how a physician thinks—considering multiple data sources—but with the advantage of quantitatively analyzing them all. Another future opportunity is global health and accessibility. The combination of more portable imaging devices (like handheld ultrasounds, portable MRIs in development) with AI could bring advanced diagnostics to remote or underserved areas. One can imagine a clinic in a rural area with a handheld ultrasound and an AI assistant that helps a nurse detect conditions (like detecting rheumatic heart disease in a remote village via echo, guided by AI). Cloud connectivity would allow specialists anywhere in the world to confirm if needed. AI can thus be a force multiplier for healthcare equality, bridging gaps where specialists are scarce.

7.4 Continuous Improvement and Community Sharing

The future will also likely involve a more open ecosystem where AI models can continuously learn from global data (with privacy-preserving methods). We may see healthcare systems contributing to shared AI models (as part of consortia) that benefit everyone. For example, a global AI network might accumulate rare disease cases so that even an isolated hospital's AI can recognize a rare condition it's never seen locally, because the knowledge was learned from elsewhere. Initiatives to create large open datasets and model zoos (with vetted medical AI models) are already underway. This collaborative model development can accelerate progress and ensure robustness.

In terms of market and adoption, one future direction is the integration of AI into imaging hardware itself. Major scanner manufacturers are embedding AI for things like auto-scan planning (the machine identifies the correct slice alignment automatically) and even for interpreting images right on the console. Perhaps future CT scanners will come with an "AI summary" out-of-the-box that gives immediate findings—not to replace radiologists but to give instant preliminary info (like "no bleed, no fracture" on a trauma CT, which an ER doc could see within a minute of scan completion). This kind of tight integration could shave critical minutes in emergency care.

Finally, the role of AI in personalized medicine extends to therapy. Theranostics is a field combining therapy and diagnostics. AI can help not just in diagnosing but in delivering therapy (for example, in radiation therapy, AI might adapt treatment plans in real-time based on daily imaging). Adaptive radiotherapy, where treatment is modified based on changes seen in imaging (like a shrinking tumor on daily CTs), will likely rely heavily on AI to quickly re-compute plans. Similarly, in image-guided robotic surgery, AI vision can guide the robot to target pathology precisely while sparing healthy tissue.

In summary, the future of AI in medical imaging is expansive. We can anticipate more powerful algorithms that are generalists across tasks, deeply integrated with clinical context and data; smarter workflows where AI handles routine burdens and allows clinicians to focus on complex decision-making and patient interaction; and a move towards truly personalized and predictive healthcare, where imaging AI is a cornerstone in modeling each patient's unique condition and tailoring treatment accordingly. As these developments unfold, it will be important to continue addressing challenges (as discussed earlier) and involve clinicians in the design to ensure these futuristic tools remain human-centric—enhancing the capabilities of doctors and improving outcomes for patients. The collaboration of AI and clinicians, each contributing their strengths, is the vision of future medicine, and medical imaging is at the forefront of this transformation.

8 Conclusion

Artificial intelligence has become a transformative force in medical imaging, evolving from early expert systems to powerful deep learning models capable of matching or surpassing human performance in specific diagnostic tasks. This chapter provided an overview of AI's foundational principles, its integration across imaging modalities such as MRI, CT, ultrasound, and X-ray, and its role in improving diagnostic accuracy, consistency, and efficiency. By automating tasks like segmentation and anomaly detection, AI helps reduce radiologist workload and supports timely and accurate medical decisions.

Real-world deployments demonstrate AI's value in clinical settings, such as triaging emergency cases or assisting in screening in resource-limited environments. These successes highlight the practical benefits of AI, yet also bring to light essential considerations. The implementation of AI in healthcare demands careful attention to data privacy, algorithmic bias, and ethical use. Ensuring AI serves as a supportive tool rather than a replacement for human clinicians is crucial. Equally important are rigorous validation procedures and compliance with regulatory standards before integrating AI tools into routine clinical practice.

As AI continues to mature, the future points toward more deeply integrated systems. Multi-modal AI models that combine imaging data with genetic, clinical, and demographic information are paving the way toward precision medicine. Such systems may provide more accurate prognoses and guide personalized treatment strategies that extend beyond the capacity of traditional workflows. This shift could transform medical imaging into a proactive, predictive, and patient-specific discipline.

Ultimately, the most effective future lies in human-AI collaboration. Rather than replacing radiologists, AI is best positioned as an intelligent assistant—handling repetitive tasks, identifying patterns at scale, and allowing clinicians to focus on complex judgment and patient interaction. Radiologists of tomorrow may oversee AI tools, verify results, and contribute more meaningfully to interdisciplinary care. With feedback-driven continuous learning systems, both AI and clinicians can evolve together, leading to better diagnostic outcomes. Embracing AI with a balanced perspective—leveraging its strengths while remaining mindful of its limits—will be key to unlocking its full potential in reshaping diagnostic medicine.

References

1. Alyoubi WL, Shalash WM, Abulkhair MF (2020) Diabetic retinopathy detection through deep learning techniques: a review. Inf Med Unlocked 20:100377
2. Bennour A, Ben Aoun N, Khalaf OI, Ghabban F, Wong WK, Algburi S (2024) Contribution to pulmonary diseases diagnostic from x-ray images using innovative deep learning models. Heliyon 10(9)

3. Buzug TM (2021) Computed tomography. In: Springer handbook of medical technology. Springer, Berlin, pp 311–342
4. Cai L, Gao J, Zhao D (2020) A review of the application of deep learning in medical image classification and segmentation. Ann. Trans Med. 8(11):713
5. Carovac A, Smajlovic F, Junuzovic D (2011) Application of ultrasound in medicine. Acta Inf Medica 19(3):168
6. Chen Y, Schönlieb CB, Liò P, Leiner T, Dragotti PL, Wang G, Rueckert D, Firmin D, Yang G (2022) Ai-based reconstruction for fast mri–a systematic review and meta-analysis. Proc IEEE 110(2):224–245
7. Chen RJ, Wang JJ, Williamson DF, Chen TY, Lipkova J, Lu MY, Sahai S, Mahmood F (2023) Algorithmic fairness in artificial intelligence for medicine and healthcare. Nature Biomed Eng 7(6):719–742
8. Choi Y, Lee MK (2020) Neuroimaging findings of brain mri and ct in patients with covid-19: a systematic review and meta-analysis. Eur J Radiol 133:109393
9. Choi KS, Sunwoo L (2022) Artificial intelligence in neuroimaging: clinical applications. Investig Magn Reson Imaging 26(1):1–9
10. Cobo M, Menéndez Fernández-Miranda P, Bastarrika G, Lloret Iglesias L (2023) Enhancing radiomics and deep learning systems through the standardization of medical imaging workflows. Sci Data 10(1):732
11. Dlamini Z, Francies FZ, Hull R, Marima R (2020) Artificial intelligence (ai) and big data in cancer and precision oncology. Comput Struct Biotechnol J 18:2300–2311
12. Eloranta S, Boman M (2022) Predictive models for clinical decision making: deep dives in practical machine learning. J Internal Med 292(2):278–295
13. Foroughmand-Araabi MH (2023) The scope of artificial intelligence applications in medicine: a review article. J Orthopedic Spine Trauma 53–58
14. Gasmi K, Ben Aoun N, Alsalem K, Ltaifa IB, Alrashdi I, Ammar LB, Mrabet M, Shehab A (2024) Enhanced brain tumor diagnosis using combined deep learning models and weight selection technique. Front Neuroinf 18:1444650
15. Hashmi MF, Katiyar S, Keskar AG, Bokde ND, Geem ZW (2020) Efficient pneumonia detection in chest xray images using deep transfer learning. Diagnostics 10(6):417
16. Hayashi Y (2019) The right direction needed to develop white-box deep learning in radiology, pathology, and ophthalmology: a short review. Front Robot AI 6:24
17. Janardhanan P, Sabika F et al (2015) Effectiveness of support vector machines in medical data mining. J Commun Software Syst 11(1):25–30
18. Kaissis GA, Makowski MR, Rückert D, Braren RF (2020) Secure, privacy-preserving and federated machine learning in medical imaging. Nature Mach Intell 2(6):305–311
19. Katti G, Ara SA, Shireen A (2011) Magnetic resonance imaging (mri)—a review. Int J Dental Clinics 3(1):65–70
20. Keskinbora KH (2019) Medical ethics considerations on artificial intelligence. J Clin Neurosci 64:277–282
21. Komatsu M, Sakai A, Dozen A, Shozu K, Yasutomi S, Machino H, Asada K, Kaneko S, Hamamoto R (2021) Towards clinical application of artificial intelligence in ultrasound imaging. Biomedicines 9(7):720
22. Larson DB, Harvey H, Rubin DL, Irani N, Justin RT, Langlotz CP (2021) Regulatory frameworks for development and evaluation of artificial intelligence—based diagnostic imaging algorithms: summary and recommendations. J Am College Radiol 18(3):413–424
23. Lebeau A, Turzynski A (2025) Pathology: diagnostics, reporting and artificial intelligence. Senologie-Zeitschrift für Mammadiagnostik und-therapie 22(01):31–42
24. Lekadir K, Frangi AF, Porras AR, Glocker B, Cintas C, Langlotz CP, Weicken E, Asselbergs FW, Prior F, Collins GS et al (2025) Future-ai: international consensus guideline for trustworthy and deployable artificial intelligence in healthcare. BMJ 388
25. Li X, Liu Y, Wu X, Huang R, Chen S, Yuan K (2025) Ultrasound meets nanomedicine: towards disease treatment and medical imaging. Microchimica Acta 192(4):215

26. Lorkowski J, Grzegorowska O, Pokorski M (2021) Artificial intelligence in the healthcare system: an overview. Best Pract Health Care 1–10
27. Lundström C, Lindvall M (2023) Mapping the landscape of care providers' quality assurance approaches for ai in diagnostic imaging. J Digital Imaging 36(2):379–387
28. Nensa F, Demircioglu A, Rischpler C (2019) Artificial intelligence in nuclear medicine. J Nucl Med 60(Supplement 2):29S–37S
29. Niaz A, Memon AA, Rana K, Joshi A, Soomro S, Kang JS, Choi KN (2020) Inhomogeneous image segmentation using hybrid active contours model with application to breast tumor detection. IEEE Access 8:186851–186861
30. Niaz A, Iqbal E, Akram F, Kim J, Choi KN (2022) Self-initialized active contours for microscopic cell image segmentation. Sci Rep 12(1):14947
31. Niaz A, Iqbal E, Memon AA, Munir A, Kim J, Choi KN (2023) Edge-based local and global energy active contour model driven by signed pressure force for image segmentation. IEEE Trans Instrum Meas 72:1–14
32. Niaz A, Amin SU, Soomro S, Zia H, Choi KN (2024) Spatially aware fusion in 3d convolutional autoencoders for video anomaly detection. IEEE Access 12:104770–104784
33. Oh SW, Park S, Chong A, Kim K, Bang JI, Seo Y, Hong CM, Lee SW (2025) Nuclear medicine imaging in differentiated thyroid cancer: summary of the korean thyroid association guidelines 2024 from nuclear medicine perspective, part-i. Nucl Med Mol Imaging 59(1):1–7
34. Papp J (2023) Quality management in the imaging Sciences-E-Book: quality management in the imaging Sciences-E-Book. Elsevier Health Sciences, Amsterdam (2023)
35. Pellicori P, Platz E, Dauw J, Ter Maaten JM, Martens P, Pivetta E, Cleland JG, McMurray JJ, Mullens W, Solomon SD et al (2021) Ultrasound imaging of congestion in heart failure: examinations beyond the heart. Eur J Heart Failure 23(5):703–712
36. Rahman H, Ben Aoun N, Bukht TFN., Ahmad S, Tadeusiewicz R, Pławiak P, Hammad M () Automatic liver tumor segmentation of ct and mri volumes using ensemble resunet-inceptionv4 model. Inf Sci 121966
37. Rajpurkar P, Irvin J, Zhu K, Yang B, Mehta H, Duan T, Ding D, Bagul A, Langlotz C, Shpanskaya K et al (2017) Chexnet: radiologist-level pneumonia detection on chest x-rays with deep learning. Preprint, arXiv:1711.05225
38. Rashidi HH, Pantanowitz J, Hanna M, Tafti AP, Sanghani P, Buchinsky A, Fennell B, Deebajah M, Wheeler S, Pearce T et al (2025) Introduction to artificial intelligence (ai) and machine learning (ml) in pathology & medicine: generative & non-generative ai basics. Mod Pathol 100688
39. Rasool N, Bhat JI, Ben Aoun N, Alharthi A, Wani NA, Chopra V, Anwar MS (2024) Resmhanet: Enhancing glioma segmentation and survival prediction using a novel deep learning framework. Comput Mater Continua 81(1)
40. Ronneberger O, Fischer P, Brox T (2015) U-net: convolutional networks for biomedical image segmentation. In: Medical image computing and computer-assisted intervention–MICCAI 2015: 18th international conference, Munich, Germany, October 5–9, 2015, proceedings, part III 18. Springer, pp 234–241
41. Seeram E, Kanade V (2024) Ai fundamentals. In: Artificial intelligence in medical imaging technology: an introduction. Springer, Berlin, pp 17–34
42. Shen D, Wu G, Suk HI (2017) Deep learning in medical image analysis. Ann Rev Biomed Eng 19(1):221–248
43. Sidey-Gibbons JA, Sidey-Gibbons CJ (2019) Machine learning in medicine: a practical introduction. BMC Med Res Methodol 19:1–18
44. Suganthi K et al (2021) Review of medical image synthesis using gan techniques. In: ITM web of conferences, vol. 37. EDP Sciences, p. 01005
45. Suman A, Suman P, Padhy S, Kumar N, Singh A (2025) Healthcare revolution: advances in ai-driven medical imaging and diagnosis. In: Responsible and explainable artificial intelligence in healthcare. Elsevier, Amsterdam, pp 155–182
46. Tong Y, Lu W, Yu Y, Shen Y (2020) Application of machine learning in ophthalmic imaging modalities. Eye Vision 7:1–15

47. Tran BX, Vu GT, Ha GH, Vuong QH, Ho MT, Vuong TT, La VP, Ho MT, Nghiem KC,P., Nguyen HLT et al (2019) Global evolution of research in artificial intelligence in health and medicine: a bibliometric study. J Clin Med 8(3):360
48. Tsapatsaris A, Thompson SA, Reichman M (2025) Review of mammography screening guidelines of the 5 largest global economies. Clin Imaging 110415
49. Yoon JH, Kim EK (2021) Deep learning-based artificial intelligence for mammography. Korean J Radiol 22(8):1225
50. Zeng Y, Liu Y, Li J, Feng B, Lu J (2025) Value of computed tomography scan for detecting lymph node metastasis in early esophageal squamous cell carcinoma. Ann Surgical Oncol 32(3):1635–1650
51. Zhang Z, Seeram E (2020) The use of artificial intelligence in computed tomography image reconstruction-a literature review. J Med Imaging Radiat Sci 51(4):671–677
52. Zhang J, Yu X, Lei X, Wu C (2022) A novel deep lenet-5 convolutional neural network model for image recognition. Comput Sci Inf Syst 19(3):1463–1480
53. Zhang X, Xu M, Qiu D, Yan R, Lang N, Zhou X (2024) Mediclip: adapting clip for few-shot medical image anomaly detection. In: International conference on medical image computing and computer-assisted intervention. Springer, pp 458–468

Fundamentals of Medical Image Analysis

Wesam Ahmed and Mohamed Hammad

1 Introduction

The field of medical imaging and image analysis emerges from the collaborative efforts of numerous disciplines, including engineering, mathematics, medicine, and fundamental sciences [1]. This interdisciplinary approach represents a sophisticated method of understanding human physiology and pathology through advanced technological means. The primary objective of medical imaging is to obtain valuable information about the body's organs and ongoing physiological and pathological processes by utilizing either internal or external energy sources [2]. The current imaging methods available for radiological imaging may utilize internal, external, or a combination of energy sources. It is sometimes necessary to examine the human body due to various physiological or pathological concerns. The first method involves directly cutting the body open through surgery. The second method involves imaging techniques or technologies that allow the physician or radiologist to observe the human body without surgery or cutting. Technologies that enable physicians to investigate the internal components of the human body in search of indications of a medical condition are referred to as diagnostic imaging. Imaging modalities are selected based on the symptoms and the body part examined. Situations may arise where the actual condition of a specific organ of interest or the localization of pathological regions necessitate integrating multiple imaging tech-

W. Ahmed (✉)
Faculty of Computers and Artificial Intelligence, Hurghada University, Hurghada, Egypt

M. Hammad
EIAS Data Science Lab, College of Computer and Information Sciences, Prince Sultan University, Riyadh, Saudi Arabia

Faculty of Computers and Information, Menoufia University, Shibin El Kom, Egypt
e-mail: mhammad@psu.edu.sa

N. Ben Aoun et al. (eds.), *AI for Medical Image Analysis*,
https://doi.org/10.1007/978-3-032-02963-8_2

niques. While numerous diagnostic imaging procedures are non-invasive, painless, and simple to administer, they may require the patient to be confined to a machine or adhere to specific conditions, such as maintaining a specific posture, performing an exercise, or holding their breath for an extended period. It is generally accepted that specific methods involving ionizing radiation are secure due to the regulation of dosage. Cameras or other devices may be inserted into the body during certain diagnostic imaging procedures. These procedures are classified as invasive and may require sedation or anesthesia.

Numerous imaging modalities are currently used to obtain anatomical, physiological, metabolic, and functional data from the human body. Using computers, it is possible to manipulate and process multi-dimensional digital images of anatomical structures to visualize diagnostic features that are difficult or impossible to detect using planar imaging methods [3]. The clinical information that multi-dimensional visualization and quantitative analysis of physiological structures provide is extremely valuable in diagnosing and treating many critical radiological applications. Early detection of breast cancer is an example of the functionality, scope, and efficacy of computer-aided diagnosis (CAD).

Medical image processing is a field of research that involves developing and implementing algorithms and techniques to interpret and analyze medical images. The primary goal of medical image processing is to extract valuable information from medical images to facilitate the planning of treatment, diagnosis, and therapeutic interventions. Image segmentation, image registration, feature extraction, classification, and visualization are among the numerous tasks that comprise medical image processing. The primary objective of medical image processing is to extract relevant information from medical images, thereby simplifying the processes of diagnosis, treatment planning, and therapeutic interventions. The images generated by various modalities may require specific processing techniques to extricate valuable information, as each modality has distinct strengths and limitations. The field of medicine has been transformed by medical image processing techniques, which offer a noninvasive method for visualizing and analyzing the internal structures and functions of the body. It has facilitated early detection and diagnosis of diseases, an accurate plan of treatment, and monitoring of treatment response. The quality of care of the patient is significantly improved, the cost of treatment is reduced, and the patient's results have improved through medical image processing. The chapter offers a comprehensive discovery of medical image analysis through several important lenses. At its core, the research therapy enters the theoretical foundation by offering a comprehensive observation of the therapy imaging principles and exposing the complex interdisciplinary approach to image analysis. From a technical point of view, the task examines the current imaging forms, tricks, advanced processing techniques, and innovative computational approaches reshaping therapy diagnosis. The practical application section focuses on displaying how this technological progress translates into real-world clinical contexts, including refined diagnosis methods, strategic treatment plans, and refined disease monitoring techniques. Recognizing the dynamic nature of medical imaging, the chapter also critically addresses current limitations in medical image analysis, explores emerging technologies, and identifies promising research opportunities that have the potential to transform future healthcare practices. By integrating theoretical insights, technological innovations, practical applications, and forward-looking perspectives, the chapter aims to provide a holistic and nuanced understanding of the rapidly evolving field of medical image analysis.

The remaining Chapter is organized as follows: Sect. 2 gives an overview of the medical image modalities. Section 3 presents the main body of the reviewed literature. Section 4 touches upon the public data repositories for Medical Imaging. Section 5 highlights the major image processing techniques on medical images. Section 6 discusses recommendations for dealing with these challenges as future directions. The article concludes in Sect. 7.

2 Overview of Medical Imaging Modalities

Medical imaging has revolutionized modern healthcare by enabling non-invasive visualization of internal anatomical structures and physiological processes. Over the past century, advancements in imaging technologies have provided clinicians with powerful diagnostic tools, improving disease detection, treatment planning, and patient outcomes. This section provides a detailed examination of the primary medical imaging modalities, including their underlying principles, clinical applications, advantages, and limitations.

2.1 X-ray Imaging

X-ray imaging, one of the oldest and most widely used modalities, relies on ionizing radiation to produce two-dimensional images of internal structures. When X-rays pass through the body, denser tissues (e.g., bones) absorb more radiation, appearing white on the resulting radiograph, while softer tissues (e.g., muscles and lungs) appear in shades of gray [4, 5]. Conventional X-rays are primarily used for diagnosing fractures, detecting lung abnormalities, and assessing dental conditions. Despite its widespread use, X-ray imaging has limitations, including poor soft-tissue contrast and exposure to ionizing radiation, which carries a small but non-negligible risk of carcinogenesis with repeated exposure.

2.2 Computed Tomography (CT)

Computed tomography (CT) has significantly advanced diagnostic images, exceeding several limitations inherent to conventional radiography. Unlike traditional x-rays that provide only two-dimensional projections, TC technology employs a rotary X-ray set set to acquire various image slices from different angles around the body. These projections are later rebuilt using sophisticated computational algorithms to produce high resolution transverse images and, in many cases, detailed three-dimensional views (3D) of internal anatomical structures [6]. This capacity of various planar images allows improved spatial resolution and improved anatomical differentiation, making CT an indispensable tool in a wide range of clinical applications. The CT image has been particularly valuable in scenarios that require precise anatomical details, such as trauma assessment, cancer detection and staging, and vascular images. The ability to detect subtle abnormalities or injuries that can be obscured or lost in standard X -ray significantly increases diagnostic trust and facilitates timely medical intervention. For example, in emergency environments, full-body computed tomography can quickly identify internal bleeding, fractures, or organs, thus supporting critical decision-making processes and potentially saving lives. Despite these benefits, the image of the TC does not fail to have its disadvantages. One of the most prominent concerns is the relatively high radiation dose associated with CT exams, usually estimated up to ten times higher than that of conventional radiography [7]. This elevated exposure enhances special concerns for weak population like children as well as patients requiring frequent follow-up scans, where cumulative radiation doses can pose long-term health risks. In response to these security concerns, the imaging community has actively pursued strategies to reduce radiation risk without compromising image quality. Recent innovations such as low-colored whistle protocols and reconstruction techniques have played an important role in achieving this balance. Low-khurak protocols adjust to reduce the amount of radiation distributed to scanning parameters, while repetition reconstruction algorithm reduces noise and enhance image clarity, causing clinically useful images to be obtained at much lower radiation levels. These technological progresses outline the ongoing commitment to patient safety and the development of CT imaging as an accurate, efficient, and rapid clinical modality.

2.3 *Magnetic Resonance Imaging (MRI)*

Magnetic Resonance Imaging (MRI) employs strong magnetic fields and radiofrequency pulses to generate high-resolution images without ionizing radiation. Hydrogen nuclei in bodily tissues align with the magnetic field, and when perturbed by radio waves, they emit signals that are processed into detailed anatomical images [8, 9]. MRI excels in soft-tissue contrast, making it indispensable for neurological, musculoskeletal, and oncological imaging. Functional MRI (fMRI) further extends its utility by mapping brain activity through blood oxygenation changes. Despite its advantages, MRI has drawbacks, including long acquisition times (often 30–60 minutes per scan), high operational costs, and contraindications for patients with metallic implants (Fig. 1).

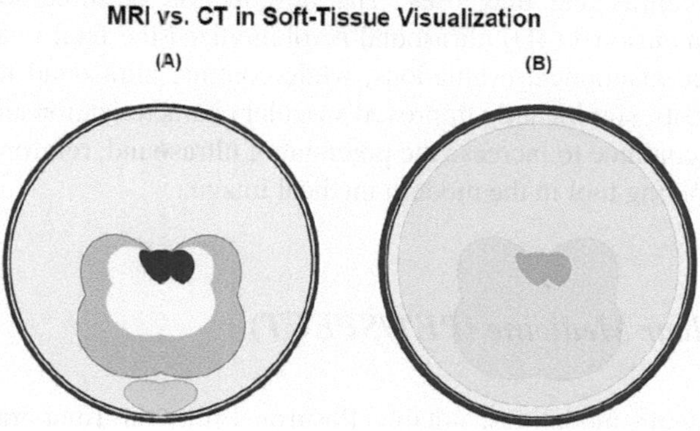

Fig. 1 MRI vs. CT in Soft-Tissue Visualization. (**a**) MRI of the brain showing detailed gray-white matter differentiation. (**b**) CT scan of the same region with lower soft-tissue contrast

2.4 Ultrasound Imaging

Ultrasound imaging, also known as sonography, leverages high-frequency sound waves–typically ranging from 2 to 18 megahertz (MHz)–to produce real-time visualizations of internal body structures. The technique involves transmitting sound waves into the body using a transducer; these waves then reflect off tissues and organs with varying acoustic impedance. The returning echoes are captured and processed by the ultrasound system to form grayscale images that depict soft tissue interfaces. One of the key innovations in this modality is Doppler ultrasound, which measures the change in frequency of the reflected sound waves to assess blood flow dynamics within vessels and the heart, offering crucial insights into hemodynamic function [10, 11]. Ultrasound's popularity in clinical practice is largely attributed to its numerous advantages: it is non-invasive, does not expose patients to ionizing radiation, is relatively cost-effective, and provides real-time feedback, which is particularly valuable in dynamic assessments such as fetal movement monitoring or cardiac function evaluation. Its portability has also made it a cornerstone in point-of-care diagnostics, especially in emergency medicine, critical care, and remote or resource-limited settings. Furthermore, ultrasound is the modality of choice in obstetrics due to its safety profile and ability to monitor fetal development across gestational stages. However, the ultrasound image is not exempt from limitations. One of the main challenges is its reduced effectiveness in patients with higher body mass index (BMI), as increased subcutaneous fat can alleviate sound wave transmission, limiting image depth and clarity. Similarly, the modality is ineffective in penetrating air-filled or dense bone structures, which restricts its application in certain anatomical regions. In addition, the quality and usefulness of the diagnosis of ultrasound images are highly dependent on the operator, with significant variability based on the technician's skill, experience, and familiarity with the clinical context. In recent years, substantial technological advances have expanded the scope and accuracy of ultrasound diagnoses. The introduction of three-dimensional (3D) and quadidimensional (4D) ultrasound revolutionized the fetal image and allowed more detailed anatomical evaluations, while contrast ultrasound techniques using microbic agents, significantly improved vascular characterization and tissues. These innovations continue to increase the potential of ultrasound, reinforcing its role as a vital and evolving tool in the modern medical image.

2.5 Nuclear Medicine (PET/SPECT)

Nuclear imaging modalities, notably Positron Emission Tomography (PET) and Single-Photon Emission Computed Tomography (SPECT), represent a unique class of diagnostic tools that provide valuable insights into the functional and metabolic processes occurring within the human body. These techniques involve the intravenous administration of radiopharmaceuticals–molecules labeled with radioactive isotopes–which localize in specific tissues based on physiological activity. Specialized detectors then capture the emitted radiation to construct images that reflect the distribution and intensity of biological functions. PET imaging, in particular, has become indispensable in the field of oncology. It frequently utilizes the radiotracer fluorodeoxyglucose (FDG), a glucose analog that accumulates in hypermetabolic cells, such as cancerous tissues. By detecting areas of increased glucose metabolism, PET scans enable clinicians to identify, stage, and monitor various malignancies with high sensitivity [12, 13]. The integration of PET with Computed Tomography (PET-CT) has further enhanced diagnostic accuracy by providing both metabolic and anatomical information in a single imaging session. This fusion allows for precise localization of abnormal metabolic activity, facilitating improved clinical decision-making in cancer management. SPECT imaging, while similar in principle to PET, employs different radiotracers and detection mechanisms. It is widely utilized in cardiology, particularly for myocardial perfusion imaging, where it helps evaluate blood flow to the heart muscle, detect ischemia, and assess the viability of cardiac tissue. SPECT is also applied in neurology for the assessment of cerebral perfusion and in orthopedics for bone scans, among other applications. Despite their strengths, nuclear imaging techniques have certain limitations. Both PET and SPECT involve exposure to ionizing radiation, which, although generally low and considered safe for diagnostic purposes, remains a concern for cumulative dose, particularly in vulnerable populations and repeated imaging scenarios. Additionally, the spatial resolution of these modalities is lower compared to anatomical imaging techniques such as Magnetic Resonance Imaging (MRI) or Computed Tomography (CT), which can sometimes limit the detection of very small lesions or subtle structural changes. Nonetheless, the unparalleled functional insights offered by PET and SPECT make them powerful complements to anatomical imaging, enabling a more comprehensive understanding of disease processes. Ongoing advancements in radiotracer development, hybrid imaging systems (such as PET/MRI), and quantitative imaging analysis continue to expand the clinical utility and precision of nuclear medicine in modern healthcare.

2.6 *Emerging Modalities and Hybrid Systems*

Recent advancements in medical imaging have increasingly focused on the integration of complementary technologies to enhance diagnostic accuracy and clinical utility. One of the most significant innovations in this regard is the emergence of hybrid imaging systems, such as Positron Emission Tomography-Magnetic Resonance Imaging (PET-MRI). These systems synergistically combine the functional imaging capabilities of PET–which highlights metabolic and molecular activity–with the superior soft-tissue contrast and anatomical detail provided by MRI. Unlike PET-CT, PET-MRI offers the added benefit of reduced radiation exposure, making it especially attractive in pediatric imaging and for repeated follow-up studies. Clinically, PET-MRI has shown particular promise in the fields of neuro-oncology, head and neck cancer, and musculoskeletal disorders, where high-resolution anatomical mapping alongside molecular profiling is critical for effective diagnosis and treatment planning. In parallel, the integration of AI into imaging workflows is revolutionizing the way images are processed, analyzed, and interpreted. AI algorithms, particularly those based on deep learning, are now capable of detecting subtle patterns in medical images that may elude even experienced radiologists. These tools can assist in tasks ranging from automated lesion detection and segmentation to predictive modeling of disease progression and therapy response. Moreover, AI enhances image reconstruction processes, enabling faster scans with reduced radiation doses or contrast agent requirements while maintaining high image quality. Together, these innovations are not just improving the technical capabilities of the image systems are also catalyzing a change toward more personalized and precision-oriented health care. By integrating anatomical, functional, and computational insights, doctors are increasingly trained to adapt the diagnoses and treatments to the unique characteristics of each patient. As these technologies continue to evolve, they have immense potential to improve results, reduce diagnostic uncertainty, and redefine the role of image in modern medicine.

3 Literature Review in Medical Image Analysis

The scenario of medical image analysis witnessed remarkable transformations in the last decade, driven by advances in computational technologies and machine learning algorithms. Researchers consistently sought innovative methodologies to improve diagnostic accuracy, improve disease detection, and develop more sophisticated image processing techniques in various medical image modalities [14].

3.1 Fundamental Research Trajectories in Medical Image Analysis

1. Image segmentation:
   The domain of medical image segmentation represents a critical nexus of computational methodology and clinical diagnosis, characterized by continuous methodological refinement and technological innovation. Traditional segmentation techniques, such as threshold-based approaches and region cultivation algorithms, initially provided fundamental mechanisms to delineate anatomical structures. However, these methods have shown significant limitations in the handling of complex medical image scenarios characterized by complex fabric interfaces, variable image qualities, and different pathological manifestations [15]. The emergence of machine learning and deep learning paradigms has fundamentally transformed image segmentation strategies. CNNs, particularly coding decoder architectures, such as U-NET, have accurately demonstrated capabilities to accurately segment medical images in various modalities. Essas arquiteturas avançadas aproveitam os mecanismos de extração de recursos hierárquicos, permitindo uma compreensão contextual sofisticada e classificação no nível de pixels com notável precisão [16]. Semantic segmentation techniques have evolved to face multifaceted challenges in medical images. The researchers developed innovative approaches, such as convolutional networks, attention, and attention mechanisms that improve spatial resolution and capture complex anatomical details. These methodological advances have been particularly transformed into complex image domains such as neurological images, cancer diagnosis, and cardiovascular structure analysis.
2. Classification and Diagnostic Algorithmic Frameworks: Development of classification algorithms represents another important research trajectory in medical image analysis. Contemporary machine learning approaches have exceeded traditional statistical classification methods, which introduce sophisticated deep learning architecture capable of extracting and creating fine clinical predictions. CNN has emerged as a major architectural structure for medical image classification. These networks show remarkable performance in various clinical challenges, including the detection of tumors, the identification of radiological discrepancies, and the monitoring of disease progression. Architectural innovation, such as residual networks and inception modules, has greatly improved the feature extraction capabilities, enabling a stronger and generalized diagnostic model [17]. Transfer teaching techniques have expanded the ability of classification algorithms by providing facilities for various imaging types and medical domains. Researchers can develop more adaptable and reference-inconceivable clinical systems by taking advantage of pre-existing models and by properly on specialized medical datasets. This approach addresses the important challenges related to limited medical imaging datasets and high computational complexity associated with the training of intensive learning models from scratch [18].

3. Multimodal Integration and Hybrid Approaches:

   The contemporary research landscape increasingly emphasizes multimodal image analysis approaches that integrate information from diverse imaging techniques. Hybrid methodological frameworks combine complementary imaging modalities to provide more comprehensive diagnostic insights. For instance, integrating MRI and CT scan data can offer more nuanced representations of anatomical structures and pathological conditions. Advanced fusion techniques, including early fusion, late fusion, and hybrid fusion strategies, enable researchers to develop more sophisticated computational models. These approaches leverage the unique strengths of different imaging modalities, creating comprehensive diagnostic frameworks that surpass the capabilities of individual imaging techniques. Table 1 shows comparative analysis of imaging modalities [19].
4. Computational Complexity and Algorithmic Efficiency: Researchers have simultaneously focused on addressing the significant computational challenges inherent in advanced medical image analysis algorithms. Optimization strategies such as model pruning, knowledge distillation, and efficient network architectures have been developed to reduce computational overhead while maintaining high diagnostic accuracy. Edge computing and distributed machine learning paradigms have emerged as promising approaches to mitigate computational constraints. These methodological innovations enable more scalable and accessible medical image analysis solutions, particularly in resource-constrained healthcare environments [15].
5. Emerging Methodological Frontiers:

   Emerging research trajectories increasingly explore probabilistic and uncertainty-aware machine learning approaches. Bayesian neural networks and ensemble learning techniques are being investigated to provide more robust and interpretable diagnostic predictions. These methodological innovations address critical challenges related to model uncertainty and generalizability in medical image analysis. Generative models, particularly GANs, represent another frontier of medical image analysis research. These techniques demonstrate potential for image synthesis, data augmentation, and advanced feature learning, offering novel computational strategies for addressing dataset limitations and enhancing diagnostic capabilities[15].

Table 1 Medical imaging modalities

Modality	Resolution	Radiation exposure	Primary applications
MRI [18]	High	None	Soft tissue imaging
CT scan [18]	Medium–High	Moderate	Bone and lung structures
X-Ray [19]	Low	Low	Skeletal diagnostics
Ultrasound [19]	Medium	None	Soft tissue and real-time

3.2 Machine Learning Integration and Deep Learning Breakthroughs

Machine learning has emerged as a transformative paradigm in medical image analysis, fundamentally reshaping diagnostic methodologies and computational approaches to medical imaging [57, 58]. The integration of advanced machine learning techniques represents a sophisticated convergence of computational intelligence and medical diagnostic expertise, enabling unprecedented capabilities in image interpretation and clinical decision support. Figure 2 shows machine learning workflow in medical image analysis [20, 21].

CNNs have revolutionized medical image analysis through their exceptional capability to automatically extract hierarchical features from complex imaging data. Unlike traditional image processing techniques, CNNs can learn intricate spatial hierarchies and representations directly from raw image data, enabling unprecedented diagnostic accuracy across multiple medical imaging modalities. The architectural sophistication of CNNs lies in their unique convolution and pooling layers, which progressively capture increasingly abstract and contextually relevant image features. These networks demonstrate remarkable performance in tasks such as lesion detection, organ segmentation, and disease classification. U-Net architectures have emerged as particularly impactful in medical image segmentation. Characterized by their symmetric encoder-decoder structure with skip connections, these networks excel at precise boundary delineation and contextual understanding. The architecture's ability to capture multi-scale contextual informa-

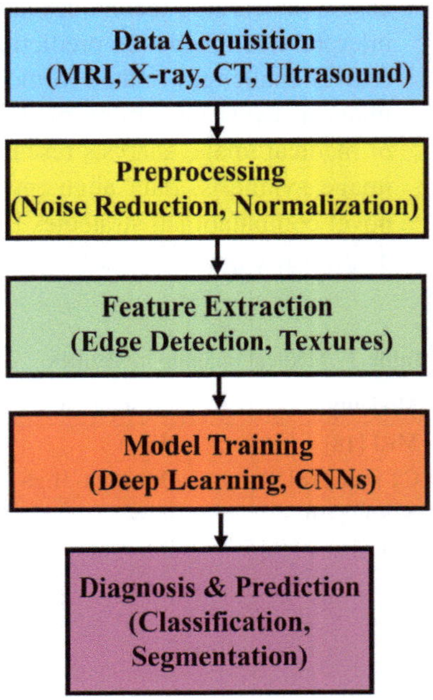

Fig. 2 Machine learning workflow in medical image analysis

Table 2 Deep learning architectures

Architecture	Key characteristics	Medical imaging applications
U-Net [22]	Symmetric encoder-decoder	Segmentation, boundary detection
ResNet [23]	Residual connections	Feature extraction, classification
Inception [24]	Multi-scale convolutions	Complex feature learning
GAN [25]	Generative modeling	Image synthesis, augmentation

tion makes it particularly suited for complex medical imaging scenarios. Residual Neural Networks address critical challenges in deep learning by introducing skip connections that facilitate more effective gradient flow. In medical imaging, ResNets enable the development of substantially deeper neural network architectures, improving feature representation capabilities and diagnostic performance. GANs represent a groundbreaking approach in medical image analysis, offering innovative solutions for image synthesis, data augmentation, and advanced feature learning. By simultaneously training a generator and discriminator network, GANs can create realistic medical images, address dataset limitations, and enhance model generalizability. Transfer learning has emerged as a critical strategy for addressing the limited availability of annotated medical imaging datasets. By leveraging pre-trained models from extensive image recognition databases and fine-tuning them for specific medical contexts, researchers can develop more robust and adaptable diagnostic algorithms. Table 2 shows the deep learning architectures.

3.3 *Probabilistic and Uncertainty-Aware Models in Medical Imaging*

The integration of probabilistic machine learning models in medical imaging has gained significant attention due to their ability to quantify uncertainty in diagnostic predictions. Unlike traditional deterministic models, which provide point estimates, probabilistic approaches offer confidence intervals and uncertainty measures, enhancing the reliability of automated decision-making systems. Bayesian neural networks (BNNs) extend conventional deep learning models by incorporating probability distributions over model parameters rather than fixed values. This probabilistic framework allows BNNs to capture epistemic uncertainty, which arises due to model limitations or insufficient training data. In medical imaging, BNNs have been applied to tasks such as disease classification, lesion segmentation, and anomaly detection, where uncertainty quantification is crucial for minimizing false positives and false negatives. By leveraging Bayesian inference techniques, such as variational inference or Monte Carlo dropout, these models provide more robust and interpretable predictions, improving clinical decision support. Ensemble learning techniques, including bagging and boosting, have also been widely employed to enhance the reliability of medical image analysis models. By aggregating predictions from multiple independently trained models, ensemble methods reduce variance and provide more stable predictions. Notably, deep ensemble models can approximate epistemic uncertainty by analyzing variations in predictions across different model instances. Additionally, these approaches help mitigate biases inherent in single-model architectures and improve generalizability to diverse patient populations. The ability to quantify uncertainty has significant implications for clinical practice. Uncertainty-aware models allow radiologists and clinicians to assess the reliability of AI-generated predictions, facilitating more informed decision-making. In high-stakes medical applications, such as cancer diagnosis or neuroimaging, understanding predictive confidence can guide follow-up testing strategies and personalized treatment plans. Furthermore, integrating uncertainty estimates into deep learning pipelines enhances transparency and fosters trust in AI-driven medical diagnostics [26].

4 Public Data Repositories for Medical Imaging

Medical image analysis has experienced tremendous growth in recent years, particularly with the advancement of deep learning techniques. However, the effectiveness of these advanced computational methods heavily depends on the availability of high-quality, well-annotated medical imaging datasets. This section provides a comprehensive examination of public data repositories for medical imaging, their significance in advancing research, and the various types of repositories available to researchers and practitioners.

4.1 Categories of Medical Imaging Repositories

Public medical imaging repositories can be categorized based on several factors, including imaging modality, anatomical region, pathology, and intended research application. This section explores these categories in detail and provides an overview of the most prominent repositories within each category [27].

4.1.1 Anatomical Region-Specific Repositories

Repositories in this category focus on specific body parts or organ systems, such as brain, chest, abdomen, or musculoskeletal structures. These specialized collections enable the development of algorithms that account for the unique anatomical characteristics and pathological manifestations in different body regions. The Alzheimer's Disease Neuroimaging Initiative (ADNI) provides one of the most extensive collections of brain imaging data, including MRI and PET scans from patients with Alzheimer's disease, mild cognitive impairment, and healthy

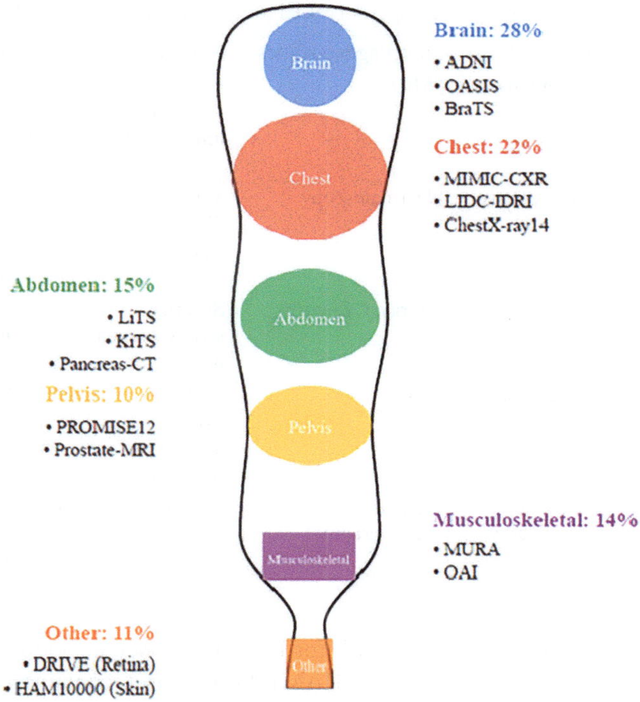

Fig. 3 Distribution of public datasets by anatomical region. Note: percentage represent proportion of publicly available datasets by anatomical region

controls. For cardiac imaging, the Cardiac Atlas Project offers a diverse collection of cardiac MRI data annotated with detailed ventricular measurements and function parameters. The LIDC-IDRI (Lung Image Database Consortium Image Collection) contains thoracic CT scans with annotated lung nodules, serving as a benchmark dataset for pulmonary nodule detection and classification algorithms. Figure 3 illustrates the distribution of available datasets across different anatomical regions, highlighting both the well-represented areas and the existing gaps in public medical imaging data [28].

4.1.2 Disease-Specific Repositories

Disease-specific repositories concentrate on particular pathologies or conditions, such as cancer, neurodegenerative diseases, or cardiovascular disorders. These repositories are invaluable for developing and validating algorithms for specific clinical applications, as they often include detailed annotations related to disease characteristics, severity, and progression. The BraTS (Brain Tumor Segmentation) challenge dataset provides multimodal MRI scans with expert-annotated tumor

Table 3 Samples of disease-specific repository used for medical image analysis applications

Repository	Disease focus	Imaging modalities	Annotations	Special features
BraTS [30]	Brain tumors	MRI	Expert segmentations, tumor grades	Multi-institutional data, annual challenge benchmark
HAM10000 [31]	Skin lesions	Dermatoscopy	Verified diagnoses, 7 categories	Includes metadata, on patient demographics
COVID-19 image collection [32]	COVID-19	X-ray, CT	Severity scores, clinical notes	Temporal series, showing disease progression
LIDC-IDRI [33]	Lung cancer	CT	Multiple expert, annotations per nodule	Includes nodule, characteristics assessment
Diabetic retinopathy dataset [34]	Diabetic retinopathy	Fundus photography	5-point grading scale	High-resolution images, quality assessment scores

segmentations, serving as a benchmark for brain tumor segmentation algorithms. For dermatological applications, the HAM10000 dataset contains over 10,000 dermatoscopic images with verified diagnoses spanning seven different skin lesion categories. The COVID-19 Image Data Collection represents a relatively recent addition, comprising chest X-rays and CT scans from COVID-19 patients with various disease severities. Table 3 provides a detailed comparison of disease-specific repositories, highlighting their clinical focus, annotation quality, and dataset characteristics [29].

4.2 *Multi-Institutional and Challenge Datasets*

Multi-institutional datasets compile medical images from various healthcare institutions, introducing valuable diversity in imaging protocols, equipment, and patient populations. These heterogeneous datasets are crucial for developing robust algorithms that can generalize across different clinical settings. Challenge datasets, meanwhile, are curated specifically for competitive evaluation of algorithms, often featuring standardized training and testing splits, as well as clearly defined evaluation metrics. The Medical Segmentation Decathlon exemplifies a comprehensive challenge dataset, encompassing ten different segmentation tasks across various organs and pathologies. The RSNA Pneumonia Detection Challenge provides chest X-rays with expert-annotated pneumonia regions, serving as a benchmark for pneumonia detection algorithms. Similarly, the Digital Mammography DREAM Challenge offers a large collection of mammograms for developing breast cancer

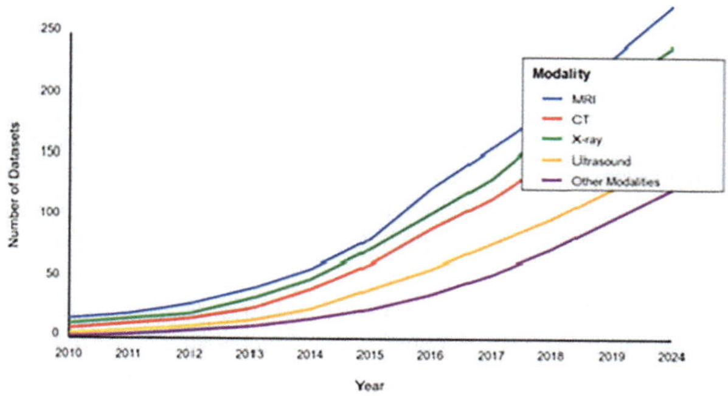

Fig. 4 Algorithm performance improvement on benchmark datasets (2015–2024)

detection algorithms. Figure 4 illustrates the performance improvement of medical image analysis algorithms over time on selected benchmark datasets, highlighting the crucial role of these challenge repositories in advancing the field [33].

4.3 *Data Formats and Annotation Standards in Medical Imaging Repositories*

The utility of public medical imaging repositories is significantly enhanced by standardized data formats and annotation protocols. This section examines the prevalent data formats and annotation standards employed across public repositories, highlighting their importance for interoperability and algorithm development [30].

4.3.1 Medical Imaging Data Formats

Medical imaging data are stored in various specialized formats designed to accommodate the complexity of medical images. For research purposes, formats such as NIfTI (Neuroimaging Informatics Technology Initiative) are commonly used, particularly for neuroimaging data. The NIfTI format offers advantages in terms of simplicity and compatibility with various analysis tools. Other formats include MINC (Medical Imaging NetCDF), ANALYZE, and more general formats like TIFF and PNG for specific applications where standard medical formats may not be necessary. Table 4 presents a comparative analysis of the primary medical imaging data formats, highlighting their features, advantages, and typical applications in research and clinical settings [31].

Table 4 Medical imaging data formats

Format	Features	Advantages	Limitations	Common applications
DICOM	Patient info, acquisition parameters, image data, comprehensive metadata	Clinical standard, widely supported, comprehensive	Complex, large file size	Clinical practice, PACS systems, multi-modality studies
NIfTI	Voxel data, orientation information, simplified metadata	Research-oriented, compact, easier preprocessing	Limited metadata compared to DICOM	Neuroimaging research, brain mapping, functional studies
MINC	Multi-dimensional data, hierarchical structure	Flexible, extensible, good for time-series	Less widespread adoption	Longitudinal studies, advanced neuroimaging research
ANALYZE	Separate header and image files	Simple structure, historical compatibility	Orientation ambiguity, deprecated	Legacy systems, older neuroimaging studies
NRRD	N-dimensional data, rich metadata	Flexible dimensions, self-describing	Limited clinical adoption	Research, multi-dimensional visualization

4.3.2 Annotation Standards and Protocols

The quality and consistency of annotations in medical imaging repositories significantly impact the development and evaluation of image analysis algorithms. Annotations in medical imaging can take various forms, including pixel-level segmentations, bounding boxes, anatomical landmarks, and diagnostic labels. Standardized annotation protocols ensure consistency across annotators and enable meaningful algorithm performance comparison. Several initiatives have emerged to standardize annotation practices in medical imaging. The Quantitative Imaging Biomarkers Alliance (QIBA) has developed profiles for standardizing the measurement of imaging biomarkers. The RadLex ontology provides a standardized terminology for radiology reporting, enhancing the consistency of text-based annotations [30, 32]. For segmentation tasks, the STAPLE (Simultaneous Truth and Performance Level Estimation) algorithm represents a widely adopted method for combining multiple expert segmentations into a consensus reference standard.

5 Image Preprocessing Techniques

Medical image analysis relies heavily on robust preprocessing pipelines to ensure data quality and consistency before quantitative analysis or machine learning applications. As noted by [35], inadequate preprocessing accounts for nearly 30% of failures in automated diagnostic systems. This section systematically examines four fundamental preprocessing operations that form the cornerstone of medical image analysis workflows.

5.1 Denoising Methods

Medical imaging plays a pivotal role in diagnosis and treatment planning, but various types of noise often compromise the quality of these images. Such noise can originate from multiple sources. For instance, in computed tomography (CT), photon starvation–a condition where insufficient photons reach the detector–leads to streak artifacts and increased noise. In magnetic resonance imaging (MRI), physiological motion such as respiration and cardiac activity introduces blurring and ghosting artifacts. Similarly, quantum noise, inherent to the physics of X-ray image formation, arises due to the stochastic nature of photon emission and detection. These noise factors degrade the visual quality and diagnostic value of medical images, necessitating robust denoising techniques. Contemporary medical image denoising methods can be broadly categorized based on their underlying principles. Table 5 provides a comparative summary of widely-used denoising algorithms, highlighting their methodological foundations and quantitative performance in terms of Peak Signal-to-Noise Ratio (PSNR) and Structural Similarity Index Measure (SSIM). These metrics are standard indicators of denoising effectiveness, with higher values indicating better preservation of image details and structural integrity.

Among these, traditional methods such as the Gaussian filter apply linear smoothing to reduce high-frequency noise but often at the expense of fine structural details. Median filtering, which leverages nonlinear order statistics, is effective against salt-and-pepper noise but can still cause blurring of edges. More advanced methods like wavelet thresholding exploit the sparsity of image representations in the wavelet domain, allowing for more targeted noise suppression. The BM3D

Table 5 Performance characteristics of medical image denoising algorithms

Method	Principle	PSNR (dB)	SSIM
Gaussian filter [36]	Linear smoothing	24.3	0.82
Median filter [37]	Nonlinear order statistics	26.1	0.85
Wavelet thresholding [38]	Sparse representation	28.7	0.91
BM3D [39]	Collaborative filtering	31.2	0.94

algorithm, regarded as a state-of-the-art technique, combines collaborative filtering with block-matching to preserve texture and structural information with high fidelity. The effectiveness of any denoising method depends heavily on the accurate estimation of noise levels and the appropriate tuning of algorithmic parameters. This process can be mathematically framed as an optimization problem:

$$\hat{x} = \arg\min_{x} \frac{1}{2}\|y - x\|_2^2 + \lambda R(x) \tag{1}$$

where y is the noisy image, x is the clean image, and $R(x)$ is a regularization term with weight λ.

Ultimately, the choice of a denoising strategy must consider both the clinical context and the specific noise characteristics of the imaging modality, ensuring that image enhancement does not inadvertently compromise diagnostic accuracy.

5.2 Normalization Strategies

In multicenter medical imaging studies, variability in scanner hardware, acquisition protocols, and site-specific calibration introduces significant inter-site differences in image intensities. These inconsistencies can hinder the reproducibility and reliability of downstream analyses, especially when using machine learning models that are sensitive to the statistical properties of input data. *Intensity normalization* is therefore a critical preprocessing step aimed at harmonizing image intensities to improve comparability across sites and subjects [40]. One of the most commonly employed techniques is **Z-score normalization**, which standardizes image intensities based on the mean and standard deviation:

$$I_{\text{norm}} = \frac{I - \mu}{\sigma} \tag{2}$$

Here, I denotes the original intensity, μ is the mean intensity, and σ is the standard deviation calculated over a defined region of interest (ROI) or the entire image. This normalization transforms the intensity distribution to have zero mean and unit variance, making it suitable for models that assume normally distributed inputs. Another widely used approach is **histogram matching**, which adjusts the intensity distribution of an input image so that it closely resembles the distribution of a reference or template image. This is achieved by aligning their cumulative distribution functions (CDFs), effectively minimizing global differences in intensity patterns. Histogram matching is particularly useful in longitudinal studies and cross-site harmonization tasks where consistency in appearance is essential. For MRI datasets, a more tailored method known as the **White Stripe** technique has been proposed [41]. This method identifies a narrow band of intensities corresponding to normal-appearing white matter (NAWM) and uses it as a stable reference for normalization. By focusing on a biologically consistent tissue type, the White Stripe method reduces variability arising from scanner differences while preserving relevant anatomical features. It has shown effectiveness in neuroimaging studies, particularly in aging and neurodegeneration research.

5.3 Contrast Enhancement

Medical images often suffer from poor contrast due to inherent limitations of the imaging hardware, suboptimal acquisition conditions, or biological constraints such as low tissue density variation. Low contrast can severely impact the visibility of critical anatomical structures or pathological regions, which in turn affects the accuracy of both manual interpretation by radiologists and automated analysis by computer vision systems. To address this, *contrast enhancement* techniques are applied during the preprocessing phase to improve the local and global visibility of structures of interest.

A widely adopted method in clinical imaging pipelines is **Contrast Limited Adaptive Histogram Equalization (CLAHE)** [42]. CLAHE is an extension of adaptive histogram equalization (AHE) that operates on small tiles or patches of the image and enhances local contrast by redistributing intensity values. Unlike traditional histogram equalization that can over-amplify noise in homogeneous regions, CLAHE introduces a *clip limit* to prevent over-enhancement and reduce the amplification of artifacts. This makes it particularly effective for enhancing subtle contrast variations in modalities such as X-rays, mammograms, and low-dose CT scans.

The implementation of CLAHE can be succinctly expressed in Python using OpenCV, as shown below:

```
def clahe_enhancement(image, clip_limit=2.0, grid_size=(8,8)):
    clahe = cv2.createCLAHE(
        clipLimit=clip_limit,
        tileGridSize=grid_size)
    return clahe.apply(image)
```

Here, `clipLimit` controls the contrast amplification threshold, and `tileGridSize` specifies the number of tiles used to divide the image. After processing, these tiles are recombined using bilinear interpolation to prevent edge discontinuities. The parameters can be fine-tuned depending on the modality and diagnostic task. While CLAHE is effective and computationally lightweight, recent research has shifted attention toward **deep learning-based contrast enhancement**, which offers the potential for more context-aware and task-specific adjustments. Miotto et al. [43] argue that the transformation of health care through big biomedical data requires models that can extract actionable insights from high-dimensional, heterogeneous, and unstructured sources such as electronic health records, imaging, and sensor data. Deep learning enables end-to-end learning from raw data, bypassing the need for manual feature engineering. Their review highlights the promise of deep learning in translating biomedical data into improved health outcomes, while also emphasizing the need for interpretability and holistic model design that bridges technical outputs with domain expertise. Montagnon et al. [44] provide a practical guide for deploying deep learning in radiology, using the case of colorectal liver metastasis imaging. Their workflow covers all stages of deep learning projects–from cohort selection to ethical considerations–underscoring the clinical potential of deep learning methods for tasks like tumor detection, segmentation, classification, and treatment monitoring. Contrast enhancement is often a critical precursor to such tasks, where improved visibility directly impacts downstream model accuracy. Wang et al. [45] contextualize deep learning as the latest stage in the evolution of AI in healthcare. They explain how earlier systems relied on explicit rule encoding by experts, whereas modern systems learn directly from raw data, such as pixel intensities in medical images. Deep learning-based contrast enhancement methods fall under this paradigm, enabling adaptive and data-driven contrast optimization that may outperform handcrafted techniques in both sensitivity and specificity. Zhang et al. [46] focus on the integration of deep learning and radiomics in oncology. They highlight that while many DL methods demonstrate efficacy in retrospective settings, prospective validation and robust clinical trials are essential for real-world deployment. Contrast enhancement plays a pivotal role here, as many predictive models rely on high-quality input features derived from enhanced images. The study advocates for stronger methodological rigor and the development of reproducible pipelines to bridge the translational gap. Van Tulder et al. [47] offer a critical review of deep learning in histopathology, acknowledging its potential to match or even surpass human-level performance in diagnostic tasks such as tumor detection. However, they caution against premature clinical adoption, citing limited deployment of these tools in actual clinical practice. Among the identified barriers are insufficient interpretability, lack of generalizability, and gaps in validation–all of which are relevant to contrast enhancement models that must perform consistently across diverse patient populations and imaging settings.

5.4 Image Registration

Image registration is a fundamental step in medical image analysis that aims to geometrically align two or more images, which may be acquired at different time points (longitudinal), from different viewpoints (multiview), or using different imaging modalities (multimodal). It is essential for tasks such as image fusion, longitudinal studies, surgical planning, and atlas-based segmentation [48].

Multimodal registration presents a unique challenge due to the inherent differences in contrast, resolution, and noise characteristics between modalities (e.g., CT vs. MRI or PET vs. MRI). These differences hinder direct voxel-wise comparisons, requiring sophisticated feature extraction and similarity measures.

The standard image registration pipeline consists of the following key steps:

1. **Feature Detection and Extraction:** Robust and invariant features are extracted from the images to establish correspondence. Common feature detectors include:
   - **SIFT (Scale-Invariant Feature Transform)**: Extracts scale- and rotation-invariant keypoints, robust to noise and illumination changes.
   - **SURF (Speeded-Up Robust Features)**: An efficient alternative to SIFT, optimized for real-time applications.
   - **ORB (Oriented FAST and Rotated BRIEF)**: A fusion of FAST keypoint detection and BRIEF descriptors, known for computational efficiency and good matching performance.
2. **Similarity Metric Optimization:** The goal is to find a spatial transformation that maximizes the similarity between the images. For multimodal registration, the following metrics are commonly used:
   - **Mutual Information (MI)**: Measures the statistical dependence between intensity distributions of two images. Particularly effective for multimodal data.
   - **Normalized Cross-Correlation (NCC)**: Suitable for mono-modal images with similar intensity distributions, but can be adapted with preprocessing for multimodal scenarios.
3. **Transformation Estimation:** A mathematical model is defined to warp one image to match the other. Common transformation models include:
   - **Rigid and Affine Transformations**: Include rotation, translation, scaling, and shearing. Useful for global alignment.
   - **Non-rigid (Deformable) Transformations**: Such as B-spline and Thin-Plate Splines, which allow local deformations, critical for aligning anatomical structures with nonlinear variations.
4. **Interpolation:** Once the transformation is applied, the pixel/voxel values at non-integer coordinates must be interpolated:
   - **Linear Interpolation**: Fast and commonly used, but may introduce artifacts in high-frequency regions.
   - **B-spline Interpolation**: Smooth and differentiable, ideal for deformable registration.
   - **Sinc Interpolation**: Provides ideal reconstruction in theory but is computationally expensive.

Advanced techniques like **elastic or deformable registration** have shown promising results in clinical applications. For example, [49] demonstrated that elastic registration achieves submillimeter accuracy (0.87 ± 0.23 mm) in brain imaging when appropriate cost functions, such as normalized mutual information, are employed.

Recent Developments Deep learning-based image registration methods are emerging as powerful alternatives to traditional optimization-based techniques. These include:

- **VoxelMorph**: A CNN-based framework that learns a spatial transformation function from training data, enabling real-time registration without iterative optimization.
- **RegNet**: A coarse-to-fine architecture that estimates both global and local deformations.
- **Adversarial Registration Networks**: Utilize generative adversarial frameworks to improve registration realism and regularization.

These models, while computationally efficient and highly flexible, still require large and representative training datasets and extensive validation before clinical deployment, particularly in multimodal settings where interpretability and robustness are critical.

Preprocessing is a foundational step in medical image analysis pipelines, but it must be approached with caution to ensure that diagnostic fidelity is not compromised. Clinical-grade image analysis systems must balance noise reduction and artifact suppression with the preservation of subtle yet clinically significant features.

Preservation of Diagnostic Features As highlighted by [50], inappropriate preprocessing—particularly aggressive smoothing or downsampling—can obscure or eliminate critical anatomical and pathological details. For instance:

- **Mammography:** Microcalcifications, which are key indicators of early breast cancer, often measure less than 0.5 mm. Excessive smoothing or compression artifacts may render them undetectable, leading to missed diagnoses.
- **Magnetic Resonance Imaging (MRI):** Subtle cortical lesions in patients with epilepsy or early-stage neurodegenerative disorders may only manifest as slight intensity variations. Overzealous denoising filters, such as bilateral or Gaussian filtering, risk suppressing these variations.
- **Computed Tomography (CT):** Small pulmonary nodules, a potential early sign of lung cancer, can be less than 3 mm in diameter. Preprocessing algorithms designed for motion artifact correction or contrast enhancement must retain the fine textural features that radiologists use for malignancy grading.

Regulatory Considerations The U.S. Food and Drug Administration (FDA) has recently tightened its regulations on AI/ML-based medical devices. According to guidance provided by [51], any preprocessing step that affects the raw image—even prior to model inference—must be explicitly documented and justified. This includes:

- **Parameter Specification:** All adjustable parameters used in preprocessing algorithms (e.g., kernel sizes, thresholds, contrast limits) must be defined and rationalized with respect to their impact on clinical output.

- **Traceability:** The pipeline must maintain full traceability from the raw input to the final model prediction, allowing independent auditors and clinical reviewers to assess how preprocessing influences model decisions.
- **Human Factors Analysis:** The FDA requires inclusion of usability studies that demonstrate the system does not mislead or reduce diagnostic confidence for clinicians due to preprocessing-induced changes in image appearance.
- **Performance Equivalence:** For software updates involving new preprocessing routines, manufacturers must show that performance metrics (e.g., sensitivity, specificity, AUC) are non-inferior to the previously approved version on an independent validation dataset.

Clinical Workflow Integration Beyond regulatory mandates, it is essential that preprocessing steps align with clinical workflows and radiological best practices:

- **Interoperability:** Preprocessing pipelines should be compatible with DICOM standards and Picture Archiving and Communication Systems (PACS), ensuring seamless integration.
- **Reproducibility:** Preprocessing algorithms should yield consistent outputs across diverse imaging systems, acquisition protocols, and patient populations.
- **Transparency and Interpretability:** Clinicians should have access to visualizations or overlays indicating what transformations were applied and where in the image pipeline, fostering trust in AI-driven decision support tools.

6 Strategies to Enhance AI Integration

The preceding sections have illuminated various challenges confronting deep learning applications in medical image analysis. This section explores comprehensive strategies and promising research avenues that offer potential solutions to these obstacles. By addressing these challenges systematically, the medical imaging community can accelerate the integration of deep learning technologies into clinical workflows and enhance patient care outcomes [52].

6.1 Addressing Data Scarcity and Annotation Challenges

The paucity of annotated medical imaging data remains a significant impediment to the advancement of deep learning applications in healthcare. Several approaches show promise in mitigating this limitation [50].

6.1.1 Advanced Data Augmentation Techniques

Conventional data augmentation techniques such as rotation, flipping, and scaling provide limited variability. More sophisticated approaches leveraging generative models offer promising alternatives. GANs and Variational Autoencoders (VAEs) can synthesize realistic medical images that preserve pathological features while introducing meaningful variations. Recent research has demonstrated the efficacy of style transfer techniques that can transform images from one modality to another (e.g., CT to MRI), thereby expanding the utility of existing datasets. Diffusion models, which have shown remarkable capabilities in general image synthesis, are increasingly being adapted for medical imaging applications with impressive results. These approaches not only increase the volume of training data but also help models become invariant to specific acquisition parameters and artifacts.

6.1.2 Semi-Supervised and Self-Supervised Learning Paradigms

Semi-supervised learning techniques effectively leverage small quantities of labeled data alongside abundant unlabeled data. Consistency regularization methods, such as Mean Teacher and FixMatch, enforce prediction consistency under different data augmentations, reducing the reliance on extensive annotations. Self-supervised learning has emerged as a particularly promising direction. By creating pretext tasks that do not require explicit labels, models can learn meaningful representations from unannotated medical images. As shown in Table 6, various self-supervised approaches have demonstrated performance comparable to fully supervised methods while requiring significantly fewer labeled examples. Contrastive learning frameworks like SimCLR and MoCo, when adapted to medical imaging contexts,

Table 6 Self-Supervised learning approaches for medical imaging

Approach	Learning paradigm	Required labeled examples	Performance vs. Fully supervised	Key benefits
SimCLR (Adapted) [54]	Contrastive	Minimal	Comparable	Effective feature representation
MoCo (Adapted) [55]	Contrastive	Minimal	Comparable	Transferable diagnostic features
Mean teacher [56]	Consistency regularization	Limited	Near-comparable	Leverages unlabeled data effectively
FixMatch [57]	Semi-supervised	Limited	Near-comparable	Enforces prediction consistency
Pretext tasks [58]	Self-supervised	None (pretraining)	Foundation for transfer	No annotations required

have yielded representations that transfer effectively to downstream diagnostic tasks [53].

6.1.3 Federated Learning for Collaborative Model Development

Federated learning offers a framework for training models across multiple institutions without sharing sensitive patient data. Each participating institution trains models locally on their data, sharing only model updates with a central server that aggregates these updates into a global model. Recent advances in secure aggregation protocols and differential privacy techniques have further enhanced the privacy guarantees of federated learning systems. Additionally, adaptive optimization strategies that account for data heterogeneity across institutions have improved convergence properties, making federated learning increasingly practical for multi-center medical imaging applications.

6.2 Enhancing Model Interpretability and Transparency

The "black box" nature of deep learning models presents significant barriers to clinical adoption. Ensuring model transparency and interpretability is crucial for building clinician trust and facilitating regulatory approval.

6.2.1 Federated Learning for Collaborative Model Development

Advanced attribution methods provide insights into model decision-making by highlighting image regions that significantly influence predictions. Techniques such as Integrated Gradients, GradCAM, and SHAP (SHapley Additive exPlanations) can generate visual explanations that align with clinical understanding. Research in attribution methods specifically tailored to 3D medical images and multi-modal inputs has yielded significant improvements in explanation quality. These methods not only enhance transparency but also serve as valuable tools for model debugging and validation against clinical knowledge.

6.2.2 Concept-Based Explanations and Semantic Disentanglement

Moving beyond pixel-level attributions, concept-based explanation methods aim to describe model decisions in terms of human-understandable concepts. Testing with Concept Activation Vectors (TCAV) and Concept Bottleneck Models enables the decomposition of complex neural representations into clinically relevant attributes. As shown in Table 7, these approaches can quantify the influence of specific radiological findings (e.g., ground-glass opacities, consolidation) on diagnostic

Table 7 Concept-based explanation methods

Method	Explanation type	Clinical relevance	Quantification capabilities
TCAV (Testing with concept activation vectors) [60]	Concept-based	High	Quantifies influence of radiological findings
Concept bottleneck models [61]	Concept-based	Very high	Decomposes predictions into clinical attributes
Semantic disentanglement [56]	Feature-based	Medium–High	Separates anatomical and pathological features
GradCAM [62]	Visual/Attribution	Medium	Highlights influential image regions
Integrated gradients [63]	Visual/Attribution	Medium–High	Precise attribution of prediction influences
SHAP [62]	Visual/Attribution	High	Quantitative feature importance

predictions. Semantic disentanglement approaches further enhance interpretability by separating different factors of variation in the data. By learning representations where different dimensions correspond to distinct anatomical or pathological features, these methods provide a natural framework for explanation and enable fine-grained control over model behavior [59].

6.2.3 Uncertainty Quantification and Calibration

Properly calibrated uncertainty estimates are essential for responsible clinical deployment. Bayesian neural networks and ensemble methods provide principled approaches to uncertainty quantification, generating predictions accompanied by confidence intervals. Recent developments in uncertainty decomposition techniques can distinguish between aleatoric uncertainty (inherent in the data) and epistemic uncertainty (arising from model limitations). This distinction provides clinicians with nuanced information about prediction reliability and helps identify cases that may require additional imaging or alternative diagnostic approaches [64].

6.3 Improving Model Robustness and Generalization

The deployment of deep learning systems across diverse clinical settings requires models that can maintain performance despite variations in imaging protocols, equipment, and patient populations.

Table 8 Multi-modal fusion architectures

Fusion strategy	Architecture	Data integration point	Performance by application	Computational requirements
Early fusion [67]	Joint input processing	Raw data level	Strong for correlated modalities	Moderate to high
Late fusion [68]	Ensemble of models	Prediction level	Robust across applications	High
Attention-based fusion [69]	Dynamic weighting	Feature level	Superior for complementary modalities	Moderate
Cross-modal transformers [67]	Self-attention	Multi-level	State-of-the-art for complex tasks	Very high
Modality-specific encoders [70]	Feature extraction	Intermediate	Good balance of performance/efficiency	Moderate

6.3.1 Domain Adaptation and Generalization Strategies

Domain adaptation techniques facilitate the transfer of models trained on source domains to new target domains with limited or no labeled data. Adversarial domain adaptation approaches, which align feature distributions across domains through adversarial training, have shown considerable promise in medical imaging applications. Domain generalization techniques take this concept further by training models that inherently generalize to unseen domains. Strategies such as meta-learning, invariant risk minimization, and style randomization encourage the learning of domain-agnostic features, improving performance on novel deployment environments without requiring adaptation data [65].

6.3.2 Multi-Modal Fusion and Complementary Information

Integrating information from multiple imaging modalities and clinical data sources can enhance diagnostic accuracy and robustness. Table 8 presents various multi-modal fusion architectures and their relative performance across different clinical applications. These approaches range from early fusion strategies that combine raw inputs to late fusion methods that integrate predictions from modality-specific models. Advanced attention mechanisms facilitate the dynamic weighting of different modalities based on their relevance to specific diagnostic tasks. These approaches can automatically emphasize the most informative modality for each case or pathology, mirroring the clinical practice of considering complementary information sources [66].

6.3.3 Continual Learning and Model Adaptation

Medical imaging practices and patient populations evolve over time, necessitating models that can adapt to shifting data distributions. Continual learning approaches enable models to incorporate new knowledge without catastrophically forgetting previously learned information. Recent advances in test-time adaptation allow models to adjust their behavior based on the statistics of individual test batches, providing an additional mechanism for addressing domain shifts without requiring retraining. These approaches are particularly valuable in clinical settings where deployment conditions may differ from training environments.

6.4 Ethical and Responsible AI Implementation

The deployment of deep learning systems in healthcare requires careful consideration of ethical implications and potential unintended consequences.

6.4.1 Fairness and Bias Mitigation

Medical AI systems must perform equitably across different demographic groups and clinical settings. Comprehensive bias assessment protocols can identify performance disparities across patient subpopulations. Techniques such as adversarial debiasing, reweighting, and representation learning with fairness constraints offer promising approaches for mitigating identified biases. Developing diverse and representative training datasets remains a fundamental strategy for ensuring model fairness. Collaborative initiatives to establish benchmarks that include diverse patient populations can help standardize fairness evaluation and drive improvements in model equity [71].

6.4.2 Privacy-Preserving Learning Techniques

Beyond federated learning, additional privacy-enhancing technologies can protect patient data while enabling model development. Differential privacy techniques introduce calibrated noise during training to provide formal privacy guarantees. Homomorphic encryption and secure multi-party computation allow computations on encrypted data, enabling collaborative analysis without exposing sensitive information [72].

7 Conclusion

Medical image analysis continues to evolve as a critical component of modern healthcare, supporting diagnosis, treatment planning, and disease monitoring across a wide array of modalities such as MRI, CT, X-ray, and Ultrasound. This chapter has provided a comprehensive overview of the foundational concepts, processing techniques, and challenges inherent to medical image analysis. We have discussed the significance of preprocessing, enhancement, segmentation, quantification, registration, and normalization strategies that contribute to robust image interpretation.

Through the exploration of various imaging modalities and processing pipelines, it has become clear that the effectiveness of computer-assisted analysis depends significantly on the careful selection and optimization of each methodological step. Additionally, the integration of deep learning has shown immense potential, although it presents unique technical and clinical challenges requiring rigorous validation, interpretability, and adherence to regulatory standards.

The chapter also highlighted the importance of publicly available datasets, which are pivotal for benchmarking and accelerating research in this field. Future advancements will likely depend on interdisciplinary collaboration, the development of interpretable models, and the clinical deployment of AI-driven solutions within ethically and technically sound frameworks.

Ultimately, this chapter serves as both an entry point and a strategic guide for researchers and practitioners aiming to contribute to this dynamic and impactful domain. By addressing current limitations and embracing innovative methodologies, the medical imaging community can drive the next generation of intelligent diagnostic tools, ultimately improving patient care outcomes.

References

1. Mienye ID, Swart TG (2024) A comprehensive review of deep learning: architectures, recent advances, and applications. Information 15(12): 755 https://doi.org/10.3390/info15120755
2. Toennies KD (2017) Guide to medical image analysis. Springer, Berlin. https://doi.org/10.1007/978-1-4471-7320-5
3. Hussain S et al (2022) Modern diagnostic imaging technique applications and risk factors in the medical field: a review. BioMed Res Int 2022(1):5164970. https://doi.org/10.1155/2022/5164970
4. Lftta JGJ et al (2024) X-rays and their uses on the human body. In: Current Clin Med Educ 2(8):91–115
5. Van Gelderen F (2004) Understanding X-rays. Springer, Berlin. https://doi.org/10.1007/978-3-642-18941-8
6. Pan X, Sidky EY, Vannier M (2009) Why do commercial CT scanners still employ traditional, filtered back-projection for image reconstruction? Inverse Probl 25(12):123009.
7. Mazrani W, McHugh K, Marsden PJ (2007) The radiation burden of radiological investigations. In: Arch Disease Childhood 92(12):1127–1131
8. Bhowmik A, Singh M, Singh R (2025) Medical imaging of the human body fluids: principles and diagnostics. In: Biofluid dynamics of human body systems. Apple Academic Press, Palm Bay, pp 621–705

9. Oppelt A. (2006) Imaging systems for medical diagnostics: fundamentals, technical solutions and applications for systems applying ionizing radiation, nuclear magnetic resonance and ultrasound. John Wiley & Sons, Hoboken
10. Revzin MV et al (2019) Optimizing image quality when evaluating blood flow at Doppler US: a tutorial. Radiographics 39(5):1501–1523
11. Hoskins PR (2008) Simulation and validation of arterial ultrasound imaging and blood flow. Ultrasound Med Biol 34(5):693–717
12. Endo K et al (2006) PET and PET/CT using 18 F-FDG in the diagnosis and management of cancer patients. Int J Clin Oncol 11:286–296
13. Hofman MS, Hicks RJ (2016) How we read oncologic FDG PET/CT. Cancer Imaging 16:1–14
14. Duncan JS, Ayache N (2000) Medical image analysis: progress over two decades and the challenges ahead. IEEE Trans Pattern Anal Mach Intell 22(1):85–106
15. Karim S et al (2023) Current advances and future perspectives of image fusion: a comprehensive review. Inf Fusion 90:185–217
16. Najjar R (2023) Redefining radiology: a review of artificial intelligence integration in medical imaging. Diagnostics 13(17):2760
17. Hussain D et al (2024) Revolutionizing tumor detection and classification in multimodality imaging based on deep learning approaches: methods, applications and limitations. J X-Ray Sci Technol 32(4):857–911
18. Mullachery V, Khera A, Husain A (2018) Bayesian neural networks. Preprint, arXiv:1801.07710. https://doi.org/10.48550/arXiv.1801.07710
19. Gómez-Chova L et al (2015) Multimodal classification of remote sensing images: a review and future directions. Proc IEEE 103(9):1560–1584
20. Hammad M et al (2022) Efficient lightweight multimodel deep fusion based on ECG for arrhythmia classification. Sensors 22(23):9347
21. Erickson BJ et al (2017) Machine learning for medical imaging. Radiographics 37(2):505–515
22. Siddique N et al (2021) U-net and its variants for medical image segmentation: a review of theory and applications. IEEE Access 9:82031–82057
23. Hammad M et al (2021) ResNet-attention model for human authentication using ECG signals. Expert Syst 38(6):e12547
24. Zhang Z et al (2020) DENSE-INception U-net for medical image segmentation. Comput Methods Programs Biomed 192:105395
25. Zhou T et al (2023) GAN review: models and medical image fusion applications. Inf Fusion 91:134–148
26. Sakr AS et al (2023) ECG-COVID: an end-to-end deep model based on electrocardiogram for COVID-19 detection. Inf Sci 619:324–339
27. Clark K et al (2013) The cancer imaging archive (TCIA): maintaining and operating a public information repository. J Digital Imaging 26:1045–1057
28. Johnson AEW et al (2019) MIMIC-CXR, a de-identified publicly available database of chest radiographs with free-text reports. Sci Data 6(1):317
29. Jack Jr CR et al (2008) The Alzheimer's disease neuroimaging initiative (ADNI): MRI methods. J Magn Reson Imaging Official J Int Soc Magn Reson Med 27(4):685–691
30. Menze BH et al (2014) The multimodal brain tumor image segmentation benchmark (BRATS). IEEE Trans Med Imaging 34(10):1993–2024
31. Tschandl P, Rosendahl C, Kittler H (2018) The HAM10000 dataset, a large collection of multi-source dermatoscopic images of common pigmented skin lesions. Sci Data 5(1):1–9
32. Cohen JP et al (2020) Covid-19 image data collection: prospective predictions are the future. Preprint, arXiv:2006.11988. https://doi.org/10.48550/arXiv.2006.11988
33. Jacobs C et al (2016) Computer-aided detection of pulmonary nodules: a comparative study using the public LIDC/IDRI database. Eur Radiol 26:2139–2147
34. Nagpal D et al (2022) A review of diabetic retinopathy: datasets, approaches, evaluation metrics and future trends. J King Saud Univ Comput Inf Sci 34(9):7138–7152
35. Demirbaga U et al (2021) Autodiagn: an automated real-time diagnosis framework for big data systems. IEEE Trans Comput 71(5):1035–1048

36. Kumar N, Nachamai M (2017) Noise removal and filtering techniques used in medical images. Orient J Comput Sci Technol 10(1):103–113
37. Chen B-Q et al (2019) Coupling denoising algorithm based on discrete wavelet transform and modified median filter for medical image. J Central South Univ 26(1):120–131
38. Jansen M (2012) Noise reduction by wavelet thresholding, vol 161. Springer Science & Business Media, Berlin
39. Danielyan A, Katkovnik V, Egiazarian K (2011) BM3D frames and variational image deblurring. IEEE Trans Image Process 21(4):1715–1728
40. Lemkaddem A et al (2012) A multi-center study: intra-scan and inter-scan variability of diffusion spectrum imaging. Neuroimage 62(1):87–94
41. Rorden C et al (2012) Age-specific CT and MRI templates for spatial normalization. Neuroimage 61(4):957–965
42. Reza AM (2004) Realization of the contrast limited adaptive histogram equalization (CLAHE) for real-time image enhancement. J VLSI Signal Process Syst Signal Image Video Technol 38:35–44
43. Miotto R et al (2018) Deep learning for healthcare: review, opportunities and challenges. Briefings Bioinf 19(6):1236–1246
44. Montagnon E et al (2020) Deep learning workflow in radiology: a primer. Insights Imaging11:1–15
45. Wang F, Casalino LP, Khullar D (2019) Deep learning in medicine—promise, progress, and challenges. JAMA Internal Med 179(3):293–294
46. Zhang X et al (2022) Prospective clinical research of radiomics and deep learning in oncology: a translational review. Crit Rev Oncol Hematol 179:103823
47. Van der Laak J, Litjens G, Ciompi F (2021) Deep learning in histopathology: the path to the clinic. Nature Med 27(5):775–784
48. Karakas AB et al (2025) From pixels to prognosis: leveraging radiomics and machine learning to predict IDH1 genotype in gliomas. Neurosurgical Rev 48(1):1–26
49. Hill DLG, Hawkes DJ (2000) Across-modality registration using intensity-based cost functions. In: Handbook of medical imaging: processing and analysis, 537–553. https://doi.org/10.1016/b978-012077790-7/50040-0
50. Sharma P (2024) Medical image processing using AI. Academic Guru Publishing House, Bhopal. ISBN: 978-81-972615-5-8
51. Johnson A et al (2024) Mimic-cxr database. PhysioNet10 13026:C2JT1Q
52. Khan S et al (2022) Transformers in vision: a survey. ACM Comput Surv 54(10s):1–41
53. Shahid MS, Imran A (2025) Breast cancer detection using deep learning techniques: challenges and future directions. Multimed Tools Appl 84:3257–3304
54. Diong ZY, Lim WY, Goh CP (2024) Self-supervised learning in medical diagnostics: an examination of simclr and byol in image classification. In: 2024 3rd international conference on digital transformation and applications (ICDXA). IEEE, pp 210–214
55. Sowrirajan H et al (2021) Moco pretraining improves representation and transferability of chest x-ray models. Med Imaging Deep Learn 2021:728–744
56. Wang K et al (2022) Semi-supervised medical image segmentation via a tripled-uncertainty guided mean teacher model with contrastive learning. Med Image Ana 79:102447
57. Zenk M et al (2022) Realistic evaluation of fixmatch on imbalanced medical image classification tasks. In: Bildverarbeitung für die Medizin 2022: Proceedings, German workshop on medical image computing, Heidelberg, June 26–28, 2022. Springer, pp 291–296
58. VanBerlo B, Hoey J, Wong A (2024) A survey of the impact of self-supervised pretraining for diagnostic tasks in medical X-ray, CT, MRI, and ultrasound. BMC Med Imaging 24(1):79
59. Wang J, Wang S, Zhang Y (2025) Deep learning on medical image analysis. CAAI Trans Intell Technol 10(1):1–35
60. Kim B et al (2018) Interpretability beyond feature attribution: Quantitative testing with concept activation vectors (tcav). In: International conference on machine learning. PMLR, pp 2668–2677

61. Koh PW et al (2020) Concept bottleneck models. In: International conference on machine learning. PMLR, pp 5338–5348
62. Hammad M et al (2025) Explainable AI for lung cancer detection via a custom CNN on CT images. Sci Rep 15(1):12707
63. Chakraborty A, Staib LH, Duncan JS (1996) Deformable boundary finding in medical images by integrating gradient and region information. IEEE Trans Med Imaging 15(6):859–870
64. Agneya DA et al (2024) Deep learning in medical image analysis: a survey. In: 2024 international conference on innovation and novelty in engineering and technology (INNOVA), vol I, pp 1–5
65. Mansur Z et al (2025) Deep learning-based brain tumor image analysis for segmentation. SN Comput Sci 6(1):1–18
66. Suzuki K (2017) Survey of deep learning applications to medical image analysis. Med Imaging Technol 35(4):212–226
67. Huang B et al (2020) A review of multimodal medical image fusion techniques. Comput Math Methods Med 2020(1):8279342
68. Khan SU et al (2023) Multimodal medical image fusion towards future research: a review. J King Saud Univ-Comput Inf Sci 35(8):101733
69. Tirupal T, Chandra Mohan B, Srinivas Kumar S (2021) Multimodal medical image fusion techniques—a review. Current Signal Transduction Therapy 16(2):142–163
70. Li Y et al (2024) A review of deep learning-based information fusion techniques for multimodal medical image classification. Comput Biol Med 108635.
71. Vrudhula A et al (2024) Machine learning and bias in medical imaging: opportunities and challenges. Circ Cardiovasc Imaging 17(2):e015495
72. Gomis-Pastor M et al (2024) Clinical validation of digital healthcare solutions: state of the art, challenges and opportunities. Healthcare 12(11):1057. MDPI

The Role of AI in Enhancing Imaging Modalities

Yazhini Karthik, M. Sujithra, and B. Senthilkumar

1 Introduction

1.1 Background on the Evolution of AI in Medical Imaging

Modern healthcare practice depends on medical imaging techniques because these methods help early diagnosis and proper treatment planning. The imaging technologies which include X-ray alongside CT and MRI and ultrasound and PET have undergone substantial advancement through technological developments. Advancements in medical imaging required facing new problems including the creation of image noise artifacts while demanding better resolution together with enhancement of interpretation precision. The medical field benefits from Artificial Intelligence (AI) because it improves both the quality of images and the automation of diagnostics together with clinical practice efficiency. Medical imaging with AI experiences distinct stages of advancement which we can divide into major phases [1].

However, integration of AI into medical imaging both improved diagnostic accuracy and contributed to decreases work load, and better clinical decision making [2, 3, 19].

Y. Karthik (✉) · M. Sujithra
Department of Computing – Data Science, Coimbatore Institute of Technology, Coimbatore, India
e-mail: 2032051mds@cit.edu.in; sujithra@cit.edu.in

B. Senthilkumar
Department of Mechanical Engineering, Kumaraguru College of Technology, Coimbatore, India
e-mail: senthilkumar.b.mec@kct.ac.in

N. Ben Aoun et al. (eds.), *AI for Medical Image Analysis*,
https://doi.org/10.1007/978-3-032-02963-8_3

1.2 Scope and Objectives of the Chapter

This chapter discusses the application of AI to improve precision, automate, and image quality of medical imaging modalities. Within the scope of the discussion the discussion extends to AI driven advancement in noise reduction, artifact removal, super resolution imaging, real time imaging. The chapter also examines AI's effect on disease detection, pattern recognition and radiologists' decision support systems. The main objectives of this chapter are:

- To examine AI integration in different imaging modalities such as MRI, CT, and ultrasound.
- To discuss AI-driven techniques for noise reduction, artifact removal, and super-resolution imaging.
- To highlight AI's role in real-time imaging guidance, optimized imaging systems, and low-dose imaging techniques.
- To explore AI-based image reconstruction methods, including deep learning and compressed sensing.
- To analyze the impact of AI on disease detection, pattern recognition, and decision-support systems for radiologists.
- To present future directions in AI-powered medical imaging, such as ultra-low-dose imaging and AI-augmented compact imaging devices..

This chapter intends to explain in detail the transformational effect of AI on medical imaging and its capability to uproot traditional diagnostic imaging in the modern healthcare in an attempt to address these objectives.

2 Overview of Imaging Modalities and Their Importance

In the current state of health care, medical imaging is a crucial part of contemporary practice, which enables visualization of the internal anatomy to facilitate a precise diagnosis, treatment observation and disease monitoring. Different imaging modalities have been designed for clinical use with advantages. This section gives a review of the importance of the modalities imaging in the practice of medicine.

2.1 Important Imaging Modalities

Magnetic Resonance Imaging (MRI) is a non-invasive imaging technique that produces detailed medical images using magnetic fields and radio waves, eliminating the need for ionizing radiation [4]. Computed Tomography (CT) technology generates cross-sectional images of the body using multiple X-ray images obtained from various angles, providing rapid and detailed imaging, making it crucial in

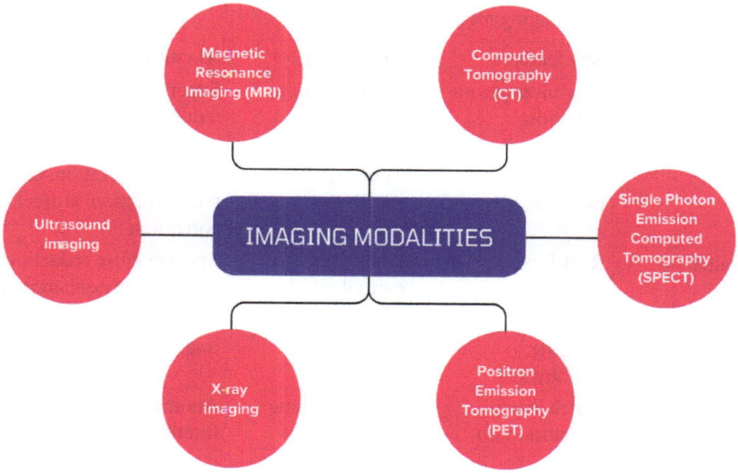

Fig. 1 Important imaging modalities

trauma and emergency medicine. Ultrasound imaging, or sonography, creates real-time pictures of internal organs and tissues using high-frequency sound waves. It is widely used in obstetrics, cardiology, and gastroenterology. X-ray imaging remains one of the most commonly used diagnostic tools, particularly useful in orthopedics, pulmonology, and dentistry for detecting fractures, infections, and lung diseases. Positron Emission Tomography (PET) and Single Photon Emission Computed Tomography (SPECT) are nuclear imaging techniques that use radiotracers to visualize metabolic and functional processes in the human body, aiding in oncology, neurology, and cardiology [5]. Figure 1 illustrates the primary imaging modalities used in medical diagnostics, including MRI, CT, ultrasound, X-ray, PET, and SPECT, each serving distinct clinical purposes with unique technological advantages.

A comparative overview of major imaging modalities, their features, clinical applications, and the role of AI enhancements is provided in Table 1.

2.2 *Importance of Imaging Modalities in Healthcare*

Imaging technologies play a significant role in disease detection, treatment planning, and patient monitoring. The integration of AI in imaging systems has further improved diagnostic accuracy and efficiency.

Table 1 Comparison of imaging modalities

Imaging modality	Key features	Applications	AI enhancements
MRI	Non-invasive, no radiation	Neuroimaging, tumors	Super-resolution, noise reduction, motion artifact removal
CT	Cross-sectional, rapid imaging	Trauma, oncology	Dose optimization, fast reconstruction, artifact correction
Ultrasound	Real-time, portable	Obstetrics, cardiology	Speckle noise reduction, image clarity enhancement
PET/SPECT	Functional imaging, radiotracers	Oncology, neurology	Radiotracer dose reduction, image segmentation
X-Ray	Quick, basic structural info	Fractures, lung exams	Anomaly detection, quality filtering

2.2.1 Early Disease Detection

Early Medical detection of diseases gives better treatment results and better survival chances. Pathological changes become visible through MRI and CT and ultrasound imaging tests that work before clinical symptoms develop. The medical procedure of mammography identifies early breast cancers during their initial stages whereas low-dose CT scans screen for lung cancer. MRI scans are used to determine the neural condition Alzheimer's disease and multiple sclerosis to get a diagnostic accuracy and prompt medical treatment strategies. AI powered image analysis enhances the detection method on account of the system being able to detect subtle anomalies that human evaluators cannot detect during the manual inspection.

2.2.2 Treatment Planning and Precision Medicine

Medical images are of vital precise nature that forms basis for designing patient specific treatments and intervention preparation. Surgeons today have detailed looks of the body structures through modern imaging tools that assist them in carrying out of complicated brain and orthopaedic surgical procedures. PET-CT imaging techniques in radiation therapy enhance both adequacy of tumor damage and damage to nearby tissue, providing oncologists with a means to create more accurate treatment plans. Real time imaging is also used in interventional radiology to perform minimally invasive procedures where procedures can be done at less risk and with shorter recovery time of surgery [6].

2.2.3 Disease Monitoring and Follow-Up

Once there is the diagnosis, but before the treatment planning has occurred; medical imaging has essential multi-functional roles that include monitoring disease through its progress and evaluating which treatments are effective. Repeated imaging scans can be used to adjust activated oncology treatments because these scans can monitor how tumors respond to chemotherapy and radiation therapy. Doctors use echocardiography with cardiac MRI to image heart function and search for structural anomalies that develop over time in cardiac patients. Imaging examinations are needed to evaluate periodic liver cirrhosis and kidness and pulmonary fibrosis. AI systems they run on medical images can help healthcare providers get more precise disease observation and predicted outcome.

2.2.4 Guiding Minimally Invasive Procedures

The advancing capabilities of image equipment was the main reason why healthcare professionals have been using these ingenious gadgets to perform minimally invasive surgery and from this they had been able to forego many open surgical procedures. Only using real-time imaging allows doctors to perform their procedures with great precision during tasks including catheter insertions and endovascular interventions along with biopsies. Medical professionals use ultrasound steering to carry out biopsies on liver and breast tissue alongside thyroid tissue by reducing patient discomfort during sample collection. The medical procedures of angioplasty and stent placements heavily depend on fluoroscopy and CT imaging applications. Medical procedures using AI-improved imaging capabilities ensure more precise surgeries that create better outcomes while protecting patient safety.

2.2.5 Improving Accessibility and Remote Diagnostics

Medical imaging solutions now have greater accessibility because of portable and AI-powered diagnostic devices that have become available. Through handheld ultrasound devices medical staff can carry out quick examinations directly at the site of care including emergency rooms and rural locations with field hospitals. Through Teleradiology healthcare professionals can provide prompt medical interpretations of remote imaging tests because this technology functions as a vital solution for distant healthcare services. Mobile imaging units that include both X-ray and ultrasound capabilities now service underserved regions to help patients screen early for diseases and get preventive healthcare measures. AI automation systems help non-specialists view medical images since they provide assistance with image interpretation to make medical diagnosis possible despite expertise shortages.

2.2.6 Enhancing Radiologists' Efficiency and Reducing Workload

Medical imaging studies continue to accumulate in large numbers which negatively affects radiologists so it becomes essential to develop AI-based workflow optimization systems. Radiologists benefit from automated algorithmic detection of normal scans through which they can dedicate their time to handle difficult cases needing expert analysis. AI triage systems use priority controls to locate and treat urgent medical situations including strokes and pulmonary embolisms so they get rapid assessment. AI-based decision-support platforms enable radiologists to receive complementary assessments from machines which decreases diagnostic mistakes as well as enhances imaging interpretations' accuracy [7, 20].

3 Limitations and Challenges of Imaging Modalities

The great advances in medical imaging have not removed some ongoing problems that lower diagnosis accuracy and reduce clinical efficiency. Technical constraints and inconsistent imaging environments and various artifacts produce obstacles that impair the detection of important diagnostic elements. Medical imaging needs these limitations solved to achieve better quality diagnosis from reliable interpretation.

3.1 Diagnostic Constraints Due to Noise and Artifacts

Medical images regularly contain noise and artifacts which weaken image quality potentially causing wrong interpretation of results. Random pixel intensity fluctuations occurring in imaging systems block essential anatomical as well as pathological information from view. Various factors like low signal-to-noise ratio (SNR) along with hardware constraints and patient movement result in the formation of this artifact. An artifact represents an image-based distortion which stands apart from actual anatomical features. The rise of artifacts during medical imaging occurs due to patient movement, suboptimal imaging protocols, metal hardware items within the body and faulty computer operations. In the case of MRIs, due to the long scan periods associated with MRIs, patient movement can induce motion artifacts, hence, beam hardening artifacts in CT occurs as a result of high-density dental materials or orthopaedic hardware.

The combination of noise with artifacts creates diagnostic uncertainty that pushes radiologists to several testing phases or add supplementary diagnostic methods to achieve better visibility. The effective potential of AI-based methods to solve noise and artifact problems exists yet these solutions need further development for clinical impacts along with prompt diagnostic performance.

3.2 Resolution Limitations and the Need for Super-Resolution Imaging

Medical imaging strongly depends on resolution quality. Image resolution determines the clarity for observing subtle details within pictures. The resolution depends on three key factors: imaging system hardware components and the speed of data collection and the computer processing power. Poor image resolution reduces visibility of critical features thus making it difficult for doctors to detect tiny tumors as well as detect fracture fragments or track subtle body changes appearing in disease progression.

Modern imaging tools have received several upgrades to reach past their natural resolution capabilities. Past technology solutions require better detectors and superior optical components yet these solutions become expensive to implement and difficult to operate. High-resolution pictures result from deep learning models that process low-resolution images thus leading to enhanced test accuracy. MRI along with ultrasound testing faces distinct challenges because of their slow data acquisition processes and weak hardware components. The combination of adversarial networks with deep learning methodologies using artificial intelligence techniques are receiving widespread attention as solutions to enhance image resolution while maintaining constant scanning time and radiation dosage levels.

3.3 Variability in Image Quality Across Different Technologies

The imaging technologies used in medical care exhibit varying abilities which results in quality image discrepancies that depend on the technology type and device along with the acquisition parameter settings. The factors that cause image quality variations include machine calibration state alongside operator expertise and patient positioning routines as well as environmental situations.

Contrast and image intensity in MRI examinations of the same patient when obtained with various machine brands creates difficulties for accurate comparative analysis between periods or healthcare facilities. The quality of ultrasound images heavily relies on the skills of the sonographer along with probe positioning and particular features of each patient including their body composition. Particle CT imaging yields various levels of image clarity as different radiation dose protocols are used because low dose settings may compromise diagnostic accuracy. AI powered image harmonization software can be incorporated in standardization techniques that output-normalize across multiple machines and health care sites in clinical practice. Through AI-powered algorithms quality control functions get automation because the programs recognize poor imaging quality and recommend methods to improve image reliability.

Common limitations in medical imaging modalities along with their AI-powered mitigation strategies are summarized in Table 2.

Table 2 Imaging limitations and AI solutions

Limitation	Cause	Impact	AI solution
Noise	Motion, low SNR	Loss of detail	Noise reduction
Artifacts	Metal, motion	Image distortion	Artifact correction, MAR[a]
Low resolution	Hardware limits	Missed small features	Super-resolution (CNNs, GANs)
Quality variance	Machine setup	Inconsistent output	Image harmonization

[a] *MAR* Metal Artifact Reduction

4 The Emergence of AI in Medical Imaging

Artificial Intelligence(AI) in medical imaging is a paradigm shift for diagnostics and clinical decision-making. AI has not only improved X-Rays for image processing, enabling the easier detection, classification, and planning of disease treatment with the help of innovative AI. Nowadays AI is not as simple as it used to be, and it has progressed from rudimentary computational techniques of AI to advanced deep learning models which improves the accuracy and efficiency of these systems in medical imaging. This section talks about the contribution of AI in imaging and AI in clinical workflows, where we discuss about the notable landmarks in historical events relating to AI in imaging.

4.1 Historical Milestones and Recent Advancements

Medical imaging AI evolution has a long history of several decades starting from early computational techniques till sophisticated deep learning models developed over time. The first applications of AI in medical imaging were expert systems, that ran on fixed rules that were modeled with statistics and decide. The base for automated image analysis was thus created by these systems enabling patterns to be detected in primary patterns based in radiographic and histologic images.

New adapted learning algorithms emerged with the advent of machine learning, and they were able to process medical datasets. Image classification tasks mostly utilized Support Vector Machines (SVM) together with decision trees and k-nearest neighbours (k-NN) algorithms to detect tumors while segmenting anatomical structures. The emergence of deep learning, particularly convolutional neural networks (CNNs), transformed medical imaging by enabling automated feature extraction and high-accuracy classification. Figure 3 illustrates the application of major deep learning architectures–CNNs for classification, U-Nets for segmentation, and GANs for super-resolution–across typical medical imaging workflows. CNN-based models such as AlexNet, VGGNet, and ResNet demonstrated superior performance in image recognition tasks, paving the way for AI-driven radiology applications. Generative AI techniques are increasingly being applied to medical image analysis and morphological assessments [34].

With advancements in computing power, AI is now being integrated into real-time imaging workflows. AI-powered ultrasound and MRI systems are enhancing image acquisition, reducing scan times, and optimizing radiation dose exposure. The future promises AI-driven automation in diagnostics, enabling faster and more precise medical decisions.

4.2 AI's Integration into Clinical Imaging Workflows

AI is increasingly being embedded into routine clinical imaging workflows, assisting radiologists, pathologists, and clinicians in multiple aspects of medical imaging. Its use is for image acquisition, pre-processing work and analysis and subsequently to offer decision support functions. Good performance in structure segmentation and disease classification was achieved in the presence of AI. Deep learning methods include CNNs and other models, automated detection of lung diseases from chest radiographs and CT scans, and brain tumor classification from MRI scans, as well as cardiovascular disease assessment using echocardiography and angiography. Figure 2 illustrates the application of major deep learning architectures in medical imaging workflows.

Automated report generation and suspicious area identification along with provide medical consultation, are some of the assistances given to the radiologists by the AI based support systems. Their operations create such systems that

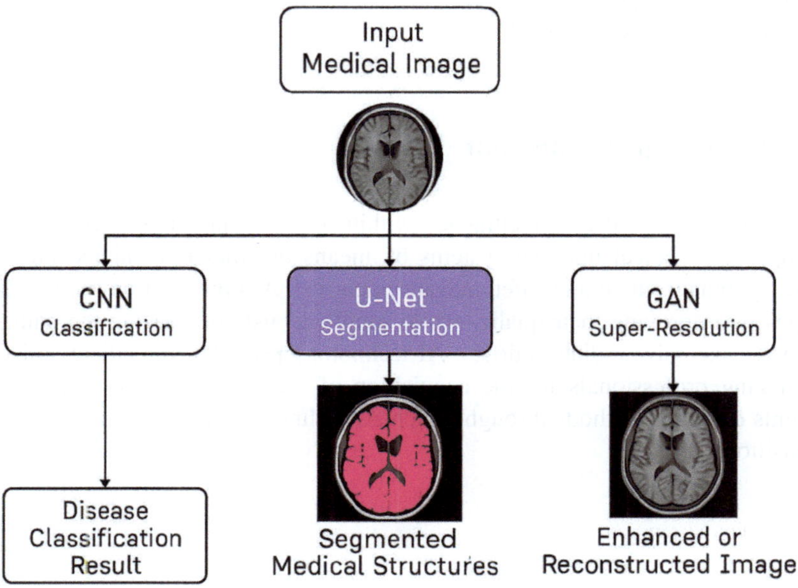

Fig. 2 Application of deep learning models in medical imaging

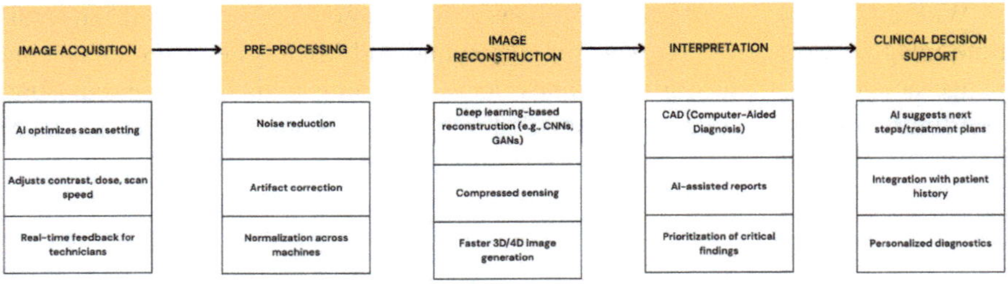

Fig. 3 AI contributions across the medical imaging workflow

build diagnostic consistency and minimize human mistakes. Radiologists' jobs are executed more easily on computational systems that carry out boring job sequences such as tumor tracking and organ partitioning jobs, as well as lesion quantity assessment jobs. Human intervention is needed in advanced medical situations, and hence, healthcare professionals pay their attention to these. Augmented intelligence systems combine human expertise with AI capabilities to optimize medical image scanning workflows [28].

Imaging technologies are enhanced through new AI driven technology to improve clinical workflows and improve diagnostic accuracy which improves patient management protocols. To ensure responsible utilization and fair distribution of AI in clinical practice, a wide scale implementation of it requires regulatory standards and ethics in guiding AI implementation in medical practice. The progressive integration of AI across different stages of medical imaging—from acquisition and preprocessing to reconstruction, interpretation, and clinical decision support—is illustrated in Fig. 2.

5 AI in Image Acquisition

The inclusion of artificial intelligence within image acquisition workflows leads to improved medical imaging systems by means of efficiency enhancement and accuracy enhancement and safety advancement [8]. AI optimization tools enhance images by improving their quality while simultaneously decreasing the danger of receiving excessive radiation doses. AI technology provides immediate assistance to imaging professionals for the acquisition of diagnostic pictures. The section presents different methods through which AI technology improves medical image acquisition.

5.1 *Optimizing Imaging Systems for Efficiency and Accuracy*

Artificial intelligence has revolutionized imaging systems by automatically selecting parameters for multitude of different imaging modalities and consequences that this entails, such as decreased time for scanning and enhanced quality of acquired images. Traditional imaging modalities depend upon adjust parameters manually, resulting in inconsistencies in images and diagnostic reliability. On the other hand, AI-powered imaging systems use real-time optimization of these parameters based on patient-specific variables.AI algorithms analyze patient characteristics and historical imaging data to fine-tune acquisition parameters such as contrast levels, exposure time, and field of view. For instance, MRI scans benefit from AI-driven pulse sequence optimization, reducing scan duration while maintaining high-resolution images. CT imaging leverages AI to adjust X-ray tube voltage and current dynamically, optimizing image quality while minimizing radiation exposure.

The AI acceleration methods parallel imaging combined with deep-learning-based reconstructions operate to decrease the process of producing high-resolution images considerably. Patient comfort remains high because these technologies decrease the duration of long scan processes used in MRI imaging.The issue of inconsistent imaging quality between different scanners and facilities has existed since a long time. Standardization of image acquisition becomes achievable through AI because it harmonizes protocols as well as minimizes inter-scanner variability to deliver consistent imaging results between healthcare facilities.

5.2 *Enabling Low-Dose Imaging Without Compromising Quality*

Medical imaging requires constant evaluation between better images and safer procedures primarily in techniques that need ionizing radiation including CT and X-ray exams. Artificial intelligence helps decrease X-ray radiation exposure while enabling superior or better than existing diagnostic imaging quality. Algorithms based on artificial intelligence use deep convolutional neural networks (CNNs) to eliminate scan noise which keeps essential anatomical details intact. Radiologists obtain high-quality image interpretation through these methods despite the implementation of low-radiation procedures. The system adjusts radiation doses automatically through AI algorithms that depend both on patient body structure and precise medical purposes. The technology combines two AI systems for adaptive exposure control to measure radiological exposure in paediatric care and vulnerable populations together with algorithms for low-dose Iterative reconstruction.

AI-controlled reconstruction methods decrease PET and SPECT radiotracer usage which results in lower exposure of radioactive materials to patients without compromising image quality.

5.3 Real-Time Guidance for Improving Image Capture Processes

Real-time patient care instruments and imaging technician support systems are provided through the implementation of AI technologies in medical image capture processes. The feature provides essential aid for image acquisition specifically within fast-changing diagnostic areas which include ultrasound and interventional radiology. The placement of the ultrasound probe receives assistance from AI-powered systems which enables technicians to achieve maximum image acquisition results. Modern robotic systems assess ongoing imaging information to enhance the image quality by making necessary adjustments thus diminishing both technical expert dependency and scan variation.

AI algorithms detect ordinary imaging artifacts (blur, beam hardening and aliasing) automatically in real time. AI alerts operators to notify them about images that need modification during the acquisition process instead of requiring additional scan attempts. Real-time image enhancements combined with overlays and segmentation occur during surgical and catheter-based medical interventions because of AI. The cooperation of AR technology with artificial intelligence powers real-time navigation systems that boost medical accuracy in minimally invasive surgery. Medical imaging in itself is becoming more efficient, precise and safer to patients with AI integrated into image acquisition workflows. The next step involves the further automation, with the help of AI powered robotics, that will further pushed the limits of real time, AI assisted imaging.

6 AI's Contributions to Augmenting Image Quality

Medical imaging stands essential for diagnostic purposes as well as treatment strategy development and health condition surveillance. Standard imaging techniques face diagnostic complexities because they confront two difficulties which include resolving noise artifacts and issues with resolution. AI functions as a strong operational tool for image enhancement by providing three crucial features for noise reduction together with artifact elimination and superior resolution capabilities. AI image quality enhancement approaches receive analysis based on their diagnostic accuracy levels in the subsequent section.

6.1 Noise Reduction and Artifact Removal Techniques

The primary limitation of medical imaging systems develops from image artifacts and noise appearance because these features reduce diagnostic precision by hiding key information. The deep learning models in AI-driven algorithms solve image clarity problems effectively by protecting complete structural information from disruptions.

Through artificial intelligence processing of MRI and CT images the operators achieve clearer images because it improves signal-to-noise ratios to eliminate the grainy appearance. The application of AI filters in ultrasound exams results in improved visual clarity of soft tissues because these filters can both enhance contrast and diminish speckle noise.

Three main sources produce artifacts in medical images between patient movements and hardware limitations together with environmental factors. AI technologies help display researchers when they need to find and correct these image distortions. AI models study movement-related image distortions to make predictions which physicians use for improving scan quality during times of patient movement. Computational methods based on deep learning systems enable CT users to reduce beam hardening artifacts by correcting CT image distortions. The solution of Metal Artifact Reduction (MAR) enables AI algorithms to process X-ray and CT images containing metallic implants therefore the surrounding tissue remains visible. Advanced AI-based encryption and steganography techniques further enhance the security of medical images during transmission and storage [18].

6.2 *Super-Resolution Imaging for Enhanced Detail*

The resolution capabilities of imaging technologies face challenges because they cannot maintain proper image quality for detecting early-stage tumors along with microcalcifications. AI-powered super-resolution imaging enhances image details beyond conventional resolution limits.

Super-resolution convolutional neural networks (SRCNNs) and GANs upscale low-resolution images, reconstructing high-quality outputs with improved spatial resolution [25]. Figure 4 illustrates the SRCNN architecture used for super-resolution imaging, where convolutional layers progressively enhance low-resolution medical inputs to produce high-quality diagnostic outputs. AI-driven super-resolution has been successfully applied in MRI, CT, PET, and ultrasound imaging to enhance finer anatomical structures, leading to more precise diagnoses [24]. This approach is particularly useful in telemedicine and remote diagnostics, where low-resolution images may be the only available data [9, 23].

In multiframe super-resolution imaging, AI integrates information from multiple low-resolution frames to generate a single, high-resolution image. This technique is beneficial in dynamic imaging scenarios, such as cardiac imaging and functional MRI (fMRI), where temporal resolution is critical. AI-driven super-resolution techniques are also being applied to enhance low-field MRI images to achieve high-field quality [26].

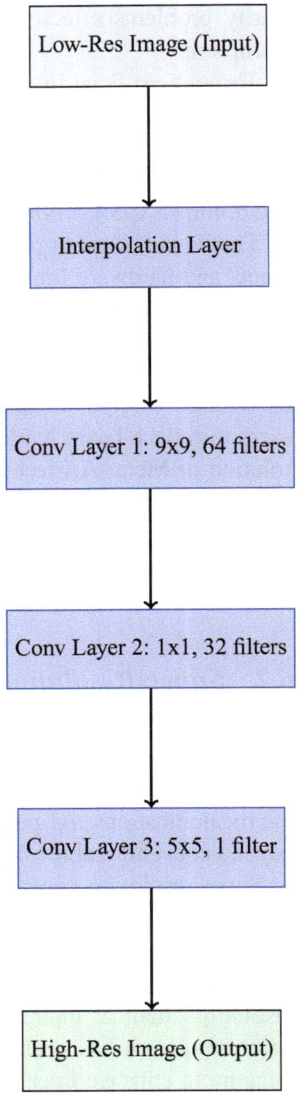

Fig. 4 SRCNN architecture for super-resolution imaging

6.3 Applications in Improving Image Clarity and Diagnostic Utility

By improving image quality, AI contributes to better visualization of anatomical structures, enhances the accuracy of automated diagnostic models, and reduces the need for repeat scans. AI-enhanced images provide radiologists with clearer and more interpretable scans, leading to increased confidence in diagnosis. The quality of medical images enables improvements of Computer Aided Diagnosis (CAD)

Table 3 AI techniques and their imaging applications

AI technique	Modality	Purpose	Example application
CNN	MRI, CT	Noise reduction	Enhancing clarity in brain scans
GAN	CT, Ultrasound	Super-resolution	Improving fetal and tumor imaging
U-Net	MRI, PET	Segmentation	Accurate tumor boundary detection
Autoencoder	X-ray, MRI	Artifact removal	Correcting metal-induced distortions

systems which enhances the performance of AI models for disease detection such as lung nodules and breast cancer and brain tumors. The implementation of AI produces CT examinations with low-dose levels yet achieves outstanding diagnostic results which lowers patient exposure to radiation. Using artificial intelligence enables nuclear medicine staff to generate high-quality PET images from less radioactive tracer exposure reducing risk exposure to patients.

The adaptation of AI enhancement methods depends on imaging modalities alongside clinical necessities for optimal optimization of different imaging applications. Artificial intelligence improves fundus photograph clarity in retinal imaging because it increases the accuracy of diabetic retinopathy screening. Medical imaging experiences a transformation through advanced AI-driven image quality improvements which increases diagnosis precision along with operational efficiency and ensures better safety for patients. Advanced medical imaging applications will obtain their highest potential during AI model evolution.

As summarized in Table 3, various AI techniques such as CNNs, GANs, and U-Nets play distinct roles in enhancing image quality across different modalities, contributing significantly to diagnostic clarity and utility

7 AI in Image Reconstruction

Medical imaging starts with unprocessed data that goes through procedures to create visible outputs for medical analysis. The traditional methods of image reconstruction lead to lengthier processing times that diminish quality in addition to performance-intensive computer procedures. AI technology in image reconstruction enabled faster processing algorithms that improved both three-dimensional and four-dimensional image results along with compressed sensing technique implementation [10].

7.1 Faster Reconstruction Algorithms for Efficient Imaging

CT and MRI systems depend on filtered back projection (FBP) and Fourier-based techniques which traditionally force users to choose between swift operation or high-resolution images. Artificial intelligence through reconstruction optimization techniques reduces computational complexities while preserving high-quality images.

Traditional reconstruction algorithms incorporate deep neural networks (DNNs) to accelerate image formation processes by eliminating artifacts and reducing noise from the images. CNNs and GANs enable widespread use for manufacturing high-quality images from sensor raw data which provides near real-time imaging capabilities [30]. AI provides multiple processing capabilities that shortens the time required for MRI and PET scan reconstruction.

AI-driven methods enable instantaneous reconstruction, reducing waiting times in critical care settings. In emergency radiology, AI-based rapid reconstruction of CT and X-ray images aids in faster diagnosis of stroke, fractures, and internal bleeding [11, 31].

7.2 *Enhancing 3D and 4D Image Quality*

The field of medical imaging now depends heavily on 3D and 4D imaging methods to generate detailed assessments of both body structures and their functions. The advanced imaging techniques receive enhanced quality and operational efficiency because of AI implementation.

The absence of information in 3D images receives AI enhancement through information completion to enhance anatomical precision. Deep learning reconstruction methods have enhanced CT, MRI and ultrasound scanning accuracy so they deliver more precise information for surgical planning and disease evaluation purposes [12]. CT angiography reconstruction based on artificial intelligence enables better blood vessel observation which helps physicians detect vascular diseases.

4D imaging, which involves dynamic imaging over time, benefits greatly from AI-enhanced reconstruction techniques. AI optimizes 4D cardiac MRI, allowing real-time tracking of heart motion and improving the accuracy of functional assessments. In radiation therapy, AI improves 4D treatment planning by refining tumor motion tracking, ensuring precise radiation delivery.

7.3 *Advanced Reconstruction Techniques, Including Compressed Sensing*

The advanced mathematical approach Compressed sensing (CS) helps medical imaging professionals generate high-quality images from reduced numbers of measurements. Through AI enhancements CS methods have gained efficiency and became suitable for use with various imaging techniques. Traditional CS relies on sparse data acquisition, requiring computationally heavy iterative reconstruction.

AI accelerates this process by learning optimal reconstruction patterns. Deep compressed sensing algorithms enable high-quality MRI scans from fewer acquired signals, reducing scan time while maintaining diagnostic accuracy. The application of AI-driven CS in PET imaging helps minimize prolonged procedures because it rebuilds images with high fidelity using restricted data.

AI uses physics-based reconstruction models to improve accuracy while maintaining the interpretative capacity of healthcare professionals on the medical outcomes. The hybrid deep learning-CS models improve the acquisition of MRI and CT data by generating images with higher quality and little artefact. AI-enhanced MBIR allows low-dose reconstruction of signals, maintaining clinical quality, while providing radiation doses to patients at lower levels. Medical imaging has also been revolutionized by AI-based image reconstruction (via daily imaging), leading to speedier, more efficient, and higher-quality images. Deep learning, compressed sensing, and hybrid models have come together to further stretch the limits of imaging capabilities. With the continuous development of artificial intelligence, future reconstruction methods will optimize imaging workflows even further, allowing for ultra-fast, high-resolution scans while minimizing the risk associated with exposed patients.

8 AI for Image Analysis and Interpretation

AI technology improves medical image assessments by establishing automated disease-diagnostic systems and pattern recognition systems and extracting essential quantitative biologic marks from medical images. Better healthcare diagnosis and shorter reading times enable medical staff to create educated clinical choices enabled by deep learning technology combined with advanced computing systems. This part details the essential ways AI brings value to image analysis together with interpretation procedures.

8.1 Disease Detection and Pattern Recognition Through AI

Medical imaging diagnostics have experienced a revolutionary change because AI systems now perform automatic disease recognition in combination with pattern recognition capabilities. Multiple models work alongside each other to assess enormous imaging databases which yield superior results in detecting irregularities better than medical experts can manage independently [29].

CNNs have become a central tool in radiology disease detection for identifying pathologies within X-rays and CT scans and MRIs. Through AI detection systems the analysis of subtle patterns achieves success in identifying lung cancer and both brain tumors and diabetic retinopathy and cardiovascular diseases at levels above human capabilities. With AI-based models healthcare professionals can recognize disease severity while performing earlier diagnosis procedures which decreases the number of wrong positive results.

Complex image patterns detected by the technology reveal diseases early before clinical symptoms become detectable to patients. Using medical image patterns as input Radiomic analysis assists doctors in foreseeing disease development and evaluating treatment effects. The identification of extraordinary and challenging pathologies becomes enhanced through AI system training that uses extensive medical datasets leading to improved diagnostic results for uncommon medical conditions.

8.2 Extracting Quantitative Imaging Biomarkers

Disease characterization and treatment planning as well as prognosis prediction utilizes objective data which medical professionals use for their analysis. AI technology improves the identification together with understanding of various biomarkers in medical analysis.

Through automation AI extracts tumour measurements, morphology, structural features and tissue distinctions from MRI and CT images for accurate cancer staging procedures. Deep learning models measure vascular density together with blood flow and tissue perfusion that doctors need to evaluate stroke patients and those with cardiovascular diseases. Bone mineral density assessment which uses X-ray and CT scans with AI-driven analysis enables medical staff to detect osteoporosis at an early stage.

AI technology extracted from medical images enables Radiomics to deliver high-dimensional features linked to disease advancement. AI-based predictive models use extracted biomarkers to estimate patient survival rates, response to therapy, and recurrence risks in oncology. AI combined with genomics (radio genomics) identifies imaging-genetic correlations, aiding in personalized treatment strategies.

8.3 Augmenting Radiologists With AI-Driven Decision-Support Systems

Through its decision-support system function AI delivers valuable support to radiologists which both accelerates workflows and cuts down diagnostic failures. These systems deliver real-time information while marking abnormalities to help medical personnel make their clinical choices. The pre-screening process through AI technology enables studies to prioritize cases with high abnormality scores that get immediate review. The operation of image annotation tools by AI software reduces manual workload allowing radiologists to focus on complex testing responsibilities [21]. Electronic health record integration facilitates the examination of patient history by imaging results to achieve holistic diagnosis. AI-augmented knowledge management systems further enhance clinical performance by integrating imaging insights with broader healthcare data [27].

AI-powered computer automated detection systems improve breast cancer and lung nodule and brain lesion identification by increasing detection accuracy. CAD applications in mammography assist radiologists in identifying microcalcifications, an early indicator of breast cancer. AI-powered CAD in colonoscopy and endoscopy aids in detecting polyps and gastrointestinal abnormalities. The explainable AI models generate visual display heatmaps which simplify the interpretation of important medical imaging areas [35]. AI-generated reports summarize findings with confidence scores, enabling radiologists to validate AI suggestions before making final decisions. AI-enhanced case reporting systems are improving the integration of imaging findings with comprehensive patient documentation [39]. Ethical AI integration ensures that radiologists remain the primary decision-makers while AI serves as an assistive tool rather than a replacement. Ensuring AI interpretability and transparency in medical imaging is crucial for clinical acceptance and trust [33].

Medical image analysis experiences transformation through AI because the technology enhances disease identification abilities and releases quantitative assessment systems for imaging biomarkers and assists radiologists with diagnostic support tools. Professional AI models reaching maturity will enable their integration into healthcare systems to enhance diagnoses and image reading as well as achieve better patient health results. Through its partnership with medical experts AI technology will create a medical imaging system that provides superior accuracy and better efficiency together with broad access.

9 Applications Across Imaging Modalities

Artificial Intelligence (AI) has significantly enhanced various imaging modalities, improving diagnostic accuracy, efficiency, and automation in clinical workflows. AI-powered systems optimize image acquisition, interpretation, and post-processing across multiple imaging techniques, including radiology, ultrasound, nuclear medicine, and hybrid imaging systems. Figure 5 highlights the distribution of AI-based applications across imaging modalities, with MRI and CT exhibiting the highest adoption of AI-enhanced solutions.

9.1 AI in Radiology

Radiology, encompassing X-ray, CT, and MRI imaging, has greatly benefited from AI integration. AI-based detection systems assist in identifying lung abnormalities such as pneumonia, tuberculosis, and lung cancer in X-rays while also improving orthopedic diagnostics by detecting fractures and bone lesions with greater accuracy. AI aids in low-dose CT reconstruction, reducing radiation exposure while preserving image quality, and deep learning models support early stroke detection and vascular abnormality identification. For MRI, AI enhances image reconstruction, reducing scan times and improving resolution, aiding in the diagnosis of neurodegenerative diseases such as Alzheimer's and multiple sclerosis. By automating image segmentation and anomaly detection, AI streamlines the diagnostic workflow and reduces the workload on radiologists [13, 14, 37].

9.2 AI in Ultrasound Imaging

AI has enhanced ultrasound imaging by improving image clarity, reducing noise, and enabling automated interpretation. It provides accurate insights into fetal anomalies and congenital conditions, making obstetric imaging more efficient. AI-powered echocardiography helps in diagnosing heart diseases by automating cardiac function analysis, ensuring precise and faster evaluations. Additionally, AI-driven elastography allows for better assessment of liver fibrosis and early detection of tumors. The integration of AI in portable ultrasound devices also enables real-time point-of-care diagnostics, expanding accessibility in remote healthcare settings [15].

9.3 AI in Nuclear Medicine

Nuclear medicine imaging, including PET and SPECT, has seen advancements with AI-driven optimization techniques. AI improves PET and SPECT reconstruction, enhancing image resolution while reducing scan times, which is crucial in reducing

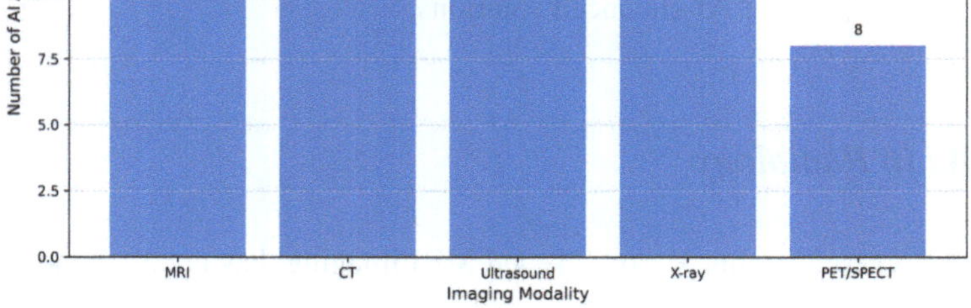

Fig. 5 AI contributions across different imaging modalities

patient exposure to radiotracers. It facilitates more accurate tumor detection and staging in oncology, assisting clinicians in planning targeted therapies. In cardiology, AI-driven segmentation of nuclear images allows for better assessment of metabolic activity and myocardial perfusion, leading to early and more precise diagnosis of cardiovascular diseases. These improvements make nuclear imaging more efficient, reliable, and clinically valuable.

9.4 AI in Optical and Hybrid Imaging

AI applications in optical and hybrid imaging systems have improved disease visualization, early detection, and treatment planning. AI-powered endoscopic imaging enhances the detection of gastrointestinal conditions, aiding in early diagnosis of cancers and inflammatory diseases. Ophthalmic imaging has benefited from AI-driven automation, allowing early identification of conditions like diabetic retinopathy and glaucoma. In hybrid imaging, AI enhances PET-CT and PET-MRI by improving image fusion and alignment, facilitating a more comprehensive assessment of both anatomical and functional data. These advancements lead to more personalized treatment strategies in oncology, neurology, and other specialties. Multimodal generative AI approaches are emerging to integrate multiple imaging modalities for comprehensive diagnostic interpretation [32].

By integrating AI into these imaging modalities, the healthcare industry is moving toward faster, more accurate, and efficient diagnostics, ultimately improving patient outcomes and clinical decision-making.

Artificial Intelligence (AI) has significantly enhanced various imaging modalities, improving diagnostic accuracy, efficiency, and automation in clinical workflows. AI-powered systems optimize image acquisition, interpretation, and post-processing across multiple imaging techniques, including radiology, ultrasound, nuclear medicine, and hybrid imaging systems.

10 Future Trends in AI-Enhanced Medical Imaging Modalities

The coming changes in the field of medical imaging come from AI. It gives better precision, fast results as well as more access. Lower imaging doses need development for achieving radiation reduction standards while maintaining picture quality standards. As a collaboration with the IMPACT group, we build specialized imaging methods that require minimal doses to produce images. Serial surgical operations gain assistance through AI by providing real-time recommendations to medical professionals. Small imaging tools that employ AI technology will provide ongoing health monitoring and personal examinations to prevent health problems before they arise. The transition of AI technologies from research to clinical adoption represents a critical pathway for realizing the full potential of AI in medical imaging [40].

10.1 Real-Time Imaging for Immediate Insights

AI-driven real-time imaging enables immediate interpretation and decision-making, reducing diagnostic delays. Faster deep learning models provide on-the-fly segmentation and classification of medical images, assisting radiologists and clinicians during procedures. AI-powered real-time anomaly detection allows for the identification of critical conditions such as stroke, cardiac arrest, and internal bleeding, facilitating faster intervention and better patient outcomes [16].

10.2 Ultra Low-Dose Imaging to Minimize Radiation Exposure

Reducing radiation exposure while maintaining high image quality is a crucial advancement in medical imaging. AI-based noise reduction techniques enhance low-dose imaging quality, allowing for diagnostic precision without excessive radiation. AI-driven dose optimization adjusts radiation levels dynamically based on patient-specific factors, ensuring optimal safety while preserving image clarity. This is particularly important for pediatric and chronic disease patients who require multiple imaging sessions over time.

10.3 Advanced Reconstruction and Multi-Modal Imaging Techniques

AI-driven reconstruction techniques such as compressed sensing and deep learning-based image enhancement accelerate MRI and CT scans without compromising diagnostic quality. AI improves data integration in PET-CT and PET-MRI, enhancing diagnostic accuracy by combining anatomical and functional imaging. Super-resolution imaging techniques powered by AI allow for improved visualization of microstructures, making it highly beneficial for applications in oncology, neurology, and cardiology. These techniques facilitate earlier disease detection and better treatment planning.

10.4 Development of AI-Optimized and Portable Devices

The development of AI-powered imaging devices is making diagnostic imaging more accessible, especially in remote and resource-limited settings. AI-driven handheld ultrasound devices enable real-time imaging at the point of care, allowing clinicians to make immediate assessments. Mobile radiography systems equipped with AI improve emergency imaging capabilities, ensuring rapid diagnosis in field settings. Wearable AI-integrated imaging devices are emerging for continuous monitoring of cardiovascular and neurological conditions, providing real-time insights into disease progression and management. Embodied AI technologies are expanding the possibilities for interactive and autonomous healthcare imaging systems [36].

10.5 Integrating AR/VR for Imaging Interpretation

Augmented reality (AR) and virtual reality (VR) are transforming the way medical images are interpreted and utilized. AI-powered AR overlays assist in surgical navigation and interventional procedures by superimposing imaging data onto a patient's anatomy, enhancing precision and reducing risks. VR-based 3D visualization of medical scans improves pre-surgical planning and medical education, allowing healthcare professionals to better understand complex anatomical structures. AI-driven AR applications also support guided procedures such as biopsies and catheter placements, making medical imaging more interactive and intuitive. With continuous advancements in AI, the future of medical imaging is moving toward higher precision, efficiency, and accessibility. These innovations will revolutionize diagnostics and patient care, leading to improved outcomes and a more streamlined healthcare system. The future of AI in medical imaging is marked by advancements that improve diagnostic precision, reduce radiation exposure, and enhance accessibility.

11 Conclusion

The introduction of Artificial Intelligence into medical imaging practices has reformed diagnostic capabilities because it increases diagnostic precision while organizing processes and lowering costs of healthcare. Artificial Intelligence addresses traditional imaging device issues through improvement of acquisition processes simultaneously with reconstruction technology and image quality enhancement practices and interpretive capabilities. The chapter examines how AI optimizes imaging systems and enables low-dose imaging as well as enhances resolution along with its support for clinical decision-making processes. The technological developments bring improvements to diagnostic potential and lead to changes in the functioning roles of radiologists and healthcare professionals in imaging.

11.1 Summary of AI's Transformative Impact on Imaging Modalities

The evolution of medical imaging through AI funnelled advancements by resolving difficulties that included noise reduction as well as artifact removal and resolution restriction issues. Radiologists obtain precise imaging scans of high-quality using AI optimization technologies during imaging operations. AI has allowed medical practitioners to create imaging procedures with low-dose contrast which decreases radiation exposure for patients and health workers simultaneously.

The recent development of AI-based image enhancement technologies produced better-quality imaging that helps identify minor medical issues that would escape standard imaging methods [17]. The use of AI-based image reconstruction technology and methods like compressed sensing and deep-learning algorithms has both sped up image creation techniques and reinforced imaging process efficiency when generating high-fidelity 3D and 4D images.

Image analysis and interpretation through AI techniques provides significant benefit because machines assist both disease detection and pattern recognition and quantitative biomarker extraction from images. Decision-support systems become more powerful when radiologists combine AI with them because it helps them improve diagnostic skills and minimize interpreter inconsistency. Portable imaging devices that use AI algorithms have extended medical diagnoses to distant populations that need high-quality healthcare services.

11.2 Implications for Future Healthcare Systems

Healthcare delivery systems worldwide will experience fundamental changes from increasing AI application in medical imaging because the methods lead to more accurate diagnoses and enhanced workflow systems and reduced expenses. Patient care improves while doctors create specific treatment approaches which focus on individual healthcare needs through implementation of these technological solutions. The implementation of AI-powered image segmentation and report generation enables healthcare employees to sustain patient care activities which drives improvements for hospital diagnostic facilities. The financial effects resulting from AI-controlled imaging analysis generate substantial impacts on hospitals and medical facilities. Healthcare expenses decline substantially when medical imaging procedures become optimized by AI technology and when AI minimizes duplicate image orders and human mistakes occur less frequently.

Remote diagnostic service linked with Artificial Intelligence enabled telemedicine expands medical care access particularly to regions that lack a sufficient number of specialists. Intelligent portable diagnostic devices built using AI technology have developed rural patient care assessment methods by implementing point-of-care systems to offer high-quality medical examinations throughout remote areas. The advancement of AI in medical imaging creates a need to resolve multiple ethical concerns while dealing with administrative and practical implementation obstacles that appear after deployment. Addressing current challenges and understanding future directions is essential for successful AI integration in medical imaging [38]. Suitable patient safety and fair clinical use require complete assessments of privacy issues and algorithmic biases as well as strict AI model validation procedures. AI-based imaging systems need standardized regulatory systems which must be built to earn the trust of medical staff and their patient populations.

References

1. Ranschaert ER, Morozov S, Algra PR (eds) (2019) Artificial intelligence in medical imaging: opportunities, applications and risks. Springer, Berlin
2. Hasani N, Farhadi F, Morris MA et al (2022) Artificial intelligence in medical imaging and its impact on the rare disease community: threats, challenges and opportunities. PET Clin 17(1):13
3. Tang X (2019) The role of artificial intelligence in medical imaging research. BJR Open 2(1):20190031
4. Karthik Y, Sruthi R, Sujithra M (2024) Polycystic ovary syndrome prediction through CNN based image analysis: a deep learning based approach. In: 2024 8th international conference on I-SMAC (IoT in Social, Mobile, Analytics and Cloud) (I-SMAC), Kirtipur, Nepal, pp 1547–1553. https://doi.org/10.1109/I-SMAC61858.2024.10714821
5. Abhisheka B, Biswas SK, Purkayastha B et al (2024) Recent trend in medical imaging modalities and their applications in disease diagnosis: a review. Multimedia Tools Appl 83(14):43035–43070
6. Zainab H, Khan ARA, Khan MI, Arif A (2025) Integration of AI in medical imaging: enhancing diagnostic accuracy and workflow efficiency. Global Insights Artif Intell Comput 1(1):1–14
7. Najjar R (2023) Redefining radiology: a review of artificial intelligence integration in medical imaging. Diagnostics 13(17):2760
8. Tanenbaum LN (2020) Artificial intelligence and medical imaging: image acquisition and reconstruction. Appl Radiol 49(3):34–35 https://doi.org/10.1109/ICAISS55157.2022.10010850
9. Su H, Li Y, Xu Y et al (2024) A review of deep-learning-based super-resolution: from methods to applications. Pattern Recogn 110935
10. Qin C, Rueckert D (2022) Artificial intelligence-based image reconstruction in cardiac magnetic resonance. In: Artificial intelligence in cardiothoracic imaging. Springer International Publishing, Cham, pp 139–147
11. Koetzier LR, Mastrodicasa D, Szczykutowicz TP et al (2023) Deep learning image reconstruction for CT: technical principles and clinical prospects. Radiology 306(3):e221257
12. Ganesan J, Azar AT, Kamal NA (2024) The AI revolution: deep learning's role. In: Proceedings of the 10th international conference on advanced intelligent systems and informatics 2024, vol 2. Springer Nature, pp 303

13. Gore JC (2020) Artificial intelligence in medical imaging. Magn Resonance Imaging 68:A1–A4
14. Flory MN, Napel S, Tsai EB (2024) AI in radiology: opportunities and challenges. In: Seminars in Ultrasound, CT and MRI. WB Saunders
15. Komatsu M, Teraya N, Natsume T et al (2025) Clinical application of artificial intelligence in ultrasound imaging for oncology. JMA J 8(1):18–25
16. Sahithya V, Sujithra M, Senthilkumar B et al (2024) A guide to ethical geospatial practices: from historical context to future scenarios. In: Ethics, machine learning, and python in geospatial analysis. IGI Global, Hershey, pp 22–52
17. Shen D, Wu G, Suk HI (2017) Deep learning in medical image analysis. Ann Rev Biomed Eng 19(1):221–248
18. Shaik SB, Devi DS, Sujithra M et al (2022) Secure image steganography technique based on hybrid transforms and enhanced AES. In: 2022 international conference on augmented intelligence and sustainable systems (ICAISS), Trichy, India, pp 01–06, https://doi.org/10.1109/ICAISS55157.2022.10010850
19. Suman A, Suman P, Padhy S et al (2025) Healthcare revolution: advances in AI-driven medical imaging and diagnosis. In: Responsible and explainable artificial intelligence in healthcare. Academic Press, Amsterdam, pp 155–182
20. Jeong J, Kim S, Pan L et al (2025) Reducing the workload of medical diagnosis through artificial intelligence: a narrative review. Medicine 104(6)
21. Lopez-Rippe J, Reddy M, Velez-Florez MC et al (2025) RADHawk–an AI-based knowledge recommender to support precision education, improve reporting productivity, and reduce cognitive load. Pediatric Radiol 55(2):259–267
22. Kocak B, Ponsiglione A, Romeo V et al (2025) Radiology AI and sustainability paradox: environmental, economic, and social dimensions. Insights Imaging 16:88
23. Veeramani N, Jayaraman P (2025) A promising AI based super resolution image reconstruction technique for early diagnosis of skin cancer. Sci Rep 15(1):5084
24. Sahoo PK, Gountia D, Dash RK, Nanda K (2025) AI based modified approach in high-resolution image restoration techniques for smart healthcare system: a technical review and analysis. J Theor Appl Inf Technol 103(6)
25. Savaliya M, Shingadiya C, Srinivasulu G (2025) Deep learning-based super resolution for medical images. In: Digital transformation and sustainability of business. CRC Press, Boca Raton, pp 124–126
26. Kofler A, Si D, Schote D, Botnar RM, Kolbitsch C, Prieto C (2025). MR imaging in the low-field: Leveraging the power of machine learning. arXiv preprint arXiv:2501.17211
27. Kumar P (2025) Artificial intelligence (AI)-augmented knowledge management capability and clinical performance: implications for marketing strategies in health-care sector. J Knowl Manag 29(2):415–441
28. Pieper M, Gleasure R (2025) How AI helps to compile human intelligence: an empirical study of emerging augmented intelligence for medical image scanning. Inf Syst J 35(5):1399–1421. https://doi.org/10.1111/isj.12585
29. Rajamani SK, Iyer RS (2025) Revolutionizing healthcare: the power of computer vision artificial intelligence. In: Convergence of antenna technologies, electronics, and AI. IGI Global, Hershey, pp 311–334
30. Weng Z, Wang J, Zhang H et al (2025) AI-enhanced X-ray spectrum reconstruction for medical imaging system. Appl Radiation Isotopes 217:111663
31. Chepelev LL, Nicolaou S, Sheikh A et al (2023) AI for Medical Image Processing: Improving Quality, Accessibility, and Safety. AI in Clinical Medicine: A Practical Guide for Healthcare Professionals, 350–364
32. Rao VM, Hla M, Moor M et al (2025) Multimodal generative AI for medical image interpretation. Nature 639(8056):888–896
33. Ennab M, Mcheick H (2025) Advancing AI interpretability in medical imaging: a comparative analysis of pixel-level interpretability and grad-CAM models. Mach Learn Knowl Extr 7(1):12

34. Singh RR, Singh BK, Sinha GR et al (2025) Introduction to intelligent medical image analysis. In Intelligent Computing Techniques in Biomedical Imaging (pp. 3–09). Academic Press
35. Garg P, Sharma MK, Kumar P (2025) Transparency in diagnosis: unveiling the power of deep learning and explainable AI for medical image interpretation. Arabian J Sci Eng 1–17
36. Liu Y, Cao X, Chen T et al (2025) A survey of embodied AI in healthcare: techniques, applications, and opportunities. Preprint, arXiv:2501.07468
37. Cheng CT, Ooyang CH, Liao CH, Kang SC (2025) Applications of deep learning in trauma radiology: a narrative review. Biomed J 48(1):100743
38. Wang W (2025) AI for medical application: current trends, challenges, and future directions. Int J Artif Intell Sci (IJAI4S) 1(1)
39. Panahi O (2025) AI-Enhanced Case Reports: Integrating Medical Imaging for Diagnostic Insights. J Case Rep Clin Images 8(1):1161
40. Shen X, Shi Z, Lu J, Li B, Yang Q (2025) Artificial Intelligence in Medical Image Diagno sis: Advances, Challenges, and Future Perspectives. Artificial Intelligence and Medicine, 1(1)

Machine Learning for Medical Image Analysis

Amira Bouamrane, Makhlouf Derdour, Akram Bennour, Abdelmadjid Benmachiche, and Mohamed Gasmi

1 Introduction

Medical image analysis plays an important role in the healthcare field, enabling non-invasive diagnosis, disease monitoring, and treatment decisions. Imaging modalities like computerized tomography (CT scan), magnetic resonance imaging (MRI), X-ray, ultrasound, and positron emission tomography (PET) scans help greatly in diagnosing and detecting several diseases [24]. Each modality has its characteristics and advantages in specific applications. However, the increasing number of patients, the shortage of experts, and the strain of long working hours have made automated diagnostic and analysis systems essential for accelerating decision-making and improving diagnostic accuracy [8]. Machine learning has demonstrated remarkable success in medical image processing over the past decades, addressing the challenges of traditional diagnosis, and resulting in enhanced accuracy. Diverse machine learning and artificial intelligence methodologies improve the quality of medical images by removing artifacts, extracting highly relevant features, and recognizing complex patterns. As a result, these developments help radiologists to make more objective and precise decisions for various diseases such as lung cancer, brain tumors, and cardiovascular abnormalities [11]. Additionally, machine learning plays

A. Bouamrane (✉) · M. Derdour
LIAOA Laboratory, University of Oum El-Bouaghi-Larbi Benmhidi, Oum El-Bouaghi, Algeria
e-mail: amira.bouamrane@univ-oeb.dz; derdour.makhlouf@univ-oeb.dz

A. Bennour · M. Gasmi
LAMIS Laboratory, Echahid Cheikh Larbi Tebessi University, Tebessa, Algeria
e-mail: akram.bennour@univ-tebessa.dz; mohamed.gasmi@univ-tebessa.dz

A. Benmachiche
Department of Computer Engineering, Chadli Bendjedid El Tarf University, El Tarf, Algeria
e-mail: benmachiche@hotmail.fr

N. Ben Aoun et al. (eds.), *AI for Medical Image Analysis*,
https://doi.org/10.1007/978-3-032-02963-8_4

a significant role in detecting and segmenting specific regions, tissues, or tumors, and optimizing the treatment process.

In this chapter, the applications of machine learning in medical image analysis are explored, commencing with the various imaging modalities used, their attributes, preprocessing techniques used, and exclusion in detection, segmentation, and registration methods. Next, we discuss the role of artificial intelligence and machine learning in the discipline, including models, contemporary challenges, and future directions. Finally, we summarize the main developments in medical image analysis using machine learning and its impact on personalized medicine.

2 Overview of Machine Learning Techniques for Medical Image Analysis

Machine learning has revolutionized medical image analysis by enhancing diagnostic accuracy and enabling early disease detection and treatments. Its applications span across various imaging modalities, including CT, MRI, X-ray, and ultrasonic imaging modalities Fig. 1. Deep learning, especially, has shown amazing progress in automating picture segmentation, classification, and anomaly detection among advanced machine learning methods. Moreover, the effectiveness of machine learning models is strongly affected by preprocessing methods, which are essential for enhancing image quality and optimizing algorithm performance.

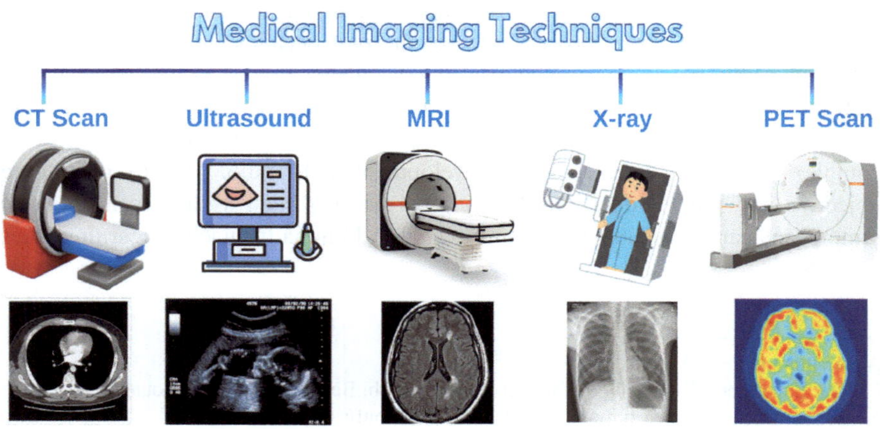

Fig. 1 Medical imaging modalities

2.1 *Success of ML-Based Medical Image Analysis*

By integrating machine learning in medical imaging, treatment times have been accelerated, diagnosis accuracy has improved, and patient outcomes have become better overall. ML approaches have demonstrated their effectiveness in many other medical imaging settings by increasing the accuracy, speed, and consistency of diagnostic processes.

Using ML models in early disease diagnosis has been one of the main innovations since ML algorithms may find anomalies at a stage when therapy is most beneficial by evaluating complicated imaging patterns. Lung cancer, breast cancer, and diabetes are among the diseases that machine learning and deep learning-based computer-aided detection (CADx) systems have shown good results and were helpful in detecting and categorizing [44].

In ML-based CADx systems for lung cancer, it is used to analyze CT scans with high sensitivity and specificity in differentiating benign from malignant nodules. These models have greatly helped to reduce false positives and enhance early detection, hence increasing survival rates [37]. Machine learning-based computer-aided diagnosis (CADx) mammography analysis for breast cancer detection detects mass lesions and microcalcifications, often outperforming diagnosis accuracy from human radiologists [37]. Studies have reported that deep learning models, particularly those with attention mechanisms, can achieve a high degree of efficiency in improving breast cancer screening by reducing recall rates and needless biopsies [32]. Moreover, in the case of diabetics, ML models examine retinal fundus images to identify early indicators of disease progression, such as hemorrhages and microaneurysms. Clinical procedures now include automated grading systems driven by machine learning to support mass screening campaigns aimed at preventing eyesight loss [41]. By integrating AI into healthcare, these models have shown similar outcomes to professional ophthalmologists, thus facilitating early intervention and good patient management. Meanwhile, ML models have further enhanced image segmentation, particularly in applications such as brain tumor segmentation, organ delineation, and lesion localization [16]. Recent architectures such as transformer-based models and U-Net offer exact segmentation that supports monitoring illness development and treatment planning [22, 53]. In medical image analysis, these automated systems have greatly raised repeatability and efficiency.

ML-powered image analysis methods offer automated feature extraction, anomaly detection, and illness categorization going beyond segmentation [16]. These features help doctors to make data-driven decisions and enable objective assessments, hence lowering variation in interpretations. Moreover, unsupervised and self-supervised learning techniques are capable of extracting significant patterns from medical images without large labeled data, therefore opening the path for more general uses in diagnostic imaging [18]. Another key success of ML is its contribution to personalized medicine. Using multi-modal imaging and combining clinical data, ML models predict disease progression and treatment response to allow tailored therapeutic strategies. In this context, the machine-learning-based assessment of Alzheimer's disease using MRI and PET has contributed to early intervention, whereas the osteoarthritis progression models have helped clinicians better manage their patients [25]. The role of machine learning during this pandemic has been critical, and it has included algorithms that distinguish patients with COVID-19 using chest X-rays or CT images from patients with other pulmonary infections, reducing reporting time and minimizing human errors, and it has enabled efficient decisions [7]. AI-based image analysis techniques standardize diagnostic procedures across institutions, allow radiologists to mark areas of concern, and prioritize patients based on urgency. Another interesting avenue is real-time analysis during surgical procedures, where algorithms provide instant feedback to the surgeons, which may in the end reduce complications and enhance surgical outcomes [27].

Effective preprocessing techniques are required, and optimum utility can be derived from ML in medical imaging. Image quality enhancement, noise reduction, and normalization of the data set format work such that the ML models receive the best possible inputs for analysis.

3 Machine Learning Workflow for Medical Image Analysis

The application of machine learning in medical image analysis has caused an evolution in the diagnosis methods, making them more accurate and efficient than before. The machine learning workflow covers several stages, as illustrated in Fig. 2, including data acquisition-preprocessing, annotation and labeling, feature engineering, and training processes followed by validation.

3.1 Data Acquisition

The stage is vital in determining the quality and diversity of data as there is a wide variety of imaging modalities such as CT, MRI, and X-rays. Major discussions include data sources, missing data handling, and issues of ethics [2].

3.2 Data Sources

Medical imaging data is collected from various sources, including hospitals and research institutions, which provide rich datasets containing real-world patient data. Access to such data must be ethically considered and strictly conform to privacy regulations. In addition, many repositories have made available open-access medical imaging datasets including, the Cancer Imaging Archive (TCIA), Chest X-

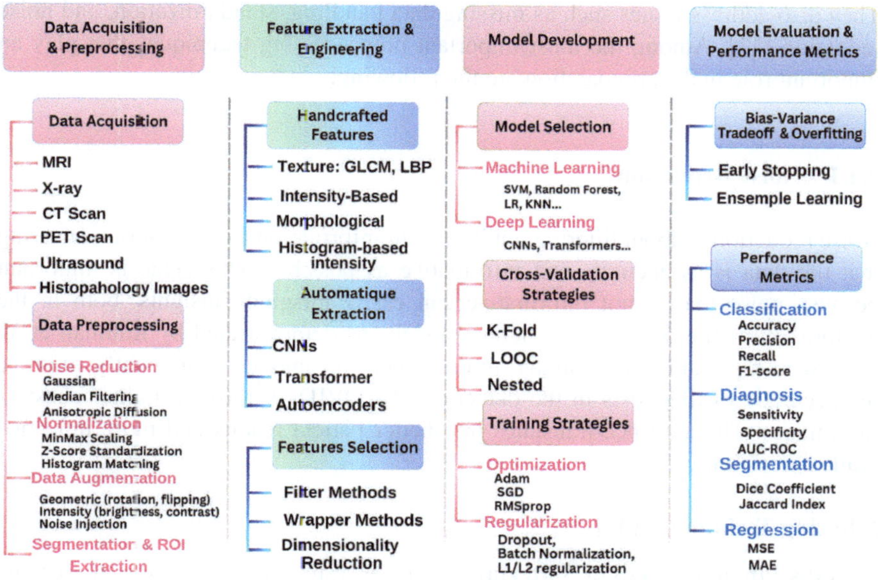

Fig. 2 Machine learning workflow for medical image analysis

ray datasets, LIDC-IDRI dataset, and LUNA-16 challenge dataset. These datasets facilitate research by providing diverse and well-annotated imaging samples [11].

3.3 Annotation and Labeling

The effective training of machine learning models will depend on key factors such as accurate labeling and annotation. Annotation can be achieved in different ways. One of the methods is manual annotation usually performed by domain experts that enables precise classifications based on clinical knowledge. However, The alternative way can also adopt automatic annotation by machine learning and deep learning techniques, which generate initial labels modified by experts [54]. This helps speed up the annotation process while keeping the accuracy.

Regardless of the method, data quality and quantity are important factors influencing model robustness and the risk of bias in decision-making.

3.4 Preprocessing Techniques

Preprocessing techniques are essential for improving the quality of the data used, thereby enhancing model performance while minimizing noise as much as possible.

They also address issues such as missing data handling, standardization, and noise reduction [11]. Among the most important preprocessing techniques that play an important role in data preparation are the following:

3.4.1 Noise Reduction

Noise reduction is about filtering out irrelevant information from a dataset, ensuring that the data is as accurate and informative as possible. This stage is important because noise that is not informative can easily misguide insights, both in the exploration of the data and predictive models, as demonstrated by Rahman et al. 4[7], who highlighted how image improvement techniques significantly improve the accuracy of diagnosis in the detection of COVID-19 through lighter chest x-ray images. This advance translates into better patient results and more informed clinical decisions.

Filtering Techniques [35]

- **Gaussian and Median Filtering:** Reduces random noise while preserving edges.
- **Wavelet Transformation and Non-local Means:** Enhances image details by removing speckles and Poisson noise.
- **Anisotropic Diffusion Filtering:** Smooth images while preserving important structures.

3.4.2 Normalization and Standardization

A critical preprocessing step that transforms image characteristics into a uniform range, as an example, between [0, 1]. This prevents variables with larger ranges from disproportionately influencing model training and ensures consistent image intensity and scale across datasets [47].

- **Normalization:** Adjusts characteristics to have an average of zero and a standard deviation of one, which is essential for statistical analysis and machine learning algorithms.
- **MinMax Normalization:** Scales pixel values to a defined range [0,1] or [1,1].
- **Z-Score Standardization:** Centers image intensity to a zero mean with unit variance.
- **Histogram Matching:** Aligns intensity distributions across different images or modalities.

3.4.3 Data Augmentation

Data augmentation is considered an essential technique for increasing the diversity of data through modified versions of preexisting images to improve the robustness, generalization capability, and reduction of overfitted models. Five genres of techniques can be used to categorize the forms of augmentation [47]:

- **Geometric Transformations**
  - **Rotation:** Simulation through different orientations of the original image.
  - **Flipping:** Horizontal and vertical flipping confined by organ structures.
  - **Cropping and Padding:** Changes image size and composition.
- **Intensity Transformations:** Modifies pixel intensity variations, such as brightness adjustment, contrast adjustment, and gamma correction.
- **Elastic Deformation:** employs techniques like random warping and deformable grids for making shapes differ realistically
- **Noise Injection and Blurring:** improves robustness by adding Gaussian or speckle-type noise (simulating the artifacts from devices) and/or using motion and Gaussian blurring.

Some researchers use augmentation techniques tailored to the specific imaging modality. For example: MRI images are augmented using shifts and normalization, while CT scans undergo changes to simulate varying exposure levels, On the other hand, X-ray images benefit from histogram equalization to enhance tissue contrast [15].

Preprocessing is an indispensable step, as it directly impacts knowledge discovery and significantly enhances the effectiveness of model decisions.

3.5 Feature Engineering

Feature engineering is considered an essential step, particularly for converting unprocessable data into meaningful representations. This stage comprises methods that optimize data quality, such as feature selection and feature fusion, which enhance model performance.

3.6 Feature Extraction in Medical Images

Feature extraction is considered an important step in medical image analysis, as it converts large image data into meaningful representations for the model. This step can be performed manually [16], known as handcrafted feature extraction, or automatically [43].

3.6.1 Handcrafted Features

In this technique, common types of handcrafted features include:

- **Texture Features:** Such as the Gray-Level Co-occurrence Matrix (GLCM) and Local Binary Patterns (LBP).
- **Shape Features:** Capturing geometric properties of structures.
- **Intensity-Based Features:** Measuring pixel distribution.
- **Morphological Features:** Extracting structural information such as edge detection and boundary descriptors.

While manual feature extraction enhances interpretability, even for small datasets, it is less adaptable to complex patterns and requires manual selection.

3.6.2 Automatic Feature Extraction

Convolutional neural networks (CNNs) provide a prime example of automatic feature extraction Fig. 3, as these models extract hierarchical features from medical images without any manual intervention. The features extracted by CNNs can be divided into Low-level features, Mid-level features, and High-level features that mainly capture intricate patterns and relationships [43]. There are certain limitations to deep learning as they entirely depend on large datasets and extensive computation to get the required outputs, along with restricting interpretation compared to the highly interpretable handcrafted feature extraction methods.

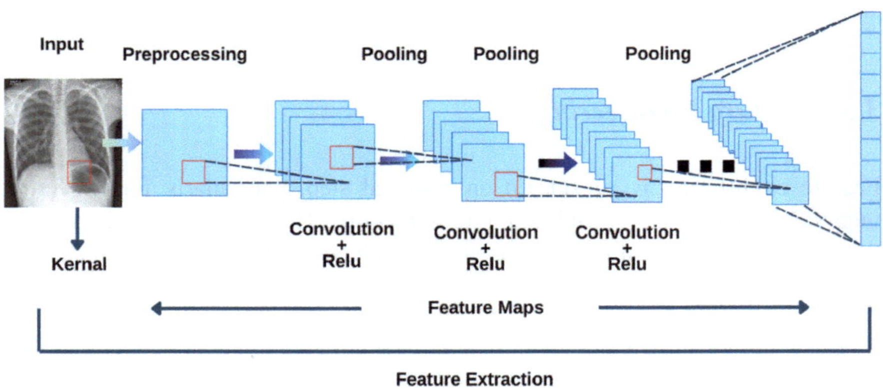

Fig. 3 Automatic feature extraction using CNN

3.6.3 Feature Selection

Different methodologies are implemented to ascertain that the training on the model features considered most relevant and effective enhance generalization and reduce training time:

- **Filter Methods:** Use statistical approaches like correlation analysis [16].
- **Wrapper Methods:** Include Recursive Feature Elimination (RFE) and Genetic Algorithms (GA) [5].

Incorporating the methods embedded into the model for itself, such as Lasso regressions and attention mechanisms based on trees, to feature selections. Hence, these acts improve model efficiency and performance by eliminating irrelevant or redundant features.

3.6.4 Feature Fusion

To improve the effectiveness of the model and the quality of data in the network, researchers sometimes resort to feature fusion, which happens in three different ways: fusing features before feeding them into the network, combining separate model predictions from different feature sets, or hybrid fusion by mixing the two previous strategies in the middle of model training. The next phase, after feature selection and processing, consists of training the model and validating it [21].

3.7 Model Training and Validation

To improve diagnostics results and clinical capability, it is important to select the most suitable, effective, and optimized architecture, implement effective training strategies, and evaluate performance to develop a robust ML model with high capability to generalize.

3.7.1 Model Selection

Model selection should depend on the data type, problem complexity, and studied task, whether for classification, detection, or segmentation, including: Traditional ML models such as SVM and Random Forest have lower complexity but are limited in the case of high-dimensional data, especially in medical imaging. In contrast, deep learning models like CNNs such as EfficientNet-V2 and Transformers are widely employed in processing such complicated images with improved accuracy and reduced processing time [22, 33]. However, they generally require huge computational power, whereas traditional ML models are more efficient in comparison

3.7.2 Cross-Validation Strategies in Medical Imaging

To ensure model reliability, especially in the case of limited datasets or imbalanced ones, cross-validation is considered an effective strategy by partitioning data into training and validation subsets, which eliminate and reduce overfitting, improving model robustness. To ensure model reliability, especially in the case of limited datasets or imbalanced ones, cross-validation is considered an effective strategy by partitioning data into training and validation subsets, which eliminate and reduce overfitting, improving model robustness [13].

- **K-Fold Cross-Validation:** The most widely used method to assess the model performance for small datasets.
- **Leave-One-Out Cross-Validation (LOOCV):** This method is most suitable for small datasets, as it applies one sample for testing while training the others, thus making it computationally expensive.
- **Nested Cross-Validation:** This technique introduces another layer of cross-validation for hyperparameter tuning to avoid data leakage.

3.7.3 Training Strategies

An effective training strategy is essential for optimizing model performance and stability by selecting appropriate optimization techniques to adjust the learning rate dynamically and incorporating regularization methods to eliminate overfitting, these strategies improve convergence. robustness and generalization.

- **Optimization Techniques:** The effectiveness of adaptive optimization algorithms, such as Adam, RMSprop, and SGD, largely depends on their learning rate programs, in particular the learning rate warm-up techniques used. learning rate warm-up strategies are implemented to gradually increase the learning rate at the beginning of training, promoting stable convergence. Adam's adaptive learning rate is particularly effective in the management of scattered gradients, while RMSprop adapts the learning rate based on the recent magnitudes of the gradient. On the contrary, Stochastic Gradient Descent(SGD) is based on a more static approach, which can significantly benefit from the learning rate warm-up, the improvement of the quality of the convergence [23].
- **Regularization technique:** to improve model generalization, and eliminate overfitting we distinguish several regularization techniques such as hyperparameters tuning, dropout, batch normalization, and L1/L2 regulation technique that control weight magnitudes [51].

3.7.4 Model Evaluation and Performance Metrics

Bias, Variance, and Overfitting in Medical Images Machine learning and deep learning models must balance bias and variance to optimize the performance as bias(underfitting) means the model does recognize key biomarkers of the disease while generalization ability, to avoid these several techniques used as early stop, dropout, and ensemble learning.

3.7.5 Performance Metrics for Medical Image Analysis

There are various evaluation metrics, choosing the suitable metric for assessment depends exactly on the kind of work involved [40]. It can be classified as follows:

- **Classification metrics:** F1-score, sensitivity, precision, and accuracy.
- **Diagnostics metrics:** sensitivity, specificity, specificity, Area Under Curve(AUC), and ROC.
- **Segmentation metrics:** Metrics like the Dice coefficient and Jaccard index are the most used metrics to evaluate segmentation models.
- **Regression metrics:** among the most commonly used models for this task are Mean Squared Error (MSE) and Mean Absolute Error (MAE).

Moreover, testing the model's generalizability and robustness is important for an accurate evaluation of its performance [11], which is why testing the model on external datasets from different demographic populations is essential. Furthermore, machine learning workflow for medical image analysis emphasizes the importance of data sources, their characteristics, and processing, as well as how to determine the features used based on the model. Additionally, selecting patterns to control the model is an important factor. Finally, it underscores the necessity of generalizing the model neutrally to indicate its real performance.

4 Supervised Learning Approaches

Supervised models play an important role in medical diagnosis. Supervised model learning refers to training the model with datasets where all input pictures correspond to specific output labels. Various supervised learning models have been described in this section.

4.1 Classification Models for Disease Diagnosis

Machine learning models with their ability to analyze complex imaging data have significantly advanced disease diagnosis, including supervised learning algorithms, such as support vector machines, random forest, and K-nearest neighbors, with high accuracy, making them essential tools in modern medical diagnostics [16].

- **Support Vector Machines (SVM):** this model widely used for tumor classification and pneumonia detection and diagnoses through X-ray and CT imaging. This model is efficient for both high-dimensional spaces and small to medium datasets.
- **Random Forest (RF):** considered robust against overfitting and widely used in disease diagnosis.
- **K-Nearest Neighbors (KNN):** a non-parametric algorithm for classification, lesion detection, and segmentation. Despite that this model is effective for small datasets, it is computationally expensive for large ones. Performance depends on distance metrics and the choice of K.

  The effectiveness of these models in accurately classifying medical images has led researchers to adopt them for diagnosing various types of cancer. Nanmaran et al. [31] developed a brain tumor classification model on SVM, KNN, and decision tree classifiers that were developed on MRI and SPECT images. SVM had the best classification accuracy of 96.8% compared to other classifiers. Similarly, Arafa et al. [4] developed a machine-learning-based model using ultrasound data from two hospitals in Riyadh (2019–2023) to predict prostate cancer risk. They employed logistic regression (LR), XGBoost (XGB), RF, and SVM with RF and XGB achieving the highest accuracy.

These models have achieved remarkable results and are highly interpretable in detecting and classifying diseases from medical imaging datasets.

4.2 Regression Models for Quantitative Analysis

On the other hand, regression models help derive quantitative evaluations for medical images. These models predict continuous output values, which can present various clinical measures, such as tumor volume prediction by estimating tumor volume for MRI, aiding in determining treatments. Therefore, disease progression forecasting includes time series regression models such as long short-term memory (LSTM). Moreover, Li et al. [28] developed multiple machine-learning models, including LR for breast nodule classification using ultrasound imaging data from 926 patients, and achieved an accuracy of 91.2%.

4.3 Example Applications: Tumor Detection, Organ Segmentation

The success achieved by these supervised models at medical levels led to their use in many diseases. Typically, as demonstrated in Fig. 4 a tumor analysis and diagnostic pipeline using medical imaging, starts from organ segmentation to nodule detection, segmentation, and diagnostic analysis. Based on the appearance,

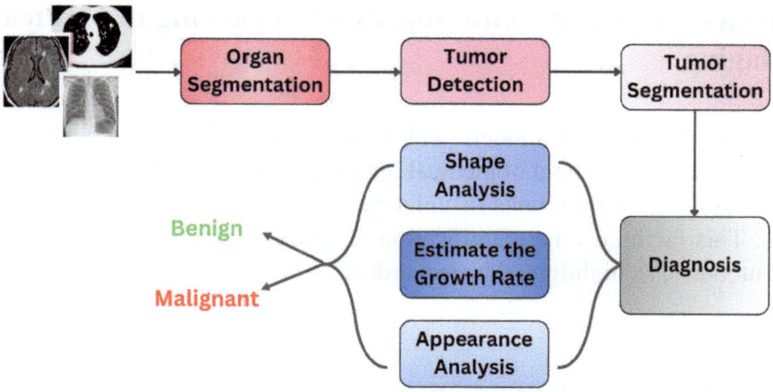

Fig. 4 Nodule analysis and diagnosis pipeline using medical imaging

shape, and estimated growth rate of the tumors, finally classify them as benign or malignant. Ozdemir et al. [33] integrated Convolutional Neural Networks (CNNs) and Vision Transformers (ViTs) for lung cancer detection using CT images. The model enhances feature extraction by incorporating InceptionNeXt blocks for multi-scale analysis and attention mechanisms (grid and block) to capture both fine-grained and global spatial relationships, it achieved an accuracy of 99.54, and 98.41% on the IQ-OTH/NCCD and the Chest CT dataset respectively. Despite these results, the model suffers from data bias because of the small size of the used dataset. Moreover, Kina et al. [25] developed a lightweight deep learning model using EfficientNet and Squeeze Attention Block for brain disease and Alzheimer's detection from MRI scans. The use of SMOTE is to balance the MRI dataset and further enhance classification performance. Grad-CAM was also used to enhance the explainability. Despite, its good performance, especially after balancing the data. However, the considered computational cost and potential ethical issues of dataset bias are limitations. Other research focused on brain tumor segmentation in MRI, Payette et al. [36] developed fetal brain segmentation algorithms using MRI data from multi-center datasets. The model achieved a white matter Dice of 89% and a Dice of: 87%. However, limitations include poor generalization for certain structures due to anatomical complexity. Brahma et al. [14] developed DeepFermi, a deep learning-based myocardial perfusion quantification model that integrates the Fermi model to improve accuracy and robustness. The model was trained using a self-supervised approach and based on a dataset of stress perfusion cardiac MRI scans, DeepFermi was compared with the classical LBFGS algorithm. The results showed that DeepFermi provided superior parameter estimation, especially in the presence of noise and outliers, while also significantly accelerating computations.

Supervised learning models play a significant role in enhancing disease diagnosis, segmentation tasks, and quantitative analysis, which enhances clinical decision analysis.

5 Unsupervised and Semi-Supervised Learning in Medical Imaging

The use of unsupervised models and semi-supervised learning techniques has significantly shaped the field of medical imaging, as these models play an important role in leveraging vast amounts of unlabeled medical data and uncovering hidden patterns. This facilitates the identification of disease subtypes and improves diagnostic outcomes, as highlighted by Eckardt et al. [18].

5.1 Clustering for Pattern Discovery

These grouping methods enable the organization of similar data points based on intrinsic characteristics, which is very fundamental in exploring and interpreting medical images. By categorizing data without prior labels to detect different patterns or clusters letting phenotype discovery and modeling the disease progression, we distinguish several techniques including [19]:

- K-means and clustering, such as clustering tumor characteristics based on imaging features such as in MRI analysis to distinguish nodules and pathological tissue
- Gaussian Mixture Models (GMM)
- Self-organizing maps (SOMs) These techniques are used to visualize high-dimensional medical data and in disease subtype identification.

5.2 Deep Learning for Medical Image Analysis

The emergence of convolutional networks and their power to automatically a high of effective features from imaging modalities has revolutionized image analysis and automatic models in healthcare. These networks have shown outstanding potential for several imaging tasks like medical detection, segmentation, classification, and prognosis. In addition, transfer learning and generative models have constantly improved developments by lessening complexity and resource requirements.

5.2.1 Convolutional Neural Networks(CNNs)

There has been a paradigm shift in medical image analysis with the advent of CNNs, which are capable of automatic feature extraction and extremely well-performing classification, detection, and segmentation tasks. CNNs handle spatial hierarchies in image data that fit the bill for medical image applications Fig. 3, such as ResNet with its deep residual networks with skip connections, encourages the training of very deep models [10], while U-Net, which uses encoder-decoder architecture with skip connections to preserve spatial information, makes U-Net one of the most popular choices for medical image segmentation [53]. DenseNet encourages feature reuse and improves gradient flow through dense connectivity between layers [9]. Additionally, CNNs are widely used to detect lung nodules in CT images, classify pneumonia in chest X-rays, and diagnose retinal diseases from fundus images, this architecture effectively segmenting different lesions or particular organs. And identify abnormal shapes in medical images for early detection of diseases [32].

Furthermore, transfer learning uses pre-trained models to enhance the performance of deep learning applications in medical imaging. Because of the small size medical datasets, transfer learning helps mitigate data scarcity issues by using knowledge from models trained on large-scale datasets like ImageNet. Moreover, feature extraction for medical image processing via pre-trained or finetuned model CNNs, such as DenseNet201, ResNet, and EfficientNet. Fine-tuning really optimizes these transformed pre-training weights for different tasks in performance. Models pre-trained on large medical imaging datasets like ImageNet can learn more of their relevant features, which would make them ready for radiology applications [12]. Disease classification from chest X-rays and histopathology images has been largely documented with transfer learning, organ and lesion segmentation improves with fine-tuned models like U-Net and DeepLab models. It has a major role within these applications for the detection of fractures in X-rays and also locating tumors within MRIs [43], thus making it a vital approach within medical image analysis.

5.2.2 Generative Models for Image Synthesis and Enhancement

Generative models play an important role in medical imaging by synthesizing realistic images, enhancing the quality of the image, and augmenting the datasets to train deep-learning models [48].

- **Generative Adversarial Networks (GANs):** A class of generative models consisting of a generator and a discriminator that compete to produce realistic images.
  - Data Augmentation: GANs generate synthetic medical images to enhance dataset diversity and improve model robustness.
  - Super-Resolution Imaging: GAN-based approaches enhance low-resolution medical images, improving clarity for diagnosis.
  - Modality Translation: Conditional GANs (cGANs) translate images from one modality to another (MRI to CT), facilitating multi-modal medical analysis.
- **Variational Autoencoders (VAEs):** A probabilistic approach for learning latent representations and generating diverse synthetic images.
- **Diffusion Models:** A new class of generative models that iteratively refine images from noise, showing promise in high-quality medical image synthesis.

Generative models, CNNs, and transfer learning continue to improve medical image analysis, enabling more accurate, efficient, and scalable AI-powered healthcare solutions.

5.3 Dimensionality Reduction for Visualization

The high-dimensional data cause increased training complexity and overfitting. Some of the dimensionality reduction techniques are given as follows [30]:

- **Principal Component Analysis (PCA):** Reduces data redundancy with variance preservation.
- **T-distributed stochastic neighbor embedding (t-SNE):** Projects high-dimensional data into 2D or 3D space to facilitate visualization.
- **Autoencoders:** Compress data into lower-dimensional representations while preserving key information.

Dehbozorgi et al. [17] developed a comparative study evaluating statistical, radiomics, and deep learning (DL) using H&E-stained for feature extraction from chest X-ray, and retina OCT datasets. They implemented statistical and radiomics feature extraction while implementing these with PCA-LDA models and also carried out a comparison against DL feature extraction using pre-trained networks (ResNet50, DenseNet121). ResNet50 improved sensitivity from 90.8% to 96.9%. While, Bouamrane et al. [9] proposed a hybrid model based on Densenet201 and multi-perceptron for pulmonary nodules diagnosis based on CT scans and achieved an accuracy of 99.22%.

5.4 Semi-Supervised Learning with Limited Labels

Semi-supervised learning (SSL) works very well for medical image analysis with limited labels, addressing the challenge of limited labeled data. It enables models to progressively improve their performance with lower complexity and without requiring a very extensive labeled dataset. This applies especially to datasets in medical imaging since most of them are scarce with annotated samples, Zhang et al. [54] have shown that pseudo-marcation and adaptive active annotation can remarkably increase the efficiency of the medical image SSL, allowing an enhanced diagnostic accuracy and reducing the dependence of labeled data sets. We distinguish several common widespread approaches in semi-supervised learning including [46]:

- **Self-training:** Models are trained on labeled data and then used to generate possible labels for the unlabeled cases.

- **Consistency regularization:** Models are trained to produce consistent predictions are consistent for different perturbations on the same type of input. The model here would generate relatively fewer variations between predictions for the different augmented versions of the same input.
- **Graph-based SSL:** It involves creating a graph in which the nodes are formed by labeled and unlabeled samples. It is a label propagation method that assigns pseudo-labels to the unlabeled ones based on the existing graph structures and makes use of the existing structural relationships present in medical images in order to extract information from unlabeled data.
- **Generative models (GANs and VAEs):** These techniques enhance classification by generating realistic medical images to address data imbalance.

Both unsupervised and semi-supervised learning significantly impact medical imaging by improving disease classification through clustering and dimensionality reduction. These techniques improve the efficiency of computation using such unlabeled datasets, addressing the challenge of limited annotating of medical data [16]. However, they may suffer from reliability issues, as errors in pseudo-labeling can propagate and degrade model performance. Such SSL models trained in different datasets only may tend to be biased towards the specific data, consequently reducing their generalizability [12]. This can be mitigated by incorporating uncertainty-aware approaches, integrating clinical records with imaging data, or developing collaborative federated SSL methods. Zhang et al. [55] developed the Graph Attention Iterative Contraction Network (GAICN) to enhance bioluminescence tomography (BLT) reconstruction. GAICN utilizes graph attention mechanisms and iterative contraction activation to improve feature aggregation and dynamic weight adjustment in a finite element mesh representation. The model enhances spatial accuracy, dual-source resolution, and generalizability by leveraging a deep-based approach with Forward-Backward Splitting (FBS). However, this model suffers from data dependence, in addition to system matrix errors in optical modeling.

6 Key Applications of Machine Learning Models in Medical Image Analysis

Machine learning (ML) emerged as a transformative force in medical image analysis, introducing significant advances in disease detection, segmentation, registration, prognosis modeling, and surgical planning. By taking advantage of the power of computational algorithms and techniques, ML facilitates improved diagnostic capabilities, allowing health professionals to detect diseases with greater accuracy and speed. Recent studies indicate substantial progress in deep learning methodologies applied to various medical image modalities, which accentuates the important role of this technology in research and clinical environments.

6.1 Disease Detection and Localization

One of the critical applications of ML in medical imaging is the detection of disease. Automated systems that employ deep learning architectures have demonstrated capabilities in identifying pathological characteristics that are usually difficult for human observers to discern. For example, convolutional neural networks (CNNS) have been particularly effective in detecting radiological image anomalies. Zafar et al. [53] trained a hybrid deep-learning model for brain tumor detection using YOLOv8 and U-Net for segmentation on MRI images from the Cancer Imaging Archive and Cancer Genome Atlas (CGA) datasets, achieving an accuracy of 98.6%. For the Modic changes (MCs) detection utilizing MRI scans, Xing et al. [52] used YOLOv8 and YOLOv5. Their results demonstrated that YOLOv8 outperformed YOLOv5 with an increased precision, recall, and F1 score.

6.2 Image Segmentation: Tumors, Lesions, and Organs

Segmentation of the image, the process of delineating structures within the images, is another area in which ML has made significant advances. The performance of segmentation methodologies has dramatically improved by implementing advanced ML techniques. The researchers explored various deep-learning-based segmentation structures that can accurately delineate complex anatomical structures for a better view and greater quantification of pathological areas. Bellmann et al. [6] developed a deep learning reconstruction (DLR) Fig. 5 model for detecting low-contrast lesions in neck CT images. They prepared nine realistic phantoms scanned in six radiation doses (0.5–5.2 mGy) on a 320-slice CT scanner. Reconstructed images using the three methods were assessed by 13 readers for lesion detection using ROC and LROC analyses. The results showed that DLR improved significantly the lesion detection and confidence of the readers compared to IR and FBP ($p < 0.05$) with the highest AUC values. Krabbe et al. [26] developed a model using 1 mm 3D T1-weighted spoiled gradient echo MRI and MRI-based synthetic CT to detect

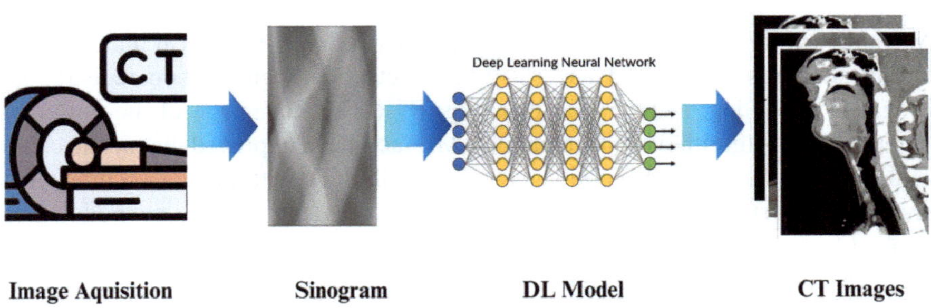

Fig. 5 Deep learning CT scan reconstruction process

structural lesions in sacroiliac joints of patients with spondyloarthritis. The study used a dataset of 19 patients, comparing these methods against conventional 4 mm T1-weighted turbo spin echo (T1w-TSE) MRI. Preprocessing involved converting T1w-GRE images into CT images using a deep learning algorithm, Bone MRI. Wan et al. [50] developed CNN models to predict overall survival (OS) in recurrent high-grade glioma (HGG) patients treated with immunotherapy. They compared DL-based classification models with radiomic signatures extracted from both manual and automated tumor segmentation. The model achieved the highest test set AUC (0.700 ± 0.101).

6.3 *Image Registration and Alignment*

With the advancements in deep learning techniques, registering medical images, where images obtained from different modalities, or patients are aligned with one another, has also undergone improvement. Automated registration frameworks were developed to help this process, reducing the manual workload on radiologists while producing a more consistent alignment of images, thereby achieving an accurate evaluation, which greatly enhances interpretability. Fu et al. [20] developed MCRAIP-Net, a deep-learning model for segmentation from multimodal MR images in 3D medical applications. The model used an attention mechanism, a dilated convolution module, and a dual-channel cross-reconstruction attention module to refine multimodal feature fusion. The inverted pyramid decoder is used for the integration of the resolution-based features. The training of the models was conducted in a semi-supervised manner on a synthetic dataset while fine-tuning on a patient dataset. Results showed that six networks significantly improved the pre-registration Dice coefficient on the synthetic dataset, while nine networks generalized well to the patient dataset. Moreover, Rahman et al. [39] developed an automated feature for segmenting liver tumors using MRI and CT images to enhance the precision of identifying liver tumor regions. The methodology involves a collection technique called ensemble ResUNet-InceptionV4, which integrates the benefits of ResNet, U-Net, and Inception architectures. And it was tested on the 3D-IRCADb-01 dataset, this model achieved an accuracy of 99.27%, a mean intersection over union of 97.74%, and a Dice score of 98.86%, outmatching conventional segmentation methods in the state of the art.

6.4 *Prediction and Prognosis Modeling*

In prognosis modeling, especially for using historical image data with corresponding clinical data, one of the major roles is played by machine learning. Several models may be developed for disease prediction and patient outcomes with the help of predictive analyses, thus helping medical professionals optimize their treatment planning [38]. These models are highly embedded in clinical workflows, allowing for better-informed decisions based exclusively on personalized risk profiles. Qiu et al. [38] developed prognosis-predictive models with MRI-based radiomics and clinicopathological features for early-stage cervical adenocarcinoma (AC) patients. A dataset of 197 patients (along with 56 patients independent validation) was used to extract 107 radiomics features from T2-weighted MRI images. Feature selection was done via Spearman correlation and RF methods. The models were trained with SVM and CNN. The combined model (radiomics + clinicopathological features) consistently outperformed the radiomics-only model, achieving AUC values up to 93.7% for disease-free survival (DFS) prediction.

6.5 Role of Machine Learning in Surgical Planning and Simulation

In conclusion, the integration of machine learning in the analysis of medical images shows a paradigm change in the field by enhancing detection, segmentation, registration, prognosis modeling, and surgical planning. The present condition of deep learning applications shows great promise as this technology progresses and hones its approach.

7 Case Studies of Machine Learning Deployment for Medical Image Analysis

By integrating machine learning models in medical image analysis, clinicians can enhance diagnostic accuracy and improve patient outcomes. Real-world case studies illustrating the useful influence of artificial intelligence-assisted radiography, automated cancer grading in histology, and artificial intelligence-assisted radiography.

7.1 AI-Assisted Radiology: Lung Nodule Detection

The advancement of artificial intelligence in radiology has completely changed the scene for pulmonary nodule detection as well as for early diagnostics and patient outcomes as a whole. The integration of machine learning techniques into imaging modalities, particularly computed tomography, has led to paradigm shifts in the way that radiologists address the evaluation of pulmonary nodules [33, 45, 49]. Table 1 compares the characteristics of malignant and benign lung nodules, highlighting differences in size, shape, growth patterns, calcification, density, location, and edge features.

Table 1 Malignant vs. Benign nodule

Characteristic	Malignant	Benign
Size	Larger, especially those greater than 8–10 mm.	Smaller, less than 8 mm in diameter.
Shape and margins	Irregular, spiculated, lobulated, asymmetric.	Smooth, round, oval, well-defined.
Growth noticeable	Growth over time.	Stable size.
Calcification patterns	Eccentric, irregular.	Central, popcorn-like, laminated.
Density and texture	Heterogeneous, varying densities, necrosis, cavitation.	Homogeneous, uniform texture.
Location	Upper lobes.	Any location, less specific.
Edge characteristics	Spiculated, irregular, spiky, hairy.	Smooth, well-defined.

Shakeel et al. [45] proposed an optimized image processing and machine learning model based on CT scans. They used a multilevel brightness-preserving method and segmenting affected regions using an improved deep neural network with an optimization hybrid model for feature selection. With a simple classifier for classification, the model showed a comparable perform, while Sori et al. [49] developed a denoising first two-path convolutional neural network (DFD-Net) to enhance lung cancer detection, this architecture was able for joint local and global feature extraction which addresses noise and complex nodule morphology. In addition to discriminant correlation analysis that improves feature representation, a retraining technique mitigates label imbalance, leading to more robust cancer prediction. Such advances have been widely documented, with systematic revisions that illustrate the effectiveness of these techniques in the diagnosis of CT-image pulmonary nodules.

Furthermore, Real-world results from detecting pulmonary nodules assisted by machine learning have so far demonstrated substantial promises to increase the accuracy of the diagnosis. Recent studies show that deep learning architectures can effectively classify and detect lung nodules, thus improving conventional diagnostic processes [11]. In addition, comparisons with traditional performances of the radiologist reveal that ML models often correspond with or exceed human accuracy, in particular in the classifications of histological images underlining that AI algorithms can achieve equal footing metrics with radiologists in the identification of pulmonary nodules using histopathology images, leading to better prognostic capabilities.

7.2 *Ophthalmology: Retinal Disease Detection Using Fundus Imaging*

AI radiology is also ready to promote workflow efficiency, a primordial consideration in the current medical assistance of increasing patient volumes and increasing administrative charges. It has been shown that the systematic integration of AI tools minimizes the time radiologists spend on preliminary evaluations, allowing more focused and fast evaluations [12]. Nithya et al. proposed a diabetic retinopathy detection approach Fig. 6 based on retinal fundus images with data augmentation and using several CNN models, including ResNet-101, VGGNet-16, and ResNet-50. The ResNet-101 achieved the best accuracy of 98.88% on many datasets (HRF, STARE, DIARETDB0, and XHO) [32]. While, Abd El-Khalek et al. developed a computer-aided diagnostic (CAD) system to detect age-related macular degeneration (AMD) early by classifying fundus images into geographic atrophy (GA), intermediate AMD, normal, and wet AMD. They record retina and optical disc local and global appearance information using weighted majority voting for better classification. The model achieved an accuracy of 96.85%, 93.72% sensitivity, and specificity of 97.89% [1]. Rasool et al. developed a glioma segmentation and survival prediction scheme that was designed to overcome problems arising from tumor heterogeneity and vague boundaries, including difficult MRI features. The proposed ResMHA-Net (ResNet Multi-Head Attention U-Net) employs ResNet residual blocks with multi-head attention to sharpen the focus on relevant areas and model long-range dependencies within 3D MRI data. It was trained and validated on BraTS 2018–2021 datasets. ResMHA-Net showed the highest segmentation accuracy on BraTS 2021, proving its robustness across diverse data. Additionally, predicted tumor masks were used to extract radiomic features. Using a voting mechanism, the ensemble achieved a 73% accuracy in predicting overall survival [42].

The implementation of AI-assisted technologies in detecting pulmonary nodules has a confluence of opportunities and challenges. Although substantial evidence supports their ability to improve diagnosis and improve workflow efficiency, careful consideration of integration strategies, continuous education, and the commitment to address technological disabilities remain imperative to perform their full potential in clinical practice. The future seems promising as the field embraces these technological advances, maintaining the promise to improve patient care in radiology.

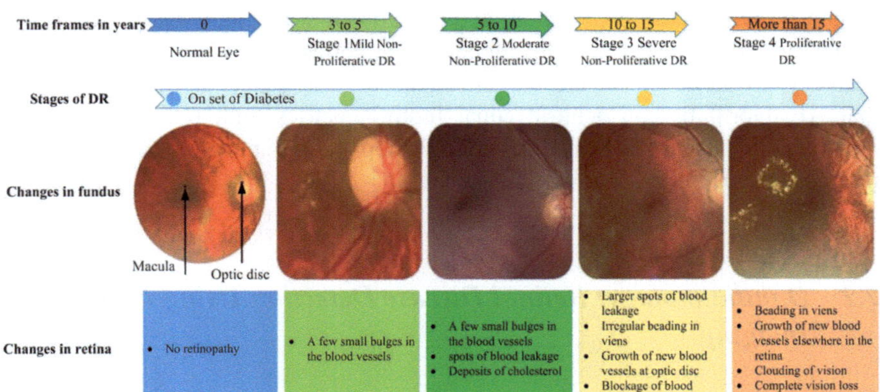

Fig. 6 Diabetic detection in retinal fundus images [32]

8 Challenges, Considerations, and Future Directions in Machine Learning for Medical Imaging

Machine learning (ML) can hold a transformable benefit when it comes to an accurate diagnosis, therapy planning, and patient outcomes in medical imaging. On the other hand, it does face certain difficulties when it comes to their practical applications: for example, data scarcity, expensive annotation, computational costs, and ethical considerations. Prominent trends such as multimodal data integration, explainable models, federated learning, real-time analysis, and personalized medicine are aimed at overcoming those challenges. This section will summarize critical issues and future directions to help scalable, ethical, and effectual deployment of ML in clinical practice.

8.1 Data Challenges: Scarcity, Annotation, and Generalizability

The lack of medical data still poses a severe impediment to research, accentuating the emphasis on privacy laws, the strength of collecting these huge sets of data, and the limited diversity of available patient data. Annotating medical images is an intensive affair involving domain experts like radiologists, resulting in increased time and cost resources in developing such technologies. To address this, techniques such as data augmentation and synthetic data generation using generative models have gained traction. These methods improve the diversity of data, meeting the objective of model generalization [29]. Also, training on heterogeneous samples and then applying regularization and adversarial training produces robustness and adaptability across clinical settings [10].

8.2 Computational Costs and Infrastructure Disparities

Advanced ML models, particularly deep learning networks like CNNs, demand significant computational resources, including powerful GPUs and high memory capacity [34]. This makes it hard for institutions with limited infrastructure, creating further disparities in the adoption of technology across healthcare settings. Efficient model optimization and cloud-based ML platforms could offer scalable alternatives to address these disparities. Therefore, federated learning allows decentralized training across multiple institutions while preserving data privacy owing to a mechanism in which only model parameters are shared. In Fig. 7. federated architecture is illustrated, where local models are aggregated at an intermediary server. Transfer learning techniques provide an increase in accuracy while upholding patient confidentiality. In addition, differential privacy and secure aggregation

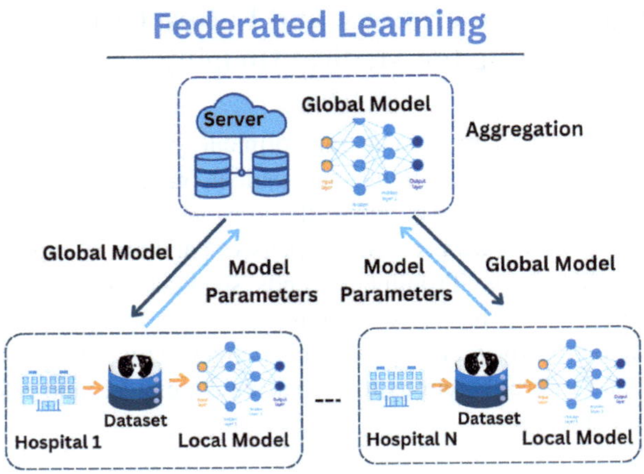

Fig. 7 Federated learning architecture

further strengthen privacy while ensuring robustness in sensitive data environments [3].

8.3 Multimodal and Personalized Medicine Integration

Combining imaging with genomic, electronic health records (EHR), and clinical data provides an almost panoramic view of the health of the patient, which enhances accuracy in diagnosis and facilitates personal treatment [20]. This multi-modal aspect improves the predictive model but makes standardization and ethical handling complicated concerning data. AI-supported predictive healthcare personalizes treatment and enhances outcomes, yet the issue of equity in access to data and that of patient trust should be considered.

8.4 Explainability and Interpretability of ML Models

In the clinical use of machine learning, a model needs to be accurate and interpretable. Explaining AI techniques such as LIME, SHAP, saliency maps, and Grad-CAM makes black box models more interpretable, highlighting the features influencing a prediction Fig. 8. For traditional models such as decision trees or logistic regression, interpretability is built-in, and deep learning methods would require post-hoc approaches for explainability or hybrid models that enable some transparency but still retain a good level of predictive performance [12].

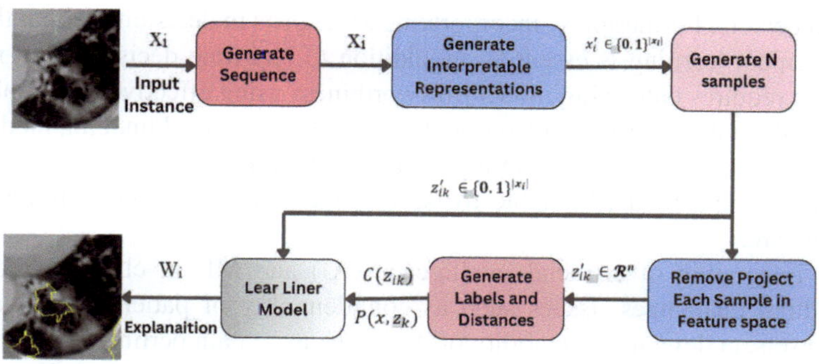

Fig. 8 Local interpretable model-agnostic explanations

8.5 *Real-Time AI and Edge Computing*

Edge computing processes data locally, reducing latency and enabling real-time diagnostics, especially vital in emergencies and time-critical applications like oncology and infectious disease detection. Using deep learning with GPU help, models such as PROTOTWIN-PET have shown great accuracy and real-time analysis [52]. Together with the Internet of Medical Things (IoMT), these developments improve adaptive care delivery and patient monitoring.

To fully realize the benefits of ML in medical imaging, concerted efforts are needed to overcome data limitations, reduce computational and ethical tenets, specifically fair equity, transparency, and accountability. Emphasizing multimodal learning, explainability, and privacy-preserving techniques–alongside real-time and personalized solutions–will be critical for sustainable, equitable, and impactful adoption of AI in clinical settings. The path forward hinges on interdisciplinary collaboration and continued innovation grounded in human-centered values.

9 Conclusion

The transformer impacts of Machine learning (ML) on medical imaging represent a significant progression of diagnostic precision and clinical results. Recent developments in ML methodologies, and deep learning, have enabled an improved analysis of complex medical images. Convolutional neural networks have proven to be very effective techniques in automating the diagnosis of various conditions with speed and accuracy, competing with traditional methods more than in the areas of detection and classification. Moreover, because of the importance of data quality and sufficiency, methods such as data augmentation, annotation, and preprocessing have become critical factors in improving model performance and robustness. In addition, exploring collaborative models while preserving patient data confidentiality, considering model complexity and resource availability in medical centers. Furthermore, incorporating specialists in decision-making through reinforcement learning is essential, in addition to real-time decisions and results. This also requires enhancing model trustworthiness using effective explainable AI. Additionally, taking into consideration the diversity of medical imaging modalities' characteristics and their availability, and developing robust and generalizable machine learning models suitable for several modalities to assess different tasks in healthcare.

The integration of artificial intelligence (AI) and ML in clinical practice is not without challenges. Issues such as confidentiality of patient data, biases in training sets, and the interpretability of AI decisions remain pertinent concerns that require debate for achieving a bigger impact. In addition, the need for rigorous validation of ML algorithms in various clinical contexts is vital to ensure their reliability and generalization. In the future, improving the accuracy of the diagnosis implies the continuous evolution of ML methods, associated with interdisciplinary collaboration between clinicians, data scientists, and ethicians. Innovations such as federated learning can allow the use of collaborative learning, and decentralized data while guaranteeing privacy. Overall, ML's progress is promising to reshape the landscape of medical imaging and considerably improve patient results.

References

1. Abd El-Khalek AA, Balaha HM, Alghamdi NS, Ghazal M, Khalil AT, Abo-Elsoud MEA, El-Baz A (2024) A concentrated machine learning-based classification system for age-related macular degeneration (amd) diagnosis using fundus images. Sci Rep 14(1):2434
2. Aktar SF, Andrei S (2023) Bias, ethical concerns, and explainable decision-making in medical imaging research. In: Data driven approaches on medical imaging, Springer, Berlin, pp 179–205
3. Albalawi E, TR M, Thakur A, Kumar VV, Gupta M, Khan SB, Almusharraf A (2024) Integrated approach of federated learning with transfer learning for classification and diagnosis of brain tumor. BMC Med Imaging 24(1):110
4. Arafa MA, Omar I, Farhat KH, Elshinawy M, Khan F, Alkhathami FA, Mokhtar A, Althunayan A, Rabah DM, Badawy AHA (2024) A comparison of systematic, targeted, and combined biopsy using machine learning for prediction of prostate cancer risk: a multi-center study. Med Principles Pract 33(5):491–500
5. Bashir S, Khattak IU, Khan A, Khan FH, Gani A, Shiraz M (2022) A novel feature selection method for classification of medical data using filters, wrappers, and embedded approaches. Complexity 2022(1):8190814
6. Bellmann Q, Peng Y, Genske U, Yan L, Wagner M, Jahnke P (2024) Low-contrast lesion detection in neck ct: a multireader study comparing deep learning, iterative, and filtered back projection reconstructions using realistic phantoms. Eur Radiol Exp 8(1):84
7. Bennour A, Ben Aoun N, Khalaf OI, Ghabban F, Wong WK, Algburi S (2024) Contribution to pulmonary diseases diagnostic from x-ray images using innovative deep learning models. Heliyon 10(9)
8. Bhavsar KA, Abugabah A, Singla J, AlZubi AA, Bashir AK, et al (2021) A comprehensive review on medical diagnosis using machine learning. Comput Mater Continua 67(2):1997
9. Bouamrane A, Derdour M, Alksas A, El-Baz A (2024) Hybrid deep learning approach with feature engineering for enhanced pulmonary nodule diagnosis. SN Comput Sci 5(7):890

10. Bouamrane A, Derdour M, Bennour A, Elfadil Eisa TA, M Emara AH, Al-Sarem M, Kurdi NA (2024) Toward robust lung cancer diagnosis: integrating multiple ct datasets, curriculum learning, and explainable ai. Diagnostics 15(1):1
11. Bouamrane A, Derdour M, Alksas A, Contractor S, Ghazal M, El-Baz A (2025) Role of artificial intelligence in early assessment of lung nodules: a brief review. Arch Comput Methods Eng 1–26
12. Bouamrane A, Derdour M, Alksas A, El-Baz A (2025) Evaluating explainability in transfer learning models for pulmonary nodules classification: A comparative analysis of generalizability and interpretability. Int J Pattern Recogn Artif Intell 25:1–33
13. Bradshaw TJ, Huemann Z, Hu J, Rahmim A (2023) A guide to cross-validation for artificial intelligence in medical imaging. Radiol Artif Intell 5(4):e220232
14. Brahma S, Kofler A, Zimmermann FF, Schaeffter T, Chiribiri A, Kolbitsch C (2024) Robust myocardial perfusion mri quantification with deepfermi. IEEE Trans Biomed Eng 72(3):1031–1044
15. Chlap P, Min H, Vandenberg N, Dowling J, Holloway L, Haworth A (2021) A review of medical image data augmentation techniques for deep learning applications. J Med Imaging Radiat Oncol 65(5):545–563
16. Chowdhary CL, Acharjya DP (2020) Segmentation and feature extraction in medical imaging: a systematic review. Proc Comput Sci 167:26–36
17. Dehbozorgi P, Ryabchykov O, Bocklitz TW (2025) A comparative study of statistical, radiomics, and deep learning feature extraction techniques for medical image classification in optical and radiological modalities. Comput Biol Med 187:109768
18. Eckardt JN, Bornhäuser M, Wendt K, Middeke JM (2022) Semi-supervised learning in cancer diagnostics. Front Oncol 12:960984
19. Ejaz K, Mohd Rahim MS, Arif M, Izdrui D, Craciun DM, Geman O (2022) Review on hybrid segmentation methods for identification of brain tumor in mri. Contrast Media Mol Imaging 2022(1):1541980
20. Fu L, Zhang Q, Lin L, Reyes R (2024) A 3d medical image segmentation method based on mcraip-net. IEEE Access. https://doi.org/10.1109/ACCESS.2024.3358897
21. Gao Y, Zou Z, Hu J, Dai J (2024) Multi-source face relighting: Pre-fusion and post-fusion approaches for improved lighting consistency and detail preservation. In: 2024 2nd international conference on computer, vision and intelligent technology (ICCVIT). IEEE, pp 1–6
22. Gasmi K, Ben Aoun N, Alsalem K, Ltaifa IB, Alrashdi I, Ammar LB, Mrabet M, Shehab A (2024) Enhanced brain tumor diagnosis using combined deep learning models and weight selection technique. Front Neuroinf 18:1444650
23. Kalra DS, Barkeshli M (2025) Why warmup the learning rate? underlying mechanisms and improvements. Adv Neural Inf Process Syst 37:111760–111801
24. Kasban H, El-Bendary M, Salama D, et al (2015) A comparative study of medical imaging techniques. Int J Inf Sci Intell Syst 4(2):37–58
25. Kina E (2025) TLEABLCNN: Brain and alzheimer's disease detection using attention based explainable deep learning and SMOTE using imbalanced brain mri. IEEE Access 13:27670–27683
26. Krabbe S, Møller JM, Hadsbjerg AE, Ewald A, Hangaard S, Pedersen SJ, Østergaard M (2024) Detection of structural lesions of the sacroiliac joints in patients with spondyloarthritis: A comparison of t1-weighted 3d spoiled gradient echo mri and mri-based synthetic ct versus t1-weighted turbo spin echo mri. Skeletal Radiol 1–10
27. Kumar A (2025) Reinforcement learning for robotic-assisted surgeries: Optimizing procedural outcomes and minimizing post-operative complications. Int J Res Publ Rev 6(31):5669–5684
28. Li L, Deng H, Ye X, Li Y, Wang J (2023) Comparison of the diagnostic efficacy of mathematical models in distinguishing ultrasound imaging of breast nodules. Sci Rep 13(1):16047
29. Maharana K, Mondal S, Nemade B (2022) A review: data pre-processing and data augmentation techniques. Global Transitions Proc 3(1):91–99

30. Muça M, Kapçiu R et al (2024) Dimensionality reduction: a comparative review using rbm, kpca, and t-sne for micro-expressions recognition. Int J Adv Comput Sci Appl 15(1)
31. Nanmaran R, Srimathi S, Yamuna G, Thanigaivel S, Vickram A, Priya A, Karthick A, Karpagam J, Mohanavel V, Muhibbullah M (2022) Investigating the role of image fusion in brain tumor classification models based on machine learning algorithm for personalized medicine. Comput Math Methods Med 2022(1):7137524
32. Nithya R, Nirmala K, Jeyakumar V, Venkateswaran N (2024) Diagnosis of diabetic retinopathy in retinal fundus images using machine learning and deep learning models. In: Internet of things and machine learning for type I and type II diabetes. Elsevier, Amsterdam, pp 63–87
33. Ozdemir B, Aslan E, Pacal I (2025) Attention enhanced InceptionNeXt-based hybrid deep learning model for lung cancer detection. IEEE Access 13:27050–27069
34. Paleyes A, Urma RG, Lawrence ND (2022) Challenges in deploying machine learning: a survey of case studies. ACM comput Surv 55(6):1–29
35. Pancholi BK, Modi PS, Chitaliya N (2022) A review of noise reduction filtering techniques for mri images. In: 2022 5th international conference on contemporary computing and informatics (IC3I). IEEE, pp 954–960
36. Payette K, Steger C, Licandro R, de Dumast P, Li HB, Barkovich M, Li L, Dannecker M, Chen C, Ouyang C, et al (2024) Multi-center fetal brain tissue annotation (feta) challenge 2022 results. Preprint, arXiv:240209463
37. Prinzi F, Orlando A, Gaglio S, Vitabile S (2024) Interpretable radiomic signature for breast microcalcification detection and classification. J Imaging Inf Med 37(3):1038–1053
38. Qiu H, Wang M, Wang S, Li X, Wang D, Qin Y, Xu Y, Yin X, Hacker M, Han S, et al (2024) Integrating mri-based radiomics and clinicopathological features for preoperative prognostication of early-stage cervical adenocarcinoma patients: in comparison to deep learning approach. Cancer Imaging 24(1):101
39. Rahman H, Ben Aoun N, Bukht TFN, Ahmad S, Tadeusiewicz R, Pławiak P, Hammad M (2025) Automatic liver tumor segmentation of ct and mri volumes using ensemble resunet-inceptionv4 model. Inf Sci 121966
40. Rainio O, Teuho J, Klén R (2024) Evaluation metrics and statistical tests for machine learning. Sci Rep 14(1):6086
41. Rajarajeshwari G, Selvi GC (2024) Application of artificial intelligence for classification, segmentation, early detection, early diagnosis, and grading of diabetic retinopathy from fundus retinal images: a comprehensive review. IEEE Access 12:172499–172536
42. Rasool N, Bhat JI, Ben Aoun N, Alharthi A, Wani NA, Chopra V, Anwar MS (2024) Resmhanet: Enhancing glioma segmentation and survival prediction using a novel deep learning framework. Comput Mater Continua 81(1)
43. Rocha MM, Landini G, Florindo JB (2023) Medical image classification using a combination of features from convolutional neural networks. Multimedia Tools Appl 82(13):19299–19322
44. Samaras AD, Feleki A, Apostolopoulos ID, Moustakidis S, Papageorgiou E, Kokkinos K, Papandrianos N (2024) Medical decision support system in nuclear medicine diagnosis for non-small cell lung cancer and coronary artery disease: a first stage prototype. In: 2024 15th international conference on information, intelligence, systems & applications (IISA). IEEE, pp 1–8
45. Shakeel PM, Burhanuddin M, Desa MI (2022) Automatic lung cancer detection from ct image using improved deep neural network and ensemble classifier. Neural Comput Appl 1–14
46. Shakya KS, Alavi A, Porteous J, K P, Laddi A, Jaiswal M (2024) A critical analysis of deep semi-supervised learning approaches for enhanced medical image classification. Information 15(5):246
47. Shorten C, Khoshgoftaar TM (2019) A survey on image data augmentation for deep learning. J Big Data 6(1):1–48
48. Islam S, Aziz MT, Nabil HR, Jim JR, Mridha MF, Kabir MM, Shin J (2024) Generative adversarial networks (GANs) in medical imaging: advancements, applications and challenges. IEEE Access 12:35728–35753

49. Sori WJ, Feng J, Godana AW, Liu S, Gelmecha DJ (2021) Dfd-net: lung cancer detection from denoised ct scan image using deep learning. Front Comput Sci 15:1–13
50. Wan Q, Lindsay C, Zhang C, Kim J, Chen X, Li J, Huang RY, Reardon DA, Young GS, Qin L (2025) Comparative analysis of deep learning and radiomic signatures for overall survival prediction in recurrent high-grade glioma treated with immunotherapy. Cancer Imaging 25(1):5
51. Wu L, Li J, Wang Y, Meng Q, Qin T, Chen W, Zhang M, Liu TY, et al (2021) R-drop: Regularized dropout for neural networks. Adv Neural Inf Process Syst 34:10890–10905
52. Xing Lp, Liu G, Zhang Hc, Wang L, Zhu S, Bao MDLH, Wang Yn, Chen C, Wang Z, Liu Xy, et al (2025) Evaluating cnn architectures for the automated detection and grading of modic changes in mri: a comparative study. Orthopaedic Surgery 17(1):233–243
53. Zafar W, Husnain G, Iqbal A, Alzahrani AS, Irfan MA, Ghadi YY, AL-Zahrani MS, Naidu RS (2024) Enhanced tumornet: Leveraging yolov8s and u-net for superior brain tumor detection and segmentation utilizing mri scans. Results Eng 24:102994
54. Zhang W, Zhu L, Hallinan J, Zhang S, Makmur A, Cai Q, Ooi BC (2022) Boostmis: Boosting medical image semi-supervised learning with adaptive pseudo labeling and informative active annotation. In: Proceedings of the IEEE/CVF conference on computer vision and pattern recognition, pp 20666–20676
55. Zhang H, Guo H, Hou Y, He X, Li S, Wang B, Yu J, Liu Y, Chu M, He X, et al (2025) GAICN: graph attention iterative contraction network for bioluminescence tomography. IEEE Trans Med Imaging 44(4):1659–1670

Deep Learning Revolution in Medical Image Analysis

Amal Jlassi, Khaoula Elbedoui, and Walid Barhoumi

1 Introduction

Medical imaging ensures a crucial and vital role in modern healthcare systems, providing valuable insights about the structure and function of every element of the human body. Nevertheless, with the increasing complexity and volume of medical data, traditional methods of medical image analysis are becoming insufficient to achieve the required accuracy and efficiency. In recent years, Deep Learning (DL) has emerged as a pivotal technology in healthcare field, particularly for medical image analysis issues. Using neural networks and large datasets, DL models have shown exceptional success in various main medical tasks such as segmentation, classification, and anomaly detection. In fact, DL has fundamentally changed the way medical images are analyzed and interpreted, by automatically learning patterns and representations from data. This potential enables more accurate diagnoses, faster processing times, and better patient outcomes. Indeed, the incorporation of

A. Jlassi (✉)
Research Team on Intelligent Systems in Imaging and Artificial Vision (SIIVA), Laboratoire de recherche en Informatique, Modélisation et Traitement de l'Information et de la Connaissance (LIMTIC), Higher Institute of Computer Science (ISI), University of Tunis El Manar, Tunis, Tunisia

University of Ibn Khaldoun (UIK), Tiaret, Algeria

K. Elbedoui · W. Barhoumi
Research Team on Intelligent Systems in Imaging and Artificial Vision (SIIVA), Laboratoire de recherche en Informatique, Modélisation et Traitement de l'Information et de la Connaissance (LIMTIC), Higher Institute of Computer Science (ISI), University of Tunis El Manar, Tunis, Tunisia

Computer Science Department, National Engineering School of Carthage (ENICarthage), University of Carthage, Tunis, Tunisia
e-mail: khaoula.elbedoui@enicarthage.rnu.tn; walid.barhoumi@enicarthage.rnu.tn

N. Ben Aoun et al. (eds.), *AI for Medical Image Analysis*,
https://doi.org/10.1007/978-3-032-02963-8_5

DL into clinical workflows has not only improved effects, but also decreased the inter- and intra-observer variability among healthcare. In this context, this chapter investigates the role of DL in healthcare, with a specific focus on its applications within the framework of medical image analysis. In the remainder of this section, we discuss how DL has been applied to different aspects of healthcare, highlighting its significant potential compared to traditional methods for medical tasks across various imaging modalities. Then, we provide a brief overview of medical image analysis, detailing the key tasks of segmentation, classification, and anomaly detection where DL models have demonstrated significant success. Section 2 is devoted to describing the fundamental architecture in DL for medical imaging, including neural networks and particularly convolutional neural networks (CNNs), followed by key achievements related to segmentation, anomaly detection, and classification. Section 3 explores DL models over medical image tasks, focusing on automated image segmentation, anomaly detection, and classification. It highlights state-of-the-art techniques such as U-Net for segmentation, autoencoders and generative adversarial networks for anomaly detection, and CNNs and transformers for disease classification, demonstrating their impact on diagnostic accuracy and clinical decision-making. Next, Sect. 4 presents some relevant real-world use cases for cancer detection, neurological disorders, and cardiovascular disease, before addressing in Sect. 5 the main challenges of exploiting DL in medical image analysis, such as data scarcity, interpretability, and generalization. Finally, Sect. 6 is dedicated to the discussion and future directions integrating DL with radiomics and personalized medicine for improved clinical impact.

1.1 Overview of Medical Image Analysis

Medical Image Analysis (MIA) is the process of extracting, refining, and interpreting meaningful information from medical images using computational methods. This process of MIA can be applied across various modalities, including Magnetic Resonance Imaging (MRI), Nuclear imaging (PET, SPECT), X-ray (2D and 3D), Computed Tomography (CT), Microscopy, Ultrasound, etc. The use of MIA is widely adopted for personalized treatment planning, monitoring disease progression, enhancing discovery of new disease markers, improving workflow efficiency and reducing diagnostic errors. The primary objectives of MIA include structure segmentation, disease classification, and anomaly detection. The segmentation task consists of splitting an image into distinct regions of interest in order to identify and delineate anatomical structures or pathological parts [1]. Accurate segmentation is a challenging task for disease management and treatment planning. For instance, in radiotherapy, precise tumor segmentation leads to targeted radiation delivery, minimizing damage to surrounding healthy tissue. Similarly, in surgical planning, detailed anatomical segmentation provides surgeons with a comprehensible understanding of the patient's anatomy, improving procedural outcomes. Regarding the classification task, it is based on assigning a label to an image

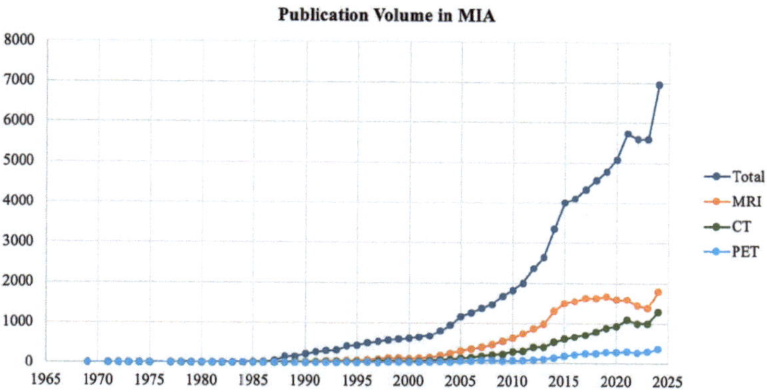

Fig. 1 Evolution of the publication volume in MIA according to PubMed (April 2025)

based on learned patterns [2]. It refers to the automated process of categorizing medical images into specific diseases, such as tumors, infections, or degenerative conditions. This task is critical to supporting clinical decision-making, allowing earlier and more accurate diagnoses, and streamlining treatment planning. Lastly, the anomaly detection task involves detecting infrequent or unusual patterns in medical images that may indicate pathological conditions [3]. In fact, it enables the identification of deviations from healthy anatomy, including tumors, lesions, or structural abnormalities, without relying on extensive labeled datasets. This is particularly valuable for rare diseases, early-stage abnormalities, or cases where labeled anomalies are scarce. It is particularly important to ensure life saving and early disease detection. Figure 1 illustrates the evolution of publication volume in MIA from 1965 to 2025 based on PubMed data. This figure shows a significant increase of interest on MIA after 2000, with an exponential surge post-2010, particularly for MRI and CT modalities, whereas PET remains less represented. This trend highlights the growing importance of computational techniques and AI-driven methods in medical imaging research.

It is important to point out that MIA result has been improved its objectives with the emergence of AI and DL techniques. This latter has made significant contributions on main medical tasks, including classification, segmentation, and anomaly detection. Overall, all these three tasks held an upward attention as shown in Fig. 2, with a notable acceleration after 2015 when DL began its real emergence. This trend, over the past two decades, highlights the field's shift toward an "intelligent medicine", driven by advances in DL, availability of large annotated datasets, and the increasing demand for precision in diagnostic imaging.

Building on these observations, the next section examines the role of DL in shaping and reshaping the healthcare landscape, particularly highlighting its effects on the MIA field in contrast to conventional machine learning techniques.

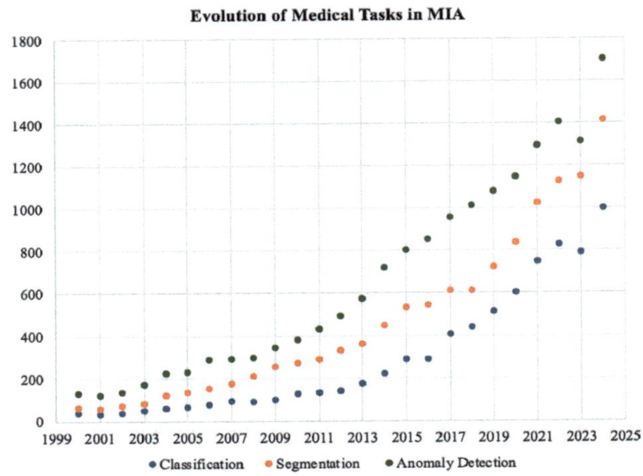

Fig. 2 Evolution of the publication volume of main medical tasks in MIA (PubMed-April 2025)

1.2 *Role of Deep Learning in Healthcare*

Deep learning has became one of the most powerful tool in healthcare to analyze and interpret complex medical data. In fact, DL allows the automatic extraction of relevant patterns from complex and large datasets, enhancing medical processes and clinical outcomes. The investigation of DL in healthcare is particularly important in the field of medical imaging, where vast amounts of data are generated across various modalities. In fact, medical imaging plays a crucial role in the diagnosis and treatment of several diseases. Traditionally, the interpretation of medical images depended totally on the expertise of radiologists and pathologists, making it a time-consuming and error-given process. However, DL models have shown exceptional potential in identifying complex patterns, segmenting challenging structures, classifying different confusing stages of disease, and detecting of rare anomalies with significant accuracy. The principal particularity of DL lies in its ability to learn and generalize from complex and large volume of medical images. Within the context of medical image exploration, DL can contribute to three main medical tasks: segmentation, classification, and anomaly detection (Fig. 3). The adoption of DL in these tasks increase the diagnostic accuracy, rate, and reliability of medical imaging, eventually improving patient outcomes. Thus, automating these tasks not only reduces the workload for medical professionals, but also ensures more consistent and objective interpretations.

Indeed, DL-based systems are increasingly being integrated into modern clinical workflows, offering clinical decision support tools that assist clinicians and healthcare professionals in detecting abnormalities and predicting disease progression. The power of DL models to continuously enhance across data augmentation and transfer learning further increases their role in modern healthcare. As the availability of annotated medical datasets increases and computational power advances, the

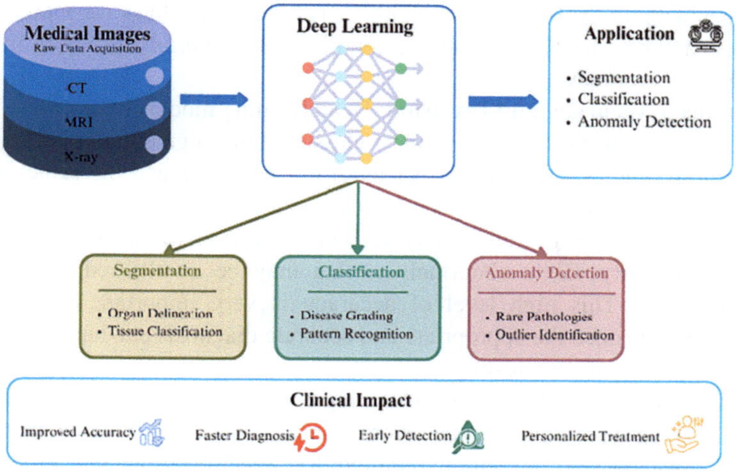

Fig. 3 Deep learning-based medical image analysis for segmentation, classification, and anomaly detection

Table 1 Key differences and transition drivers between ML and DL

Aspect	Machine learning (ML)	Deep learning (DL)
Feature extraction	Manual, expert-driven	Automatic, data-driven
Performance	Good with clear, simple features	Superior with complex, high-dimensional data
Data requirements	Effective with small datasets	Excels with large annotated datasets
Flexibility	Limited to predefined features	Learns new, complex patterns
Clinical impact	Assists in routine tasks	Enables new applications, higher accuracy

potential of DL to transform medical imaging and personalized medicine continues to grow. For instance, convolutional neural networks have been successfully employed for tumor detection, tissue classification, and disease grading. Unlike traditional Machine Learning (ML) models that require hand-crafted features, DL models automatically learn feature representations from input sample data, enabling more accurate and efficient analysis [4]. The key differences and transition drivers between ML and DL are presented in Table 1.

Overall, knowing that the ability to process large volumes of data not only enhances diagnostic accuracy but also accelerates the pace of innovation in medical imaging applications [5], key advantages of DL include:

- **Automated Feature Learning**: A significant benefit of deep learning lies in its capability to intuitively extract reliable features from raw data. Traditional methods often rely on manual feature extraction, which can be time-consuming and prone to human error. In contrast, deep learning algorithms, particularly CNNs, can automatically identify and extract relevant features from raw medical images without explicit programming. This capability allows for more nuanced understanding and interpretation of complex data patterns, leading to improved diagnostic accuracy.

- **Enhanced Accuracy and Precision**: Deep learning models have proven noticeable accuracy in tasks such as image classification, segmentation and anomaly detection. Studies have shown that these models can reach the same accuracy or even exceed those of experienced radiologists. For instance, in skin cancer detection and diabetic retinopathy screening, deep learning models have been able to identify subtle abnormalities that may be overlooked by traditional methods [6]. This high level of accuracy is very important in the clinical environment, since the appropriate and accurate diagnosis can have a significant impact on the patient's results.
- **Scalability and Efficiency**: Deep learning excels in addressing large volumes of data, making it particularly well recommended for medical imaging applications where vast datasets are often required for generalization and validation of medical insights. In fact, traditional methods may fail to address scalability due to their reliance on hand-crafted features. The ability of DL models to handle scalability not only improves diagnostic throughput, but also enables healthcare facilities to accommodate more patients and reduce waiting times for imaging services.
- **Reduction of Human Error**: The integration of deep learning into medical imaging workflows reduces obviously the risk of human errors. By automating repetitive tasks such as image segmentation or anomaly detection, deep learning models exempt clinicians from workload that exhausts their efforts to focus on vital and crucial clinical decisions. Thus, this automation leads to more rational and well-considered decisions.
- **Early Disease Detection**: Deep learning models excel also in the early detection of diseases, which is crucial for human life saving. This early detection capability leads to anticipated decisions and better treatment outcomes to prevent any adverse disease progression.
- **Multimodal Integration**: Deep learning models allows the integration of different data type to perform any desired task. In the context of medical imaging, this can be done from multiple imaging modalities (e.g., MRI, CT scans), given that combining information from different sources can improve DL model performance, while providing more comprehensive analysis of patient conditions. This multimodal approach provides a comprehensive view of the patient's health. This is very important for precise and personalized treatment planning.

Given the critical role of DL in healthcare, it is essential to examine the fundamental principles that support these advancements. The following section explores fundamental architectures of DL in medical imaging.

2 Fundamental Architectures in Deep Learning for Medical Imaging

Analyzing medical image involves deriving significant insights from medical scans, frequently employing computational techniques. that are achieved through a combination of AI models and computer vision techniques. These methods are mainly based on DL models, even if they are difficult to understand. This section explores this incorporation and highlights the deployment of neural networks, CNN, RNN, and GAN, in key medical investigations such as classification, segmentation and anomaly detection. Furthermore, we underline the growing adoption of multimodal deep learning models, which enhance learning potential via diverse medical imaging modalities. This multimodal approach not only improves model performance but also capitalizes the complementarity of medical information across different sources.

2.1 *Artificial Neural Network*

The history of DL in medical image analysis dates back to the early days of machine learning, with seminal works such as Vannier et al.'s (1985) multispectral tissue classification report using statistical pattern recognition techniques [7]. Since then, DL approaches have become the main target for medical imaging. Despite their successes, DL models for medical imaging often rely on relatively small datasets when contrasted with broader computer vision activities [8]. However, the emergence of new datasets and trends, such as the adoption of end-to-end trained models, has the potential to overcome these limitations. Indeed, the development of DL in medical imaging has evolved significantly over the past decade, marked by key milestones and innovations. Below is a chronological overview of this progression:

- **2012**: Deep learning gained prominence when a convolutional neural network has achieved remarkable success in the ImageNet classification challenge. This event presents an important pivot highlighting the importance of DL in medical image application.
- **2013**: Deep learning has been recognized as one of the "10 breakthrough technologies" by the MIT Technology Review, showing its approach to change in different fields, including healthcare [5].
- **2015–2016**: The introduction of transfer learning became a significant enabler for DL in medical imaging. Researchers began exploring whether networks pre-trained on large natural image datasets could be fine-tuned for medical tasks, demonstrating that this approach could enhance training efficiency and accuracy.
- **2017–2018**: Synthetic data augmentation emerged as another innovative solution to address the data scarcity challenge in medical imaging. Techniques such as

generative adversarial networks were developed to synthesize realistic medical images, which were shown to improve model performance by providing additional training examples.
- **2018**: The U-Net architecture was introduced for image segmentation tasks, particularly for biomedical applications. Originally designed for microscopic cell segmentation, U-Net has become widely adopted for various medical image segmentation challenges due to its effectiveness and robustness.
- **2020**: Advances in DL methodologies continued with an increased focus on interpretability and uncertainty quantification. Researchers began addressing the challenges of understanding how DL models make decisions, which is crucial for clinical applications where trust and transparency are paramount.
- **2022**: A review highlighted ongoing developments in DL applications across various medical imaging domains, including classification, detection, segmentation, and registration. The integration of Electronic Health Records (EHR) with imaging data using DL techniques also gained attention as a means of improving diagnostic capabilities [9].
- **2024-**. . .: Recent literature continues to explore the evolution of artificial intelligence in medical imaging, emphasizing the transition from classical machine learning approaches to more sophisticated DL models. This includes discussions on the challenges faced and future directions for research in this rapidly advancing field.

In this context, many architectures of DL, particularly convolutional neural networks have been widely used for different medical image tasks. In fact, each type of network tends to excel in specific applications (segmentation, classification, and/or detection). The next section will detail this main DL model and explain how it performs the required goal.

2.2 Convolutional Neural Network

Convolutional neural networks are frequently employed across various medical imaging applications, demonstrating their adaptability and efficacy in meeting diverse clinical needs. Their capability to autonomously acquire pertinent characteristics from samples of image data, eliminating the necessity for manual feature extraction, renders them especially ideal for examining intricate medical images, including those captured through MRI, CT, and X-ray techniques. CNNs have been successfully applied to tasks ranging from disease detection and segmentation to image registration and computer-aided diagnosis, contributing to improved diagnostic accuracy and more efficient clinical workflows. The architecture of CNNs allows them to capture intricate patterns within medical images, facilitating accurate diagnoses and treatment decisions. The layered structure of CNNs begins with initial layers, which detect basic features such as textures and contours, progressing to deeper layers that identify more complex structures. This hierarchical learning process enables CNNs to autonomously extract pertinent information from diverse medical imaging modalities, including X-rays, MRIs, and CT scans. The use of CNNs has been validated through numerous studies demonstrating their effectiveness in identifying anomalies and assisting healthcare professionals in clinical decision making. Furthermore, CNN features have been shown to be effective in DL-based medical image fusion (DLMIF), allowing for the seamless integration of facilitating the smooth amalgamation of data from various imaging techniques to deliver a more thorough and insightful evaluation of the patient's status. By leveraging the ability of CNNs to extract salient features from each modality, DLMIF techniques can generate fused images that highlight complementary information and enhance the visualization of subtle abnormalities. This approach has proven particularly useful in scenarios where the diagnosis requires the integration of anatomical and functional information, such as in the assessment of cardiac ischemia or the detection of cancer metastases. CNNs have demonstrated remarkable efficacy in identifying fractures in various anatomical locations, offering a potential solution to the challenges associated with manual fracture detection, which can be time-consuming and prone to human error. By training CNNs on large datasets of labeled fracture images, researchers have developed models capable of accurately detecting fractures in a variety of imaging modalities, including plain radiographs, CT scans, and MRI scans. These models have the potential to assist radiologists in the interpretation of complex fracture patterns and improve the speed and accuracy of fracture diagnosis, leading to better patient outcomes.

2.3 Recurrent Neural Network and Variants

Framework based on RNN is used in the generation of a diagnostic report, which serves as a way of automatically generating deep and detailed reports from medical images. Through taking advantage of the fact that RNNs are clearly expressed in a step-by-step manner, these frameworks have the ability to show the continuity of one region with others in different parts of a picture and then summarize the most important of them in a report, thus producing coherent and grammatically correct sentences. The radiologist's time and effort can be greatly reduced with the help of this development in technology and consistency in diagnostic work will also be greatly improved. The Long Short-Term Memory (LSTM) models, which are a form of recurrent neural network, are commonly used in the arising problems of medical image analysis, highlighting the ability to maintain sequential data progress and extract long-distance dependencies among medical images. Furthermore, the deep learning-based medical imaging report generation approach involves hierarchical RNNs that support multi-tiered report generation providing a concise record of the salient features of the tissue and at the same time all the necessary details of the triggered areas to the reader. These structured models usually include various layers of RNNs that, where the top layer is responsible for writing a high-level general and easily understandable diagnosis and the layers below are able to elaborate on the details of the problem and its clinical meaning. It is possible, therefore, that the hybridization of a model of this type results in easy-to-understand and informative reports that meet the requirements of the expert radiologist and the less experienced clinician at the same time.

2.4 *Generative Adversarial Network*

Generative Adversarial Networks (GANs) have found extensive application for medical image analysis and have displayed their power of not only creating synthetic images but also generating realistic and performing image-to-image translation tasks. GANs are made up of two neural networks, the generator and the discriminator, which work together in opposition the two neural networks are one, that have been trained in a manner they are adversarial to each other. On the one hand the generator tries to synthetically produce images that are similar to the real ones while on the other hand the discriminator is doing its best to distinguish between real and artificial images. This process becomes combative leading to the generation of realistic-looking images which are proper not only for the configuration of data but also for the recognition of symptoms, and other medical imaging applications. The use of GAN models in the segmentation tasks has shown some very outstanding results, and hence it constitutes a potential potentially solving the problem which comes with the manual image segmentation such as being very slow and subjective. By teaching GANs, to draw the segmentation masks that show the true edge of bodies of organs or areas of diseases, scientists have been able to create models that can easily automatically segment medical images with high precision and speed. Those models signify a remarkable step towards radiology and display the potential to reshape job demands for radiologists and improve the stability of results of image segmentation. Generative Adversarial Networks (GANs) are incredibly versatile and adaptable tools. They have applied their abilities and have been utilized in interesting ways such as the generation of 3D objects, medicine, pandemics, processing, face detection, texture transfer, and traffic controlling, where they indeed show their versatility and adaptability. In the area of medical imaging, GANs have been used to make 3D models of anatomical structures from 2D images that are realistic, thereby, the model can be of great use in surgical planning, medical education, and similar areas. Besides, GANs have been found to be effective in the synthesis of medical images to be fed into deep learning models, especially when the availability of real medical images is a dilemma, due to privacy concerns or the disease being rare.

2.5 Multimodal Deep Learning in Medical Imaging

Within the context of medical imaging, Multimodal Deep Learning (MMDL) represents a significant advancement in the analysis and interpretation of complex biomedical data. In fact, it integrates information from various imaging modalities to provide a comprehensive analysis of medical conditions. This approach capitalizes on the strengths of different imaging techniques, such as combining MRI with PET scans, to improve diagnostic capabilities and treatment planning. Indeed, multimodal DL offers several advantages in medical image analysis. By integrating data from multiple sources, it provides a more comprehensive analysis, capturing complex medical conditions that might be missed when relying on a single imaging modality. This approach has been shown to enhance diagnostic performance, as multimodal techniques often surpass single-modality methods in tasks such as tumor detection and characterization. Additionally, the combination of diverse imaging data enhances the accuracy and individualization of treatment approaches, empowering healthcare practicians to make informed choices that consider every facet of a patient's wellbeing. Thus, within the framework of analyzing medical images, MMDL plays a pivotal role in several key applications. One of the most significant applications is tumor segmentation, where studies have demonstrated that DL models trained on multimodal images outperform those relying on single modalities. For instance, a model integrating MRI and CT data has shown superior performance in delineating soft tissue sarcomas compared to models using only one imaging type. This improvement is attributed to the complementary nature of different imaging modalities, where one may provide enhanced soft tissue contrast while the other offers better anatomical details [10]. Another essential application of MMDL is disease prediction and classification, particularly in complex medical conditions requiring diverse data sources for accurate assessment. In liver cancer diagnosis, for example, MMDL techniques that integrate imaging data with clinical parameters from electronic health records have significantly improved the accuracy of diagnosing HepatoCellular Carcinoma (HCC) and predicting treatment responses. Moreover, the fusion of imaging data and non-imaging data allows for a more comprehensive understanding of disease progression, enabling personalized and effective treatment planning [11]. MMDL also enhances cross-modal retrieval, facilitating the correlation of medical images with other relevant patient information, such as laboratory results or clinical history. This capability is vital for comprehensive patient management, as it ensures that clinicians have access to all relevant data points when making diagnostic and treatment decisions. By aligning imaging findings with patient records, MMDL contributes to a more holistic and informed approach to medical care. Furthermore, MMDL is revolutionizing report generation by leveraging both imaging data and associated textual information. Automated diagnostic report generation not only streamlines the workflow for healthcare professionals but also minimizes the risk of human error. By integrating Natural Language Processing (NLP) with medical imaging analysis, these systems can generate structured, consistent, and detailed reports, ultimately improving efficiency in clinical settings [12]. Recent advancements in MMDL have shown promise in areas like cancer detection and neurological disorder diagnosis, where integrating various imaging modalities leads to better outcomes for patients [4]. The implementation of MMDL often involves the following architectural strategies:

- **Feature Fusion**: Combining features extracted from different modalities at various stages of the network enhances the model's ability to learn complex relationships within the data.
- **Classifier Fusion**: Different classifiers can be trained on individual modalities, with their outputs combined to improve overall predictive performance.
- **Decision-Level Fusion**: Final decisions from multiple models can be aggregated to achieve a consensus prediction, which is particularly useful in clinical settings where accuracy is paramount.

Nevertheless, despite its immense potential, multimodal deep learning still grapples with significant challenges. One major barrier is data integration, since combining diverse data types effectively demands advanced methodologies to harness meaningful insights while minimizing noise and bias. Another critical issue is interpretability; like many deep learning models, understanding the decision-making process remains difficult, yet it is essential for earning clinicians' trust. Compounding these challenges is the scarcity of labeled multimodal datasets, which often restricts the development of robust and reliable models. Thus, research should focus on enhancing model interpretability, developing techniques for effective data integration, and creating larger annotated multimodal datasets to facilitate training. In addition, exploring self-supervised learning approaches may help mitigate the need for extensive labeled data.

As research continues to evolve, addressing ethical considerations and ensuring robust validation will remain crucial for the successful implementation in clinical settings. This evolution is further detailed in Table 2 which highlights key developments in DL and MIA. As we can notice, over the past decade, the synergy between advancements in DL and MIA has been increasingly explored and exploited.

3 Deep Learning Models over Medical Image Tasks

Medical image processing has made many important advances over the last decade. This is mainly related to the increasing use of DL models. These advances have ensured more accurate diagnosis, personalized treatment planning, and real-time clinical decision-making. Indeed, DL models have improved the medical image analysis process mainly through the automation of many challenging medical tasks. This chapter explores three key areas where DL has made significant contributions: image segmentation, anomaly detection, and image classification.

Table 2 Timeline of DL and MIA advances

Date	Deep learning (DL) advances	Medical image analysis (MIA) advances
2012	AlexNet wins ImageNet [13].	CNNs introduced for tumor detection and segmentation [14].
2014	CNNs outperform in skin lesion classification [15].	Adoption of CNNs in dermatology imaging [16].
2015	U-Net introduced for segmentation [17].	U-Net becomes gold standard in medical segmentation.
2016	Inception-v3 excels at diabetic retinopathy detection [18].	AI systems begin outperforming traditional methods.
2017	Arterys Cardio AI approved by FDA.	First FDA-approved AI for cardiac MRI analysis.
2018	IDx-DR FDA-approved for diabetic retinopathy diagnosis [19].	First autonomous AI system deployed clinically.
2020	Vision Transformers (ViT) proposed [20].	ViTs applied to medical imaging tasks [21].
2021	Multi-modal DL models integrate imaging and genomics [22].	AI systems for personalized medicine developed.
2022	SimCLR and BYOL enable self-supervised learning [23, 24].	Self-supervised learning used for medical imaging [25].
2023	Federated Learning enables secure model training [26].	Hospitals adopt Federated Learning for collaboration.
2024	Diffusion models widely adopted for image generation and reconstruction [27].	Diffusion models improve MRI reconstruction and data augmentation [28].
2024	Foundation models trained specifically for healthcare (BioMedGPT, Med-Flamingo) [29].	Foundation models used for multi-modal medical diagnostics (imaging + text).
2024	Advanced XAI techniques developed for diffusion and foundation models [30].	XAI frameworks integrated into diagnostic pipelines to explain predictions to clinicians.
2025	Causal DL methods applied to medical imaging tasks [31].	Clinical use of causal AI models improves robustness and fairness of diagnosis.

3.1 *Automated Image Segmentation*

Automated image segmentation has significantly enhanced efficiency and rigor of medical diagnosis. For instance, the automation of brain tumor segmentation has reduced the time required for radiologists to identify tumor areas, and thus allowed them to maintain faster and more accurate surgical planning. Similarly, automated lung nodule segmentation has improved early detection rates of lung cancer. Overall, in order to deal with the challenging issue of automated segmentation, deep learning models have shown exceptional performance in medical image segmentation, outperforming traditional methods based on manual annotation and classical computer vision techniques. In the following, we briefly describe the most emerging segmentation models based on DL:

- **U-Net Architecture** The U-Net model, introduced by Ronneberger et al. [32], remains a cornerstone in medical image segmentation. Its encoder-decoder structure enables precise localization and accurate boundary detection, even with limited training data. Recent variants such as Attention U-Net and Residual U-Net have introduced attention mechanisms and skip connections, allowing to enhance the feature extraction process, while reducing the overfitting risk [33].
- **Transformer-Based Models** Vision transformers (ViTs) have been recently investigated within the framework of medical image segmentation. Moreover, models like TransUNet [34] combine the local feature extraction capabilities of CNNs with the global attention mechanisms of transformers, improving segmentation accuracy for complex medical images, such as brain MRIs and CT scans.
- **3D Segmentation Models** For volumetric data, such as 3D MRI and CT scans, 3D U-Nets and V-Net [35] architectures have been developed to capture spatial relationships between slices. This has led to improved accuracy in brain tumor segmentation, lung nodule detection, and cardiac structure delineation. However, since most of them are relying on local convolutional operations, 3D segmentation models struggle to capture long-range spatial relationships, and they may not fully compensate for the lack of global attention mechanisms.
- **Self-Supervised Learning** Self-supervised learning techniques [36] have emerged to address the challenge of limited annotated medical data. Models are pre-trained on large, unlabeled datasets using contrastive learning or predictive coding, and then fine-tuned on task-specific datasets for segmentation.

Table 3 catalogs DL-based segmentation methods, while emphasizing their technical innovations and practical benefits (e.g., surgical planning, reduced annotation dependency, etc.) to show their superiority over traditional methods.

3.2 Anomaly Detection

Anomaly detection focuses on identifying rare or abnormal patterns within medical images, which is crucial for early diagnosis of diseases such as cancer, neurological disorders, and cardiovascular diseases. Deep learning models have enhanced anomaly detection by learning complex patterns from large datasets and identifying subtle deviations from normal anatomy. In fact, DL-based anomaly detection has improved early diagnosis and treatment of various conditions. For instance, early detection of Alzheimer's disease through MRI-based anomaly detection has enabled earlier intervention and better patient outcomes. Similarly, automated detection of lung nodules has reduced false-negative rates in lung cancer screening. In the following subsections, we provide a concise overview of the latest anomaly detection architectures that leverage DL:

- **Autoencoders** Autoencoders have been widely used for unsupervised anomaly detection. These models are trained to reconstruct normal medical images,

Table 3 Summary of deep learning techniques for automated medical image segmentation

Model/Technique	Key features	Recent applications	Clinical impact
U-Net and variants [17]	Encoder-decoder structure with skip connections that preserve spatial details across layers	Brain tumor segmentation, blood vessel delineation [37]	High accuracy in localizing complex anatomical structures
Attention U-Net [38]	Integrates attention mechanisms to enhance focus on critical features	Liver tumor segmentation, retinal blood vessel extraction [39]	Improved weighting of relevant features and enhanced focus on regions of interest
3D U-Net/V-Net [40]	Captures volumetric spatial context, allowing analysis of 3D medical imaging data	Segmentation of brain MRI, lung CT, and cardiac anatomical structures [41]	Accurate 3D segmentation that supports surgical planning and treatment guidance
Transformer-based models [34]	Fuses convolutional layers with self-attention modules for better global context understanding	Brain and abdominal CT segmentation (e.g., TransUNet)	Enhanced performance on anatomies with complex or large spatial distributions
Self-supervised learning [25, 42]	Uses pre-training on unlabeled data and fine-tunes for downstream segmentation tasks	Anatomical structure segmentation with limited ground-truth labels	Reduces dependency on large annotated datasets, enabling broader applicability

and anomalies are detected based on high reconstruction errors. Variants such as Variational AutoEncoders (VAEs) and Convolutional AutoEncoders (CAEs) have shown promise in the detection of brain lesions and lung abnormalities [43].

- **Generative Adversarial Networks** GANs have been used for anomaly detection by learning the distribution of normal data. Anomalies are identified when the model fails to generate a realistic output. Deep Convolutional GANs (DCGANs) and CycleGANs have been particularly effective in detecting brain tumors and retinal abnormalities [44]. However, GANs suffer from instability with limited training data, often producing false detections on rare anomalies. They also lack interpretable decision limits, making clinical validation difficult.
- **Contrastive Learning** Contrastive learning approaches have been applied to anomaly detection by training the model to distinguish between normal and abnormal samples. This has improved the sensitivity and specificity of anomaly detection in mammography and MRI scans [45]. Nevertheless, the main drawback of contrastive learning for medical anomaly detection is its heavy reliance on large and diverse datasets of normal samples to learn effective feature representations, which can be challenging given data scarcity in medical imaging.
- **Transformers** Transformer-based models have shown promise in anomaly detection by capturing long-range dependencies and contextual information

within medical images. In particular, vision transformers have been applied to retinal OCT images for early detection of diabetic retinopathy [46]. It is worth noting that the lack of inherent spatial inductive bias within transformers can make them less effective than CNNs for detecting subtle and localized anomalies in medical images without extensive pre-training or architectural adaptations.

Overall, DL-based anomaly detection has improved early diagnosis and treatment of various conditions. For instance, early detection of Alzheimer's disease through MRI-based anomaly detection has enabled earlier intervention and better patient outcomes. Similarly, automated detection of lung nodules has reduced false-negative rates in lung cancer screening.

3.3 Image Classification

Image classification is one of the most widely studied applications of deep learning in medical image analysis. Classification models aim to assign a diagnostic label to a medical image, such as identifying cancerous versus non-cancerous tissue or classifying different types of brain tumors. In the following, we briefly describe the most relevant classification approaches based on DL:

- **Convolutional Neural Networks** CNNs have dominated medical image classification due to their ability to extract spatial features. Pre-trained models such as VGG16, ResNet, and EfficientNet have been effectively fine-tuned on medical datasets to classify diseases with high accuracy [47].
- **Transfer Learning** Transfer learning consists to use models pre-trained on large datasets of natural images (e.g., ImageNet) and adapting them to medical image classification. This approach reduces the need for large labeled medical datasets and improves convergence speed and accuracy. But, the domain gap between the source data and medical images can lead to mismatched features, since pretrained models may prioritize irrelevant features (e.g., textures, shapes, colors) over medically relevant patterns (e.g., subtle lesions) [48].
- **Transformers** Vision transformers have also shown competitive performance in medical image classification. Models like DeiT and Swin Transformer have been adapted for medical imaging tasks, providing enhanced feature representation and improved accuracy. However, unlike CNNs, which excel at capturing local patterns even with limited data, ViTs require extensive pretraining (often on non-medical datasets like ImageNet) due to their lack of inherent inductive biases for spatial locality and translation invariance [49].
- **Hybrid Models** Hybrid models that blend CNNs and transformers have come into play to profit from the strengths of both architectures. These models use CNNs for low-level feature extraction and transformers for high-level contextual understanding, leading to improved classification performance [50].
- **Few-Shot and Meta-Learning** Few-shot learning and meta-learning techniques have been developed to address the problem of limited training data. Models

are trained to generalize from a small number of samples, enabling efficient classification of rare diseases and rare cancer subtypes [51].

Table 4 summarizes recent key advancements in medical image processing, highlighting innovative techniques and their impact on improving diagnostic accuracy, model efficiency, and clinical adoption.

4 Key Applications of Deep Learning in Medical Image Analysis

DL has revolutionized medical image analysis by enabling an automated and highly accurate interpretation of complex medical data. The ability of deep learning models to extract intricate patterns from imaging modalities such as MRI, CT, PET, and ultrasound has led to significant improvements in diagnosis, prognosis, and treatment planning. This section explores key applications of deep learning in identifying and diagnosing cancer, neurological disorder analysis, and cardiovascular disease assessment.

4.1 Cancer Detection and Diagnosis

Cancer detection and diagnosis have greatly benefited from deep learning-based medical image analysis. Convolutional neural networks and their variants have demonstrated remarkable performance in identifying malignant lesions and classifying cancer subtypes across various imaging modalities, including mammograms, histopathological slides, and PET-CT scans.

- **Breast Cancer:** CNNs and transfer learning techniques have been used to classify breast lesions from mammograms [52], achieving performance comparable to or exceeding that of radiologists. Models such as ResNet and EfficientNet have been particularly effective in identifying microcalcifications and architectural distortions.
- **Lung Cancer:** DL models have been applied to detect lung nodules from chest X-rays and CT scans [53], with the objective of improving early detection rates. Moreover, multi-scale feature extraction and 3D CNNs have been adopted for reducing false positives and enhancing localization accuracy.
- **Colorectal Cancer:** Histopathological image analysis using deep learning has led to improved classification of colorectal cancer stages and differentiation between benign and malignant polyps [54]. Moreover, attention-based models have enhanced interpretability and diagnostic precision.

Table 4 Summary of key advancements in medical image analysis***

Domain	Techniques	Recent advances	Challenges	Clinical impact
Image segmentation	– CNN – U-Net – FCN – Transformer-based models	– Attention U-Net for better localization – Multi-scale fusion networks – Transformer-based segmentation	– Class imbalance – Poor generalization – High computational cost	– Better anatomical delineation – Faster processing – Improved localization
Anomaly detection	– Autoencoders [43] – GAN [44] – One-Class CNN – Transformer-based models [46]	– VAE for unsupervised detection – GANs for rare anomaly synthesis – CNN–Transformer hybrids	– Scarce labels for rare diseases – Overfitting on small data – Low explainability	– Earlier detection – Reduced false positives – Better robustness
Image classification	– ResNet – EfficientNet – Vision transformers [49] – Capsule networks	– Self-supervised learning – ViT for high-resolution images – Transfer learning on small data [48]	– Domain shift across institutions – Low-quality imaging – Patient data variability	– Faster diagnosis – Improved grading – More consistent outcomes

Furthermore, DL's ability to handle multi-modal data (e.g., combining radiological and genomic data) has further improved predictive accuracy and personalized treatment strategies.

4.2 Neurological Disorder Analysis

DL has enabled breakthroughs in the diagnosis and monitoring of neurological disorders through advanced image analysis of MRI, CT, and PET scans. These models have been particularly effective in detecting structural and functional abnormalities associated with neurological diseases.

- **Alzheimer's Disease:** CNNs and Recurrent Neural Networks (RNNs) have been widely used to detect early signs of Alzheimer's disease from structural MRI (sMRI) and functional MRI (fMRI) scans [55]. These models were trained to improve the accuracy of disease progression prediction.
- **Epilepsy:** Many DL models were used to ensure an automated detection of epileptic seizure. These models were performed from EEG and MRI to obtain an accurate localization [56]. Moreover, some hybrid models combining CNNs and transformers have enhanced the temporal and spatial resolution of seizure detection in order to maintain any anticipatory action.
- **Autism Spectrum Disorder (ASD):** DL models have been also used to analyze brain connectivity and structural differences in ASD patients [57]. This was improved by combining radiomics with deep learning to enhance ASD classification accuracy and to well identify biomarkers for early diagnosis.

Furthermore, DL models have recently played a significant role in advancing Brain-Computer Interfaces (BCIs) for real-time monitoring and intervention in neurological conditions.

4.3 Cardiovascular Disease Assessment (CDA)

The assessment of cardiovascular disease was reshaped by the use of DL models which performed very well the analysis of echocardiograms, cardiac MRIs, and CT angiograms. These models have enhanced the accuracy of diagnosis, the risk stratification, and mainly the treatment planning.

- **Coronary Artery Disease (CAD):** Many CNN-based models have been used to detect coronary artery stenosis from Coronary CT Angiography (CCTA). These models provide automated plaque analysis and risk prediction [58].
- **Heart Failure:** Some DL models have been also applied to echocardiograms and cardiac MRI scans to evaluate ejection fraction and myocardial strain, which helps clinicians in early detection and prognosis of heart failure [59].

Table 5 Key applications of deep learning in medical image analysis

Medical area	DL techniques employed	Main applications	Clinical contributions
Cancer detection and diagnosis	CNNs, transfer learning, attention models, 3D CNNs	Breast cancer classification, lung nodule detection [53], histopathological staging of colorectal cancer [54]	Enhances early diagnosis, reduces false positives, improves treatment personalization
Neurological disorder analysis	CNNs, RNNs, transformer-CNN hybrids	Detection of alzheimer's from MRI/fMRI [55], epilepsy localization from EEG and MRI [56], ASD biomarker identification [57]	Supports early intervention, accurate prognosis, and brain–computer interface integration
Cardiovascular disease assessment	CNNs, RNNs, transformers	Coronary stenosis analysis from CCTA [58], heart failure detection via echocardiograms and cardiac MRI [59], arrhythmia classification using ECG [60]	Improves risk stratification, enables real-time monitoring, supports personalized cardiac care

- **Arrhythmia Detection:** The analysis of electrocardiograms (ECG) have be done via relevant DL models to improve the detection of arrhythmias such as atrial fibrillation and ventricular tachycardia. Particularly, recurrent neural networks and transformer models have been investigated for handling time series data for arrhythmia classification [60].

Moreover, DL has been integrated into wearable technology, enabling real-time monitoring of heart health and early intervention in cardiovascular events. Table 5 illustrates overall view of the main medical areas where DL is applied to MIA.

5 Challenges of Deep Learning in Medical Imaging and Potential Solutions

Deep learning has considerably advanced the analysis of medical images, but it also faces several challenges that can hinder its effectiveness and adoption in clinical settings. Here are the Here are the main challenges recognized in the literature.

5.1 Data Scarcity and Imbalance

Data scarcity and imbalance are critical bottlenecks in medical image analysis, directly impacting the generalizability, reliability, and clinical adoption of deep learning models. Key challenges are as follows:

- Limited Annotated Data: Medical imaging datasets are often small due to the labor-intensive, expert-driven annotation process. For example, pixel-level segmentation labels for pathologies like tumors require hours of radiologist effort per case [3]. This scarcity restricts model training, particularly for rare diseases.
- Class Imbalance: Most datasets exhibit severe imbalance, with healthy cases vastly outnumbering pathological ones. For instance, in diabetic retinopathy screening, over 90% of retinal scans may belong to non-referable cases, biasing models toward the majority class [61].
- Cross-Modal and Cross-Site Variability: Differences in imaging protocols (e.g., MRI field strengths, CT reconstruction kernels) and patient demographics reduce model generalizability. Studies show performance drops of 15–30% when models trained on one hospital's data are tested on another's [62].
- Overfitting: Small datasets exacerbate overfitting, where models memorize noise instead of learning generalizable features. For example, CNNs trained on less than 1000 chest X-rays achieved 99% training accuracy but less than 70% on external validation [63].

Overall, some possible solutions may be applied to overcome these challenges, such as:

- Data Augmentation: Geometric transformations (rotation, scaling) and advanced methods like generative adversarial networks synthetically expand datasets. For instance, liver lesion classification has been improved by 12% in [64], using GAN-generated synthetic CT patches.
- Transfer Learning: Pretraining on large natural image datasets and fine-tuning on medical data mitigates data scarcity. For example, Tajbakhsh et al. (2016) have demonstrated that pretrained CNNs require $10\times$ less medical data to match task-specific model performance [48].
- Few-Shot and Self-Supervised Learning: Few-shot learning as meta-learning frameworks like prototypical networks classify novel diseases using less than 10 labeled examples [65]. Additionally, self-supervised learning may be used. So, models pretrained on pretext tasks (e.g., predicting image rotations) reduce dependency on labeled data. For instance, authors in [5] have achieved 92% accuracy in pneumonia detection using 80% fewer labeled chest X-rays.
- Federated Learning (FL): FL enables multi-institutional collaboration without sharing raw data. For example, the MONAI framework achieved 94% tumor segmentation accuracy across 20 hospitals while preserving patient privacy [66].
- Synthetic Data Generation: GANs and diffusion models generate anatomically plausible medical images. Within this context, the SYNTHRAD2023 challenge

has showed synthetic MRI data improved tumor detection sensitivity by 18% in low-data regimes [67].

Addressing data scarcity and imbalance is pivotal for deploying robust DL models in clinical practice. Hybrid strategies combining transfer learning, self-supervision, and federated frameworks show promise in leveraging limited data effectively. Future work must prioritize standardization (e.g., the Medical Imaging and Data Resource Center (MIDRC)) and ethical AI practices to ensure equitable, generalizable solutions.

5.2 *Interpretability and Trust*

Interpretability is a cornerstone for deploying deep learning models in clinical workflows, ensuring trust, safety, and compliance. This section synthesizes the challenges, advancements, and future directions in making medical AI transparent and actionable. This issue matters for many reasons, such as clinical decision-making, patient safety, and regulatory compliance. In fact, clinicians require intuitive explanations to trust AI recommendations. For instance, in lung cancer screening, models highlighting suspicious nodules via Grad-CAM improved radiologists' diagnostic accuracy by 18% compared to unaided decisions [68]. Furthermore, opaque models risk misdiagnoses. A 2020 study found that 32% of AI errors in mammography could have been prevented with interpretability tools [69]. Finally, regulatory bodies like the FDA now mandate model transparency for approval. The 2021 EU Medical Device Regulation (MDR) explicitly requires "explainable outputs" for AI-based diagnostics [70]. Thus, it is important to overcome the following challenges:

- Black-Box Complexity: DL models like vision transformers involve non-linear interactions across thousands of parameters, complicating post-hoc explanations.
- Lack of Standardization: Over 40 distinct XAI methods exist (e.g., SHAP, LIME), but none are universally accepted for medical imaging, leading to inconsistent clinical adoption [71].
- Medical Data Complexity: Subtle features (e.g., microcalcifications in breast cancer) are often critical for diagnosis but challenging for XAI methods to surface meaningfully [8].

Some possible solutions may be applied to overcome these challenges, such as:

- Human-Centered XAI: Co-designing interpretability tools with clinicians improves usability. For example, interactive dashboards for pathologists increased trust by 44% in a prostate cancer study [72].
- Workflow Integration: Embedding XAI into PACS/RIS systems reduces cognitive load. The IBM Watson Imaging AI Suite demonstrates real-time saliency maps during radiology workflows.
- Continual Learning: Models that update explanations dynamically as new data arrive (e.g., emerging disease variants) maintain trust over time.

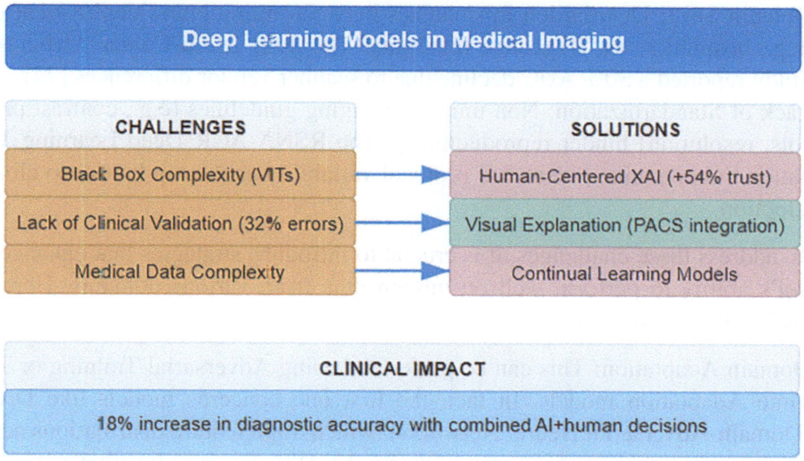

Fig. 4 Interpretability framework for medical AI

Interpretability is not optional but foundational for ethical AI in medicine. By aligning XAI methods with clinical needs, through human-centered design, standardization, and rigorous validation, researchers can bridge the trust gap and accelerate AI adoption in healthcare (Fig. 4).

5.3 *Generalization Across Diverse Populations*

Deep learning models may struggle to generalize across different patient populations and imaging modalities. Variability in patient demographics, imaging equipment, and acquisition protocols can affect model performance. For instance, a model developed using images from a specific hospital might struggle to achieve good performance when deployed on images from a different institution because of variations in imaging protocols or patient demographics. Thus, the challenges can be summarized as follows:

- Data Heterogeneity: Variability in imaging protocols (e.g., MRI field strengths, CT slice thickness) and patient demographics (age, ethnicity) degrades model performance. A 2022 multicenter study found a 15–25% drop in lung nodule detection accuracy when models trained on U.S. data were tested in India and Nigeria.
- Demographic Biases: DL models often exploit spurious correlations between demographics and outcomes. For example, a widely used chest X-ray model falsely linked race to disease risk, misdiagnosing black patients 1.5× more often than white patients [73].

- Domain Shift: Distribution mismatches between training and deployment data (e.g., hospital A vs. B) reduce reliability. The 2021 Multi-Center Alzheimer's Study reported a 30% AUC decline due to scanner vendor differences [74].
- Lack of Standardization: Non-uniform imaging guidelines (e.g., contrast protocols, resolution) hinder reproducibility. The RSNA-ACR Deep Learning Validation Subcommittee identified protocol variability as the top barrier to clinical adoption.

To address these challenges, it is crucial to introduce strategies that enhance the model's ability to perform well on unseen data from various domains. Here are several strategies for improvement:

- Domain Adaptation: This can be performed using Adversarial Training or Test-Time Adaptation models. In fact, the first one concerns models like DANN (Domain-Adversarial Neural Networks), which align feature distributions across domains, reducing performance gaps by 12–18% in cross-hospital mammography trials [75]. The second one updates batch normalization layers during inference to adjust to new domains dynamically.
- Transfer Learning: Pretraining on large, diverse datasets (e.g., RadImageNet with 1.35 million images from 104 global sites) improves out-of-distribution robustness [76].
- Multicenter Collaboration: Initiatives like the Medical Imaging and Data Resource Center (MIDRC) aggregate data from 200+ institutions, reducing geographic and demographic biases [77].
- Bias Mitigation: This may concern the Reweighting i.e. assign higher weights to underrepresented groups during training. A diabetic retinopathy model reduced racial disparities by 40% using this approach [78]. The bias mitigation may be also ensured via an adversarial debiasing which aims to penalize models for learning demographic correlates. This improved fairness in skin cancer diagnosis across skin tones by 22% [79].
- Continuous Monitoring: Deployed models should undergo routine audits using frameworks like Fairlearn or AI Fairness 360 to detect performance drift [80].

Thus, the generalization is not merely technical but ethical. By adopting domain adaptation, multicenter collaboration, and bias-aware training, the field can mitigate disparities and ensure DL models serve all populations equitably. Regulatory bodies must mandate rigorous generalization testing as part of AI certification (e.g., FDA's SaMD guidelines) to enforce accountability.

5.4 Adversarial Robustness, Ethical Concerns, and Computational Constraints

Adversarial attacks and noise can compromise the reliability of DL models within the framework of medical image analysis, raising ethical and privacy concerns in sensitive healthcare applications. Additionally, the high computational demands of deep learning models and the need for continuous learning pose practical limitations. Addressing these issues is crucial to ensuring the safety, fairness, and efficiency of AI-driven medical imaging systems. On the one hand, medical images are susceptible to various types of noise and artifacts that can adversely affect model performance. Adversarial attacks, where malicious inputs are designed to deceive models, pose a significant risk in clinical settings. Moreover, common issues such as motion artifacts in MRI scans or noise in X-ray images can lead to misclassifications if not properly addressed during preprocessing. Furthermore, the use of medical data for training deep learning models raises ethical concerns regarding patient privacy and data security. Ensuring that sensitive health information is protected while still allowing for effective model training is a critical challenge that must be addressed to gain public trust. On the other hand, DL models require substantial computational resources for training and inference, which can be a barrier in resource-constrained environments. The need for high-performance hardware (e.g., GPUs) may limit the accessibility of these technologies in smaller clinics or hospitals that cannot afford advanced computing infrastructure. Furthermore, medical knowledge and practices evolve over time, necessitating continuous updates to AI models. However, retraining models with new data while maintaining performance on previously learned tasks (known as catastrophic forgetting) poses a significant challenge.

Table 6 provides an overview of the main challenges and potential solutions for DL in MIA.

6 Discussion and Future Directions

The advancements in DL have significantly transformed the field of medical image analysis, enabling more accurate, efficient, and automated diagnosis and treatment planning. Despite these advancements, several challenges and opportunities remain. This section explores the integration of DL with other powerful techniques, such as radiomics and computer vision, the impact on real-world clinical applications, and the potential shift toward AI-driven personalized medicine.

6.1 Combining Deep Learning with Radiomics and Computer Vision

Radiomics and computer vision represent two complementary fields that, when combined with DL, can enhance the interpretability and diagnostic accuracy of medical imaging. Radiomics implies extracting a large number of quantitative characteristics from medical images, which can capture complex tissue characteristics that are not visible to the human eye. Deep learning models, especially

Table 6 Challenges and potential solutions for DL in medical image analysis

Challenge	Description	Potential solutions
Data scarcity and imbalance	Limited annotated datasets, especially for rare diseases; class imbalance favoring healthy cases.	Data augmentation, transfer learning, few-shot learning, synthetic data generation (GANs), federated learning.
Interpretability and trust	DL models often behave as "black boxes" making it hard for clinicians to understand predictions.	Explainable AI (XAI) methods, human-centered XAI tools, saliency maps, model visualization, clinical workflow integration.
Generalization across populations	Performance drop across different sites, demographics, and imaging protocols.	Domain adaptation, transfer learning, multi-center data aggregation, bias mitigation techniques.
Adversarial vulnerability	DL models are sensitive to noise, artifacts, and adversarial attacks.	Adversarial training, robustness testing, noise-robust architectures, data preprocessing techniques.
Computational constraints	High computational demands limit deployment in resource-constrained settings.	Model compression, efficient architectures (e.g., MobileNet, lightweight transformers), hardware optimization.
Ethical and privacy issues	Risks of patient data leakage and biases in diagnosis models.	Federated learning, secure model training (differential privacy), regulatory compliance (GDPR, HIPAA).
Continuous learning	Need for models to adapt to evolving medical knowledge without catastrophic forgetting.	Continual learning methods, dynamic model updating, incremental retraining strategies.

convolutional neural networks, can automatically learn complex patterns from imaging data, but they often lack interpretability. Combining DL with radiomics creates a hybrid approach that takes advantage of the strengths of both methods: the feature extraction power of radiomics and the pattern recognition capacity of DL. Thus, several studies have demonstrated that integrating radiomic features with DL models improves diagnostic performance. For instance, radiomics-based texture analysis combined with CNNs has been used to enhance tumor classification and grading in MRI and CT scans. Transformer-based models have also shown promise in processing radiomic data alongside raw imaging data, providing a more comprehensive understanding of tissue characteristics. Furthermore, computer vision techniques; such as edge detection, contouring, and feature matching; can refine the output of DL models, particularly in segmentation and anomaly detection tasks. For example, UNet architectures combined with computer vision-based post-processing steps have improved the accuracy of organ delineation and tumor segmentation in MRI and CT scans.

6.2 Real-World Applications

Although DL models have demonstrated remarkable performance in research environments, their integration into real-world clinical practice remains challenging. Factors such as regulatory approval, data privacy, and the necessity for interpretability and reliability pose significant obstacles to large-scale adoption. Despite these challenges, DL has already found its way into several clinical workflows. Automated tumor segmentation tools powered by CNNs are now assisting radiologists in achieving faster and more precise diagnoses. Similarly, DL-based image classification models have been implemented in fields like dermatology, where they aid in melanoma detection, and ophthalmology, where they improve screening for diabetic retinopathy. However, real-world deployment is complicated by the variability in medical imaging data, which differs across hospitals, imaging machines, and acquisition protocols. To mitigate this issue, researchers have explored domain adaptation and transfer learning techniques, allowing models to generalize more effectively across diverse datasets. Another critical challenge is the lack of explainability, as medical professionals require transparency in understanding how an AI model reaches a specific diagnosis. Ensuring that DL models are both accurate and interpretable remains a key priority for their successful clinical adoption.

6.3 Toward AI-Driven Personalized Medicine

The future of medical imaging is moving toward AI-driven personalized medicine, where DL models are designed to cater to individual patients by integrating their genetic, clinical, and imaging profiles. These models enhance diagnostic accuracy and treatment precision by incorporating multimodal data, including genomic information and medical history. In oncology, radiogenomics-based DL has demonstrated its potential to predict patient-specific responses to cancer treatments, leading to improved therapeutic strategies. Additionally, adaptive learning techniques, such as reinforcement and continual learning, are being explored to ensure that models evolve with new data, an essential feature in fields like oncology where tumor characteristics can change over time. Another significant application lies in predictive modeling, where DL is used to anticipate disease progression and patient outcomes. Recurrent neural networks and transformer-based architectures have already shown promise in forecasting the development of neurodegenerative diseases by analyzing longitudinal imaging data. Through these advancements, AI-driven DL continues to shape the future of personalized medical imaging, offering more precise and dynamic diagnostic and treatment solutions.

7 Conclusion and Takeaways

Deep learning has had an enormous impact on the field of medical image analysis, causing big innovations in the diagnostic precision of the whole clinical process, clinical workflow automation and personalized patient care. Its ability to extract complex patterns from multimodal imagery autonomously paves the way for the faster, earlier, and more accurate detection of diseases which were heretofore impossible to achieve. It marks an era of AI-driven healthcare that leads to more systemic, individual, and pluralistic styles of living. Not to mention the potential of not only for the development of segmentation, classification, and anomaly detection but also real-time monitoring, predictive modeling, and the integration of imaging with genetic and clinical data. This helps towards personalized medicine concepts. Nevertheless, one major point of consideration in obtaining the full benefits of these changes is to deal with these topics that are of ethical nature and how exactly AI will be used to develop them. The aforementioned issues such as bias and fairness, interpretability, data privacy, regulatory compliance, and human oversight are the key problems to be solved so that DL models may be fairly and transparently served to the broad population throughout the world. By this, we mean that trust in the AI must be built; data about a patient's privacy must be kept while federated learning privacy-preserving techniques are in place and the participation of a doctor should continue in the decision-making process. Generally speaking, the future of DL in medical imaging will rely not solely on technical innovation but in parallel with that, on our AI systems development that are trustworthy, including collecting the ethical behavior, and the patient-centered issue as also dried over the years.

References

1. Jlassi A, ElBedoui K, Barhoumi W, Maktouf C (2020) Unsupervised method based on superpixel segmentation for corpus callosum parcellation in MRI scans. In: Mokhtari M, Abdulrazak B, Aloulou H (eds) The impact of digital technologies on public health in developed and developing countries. ICOST 2020. Lecture notes in computer science, vol 12157. Springer, Cham, pp 114–125. https://doi.org/10.1007/978-3-030-51517-1_10
2. Jlassi A, ElBedoui K, Barhoumi W (2023) Glioma tumor's detection and classification using joint YOLOv7 and active contour model. In: 2023 IEEE symposium on computers and communications (ISCC). IEEE, pp 1–5. https://doi.org/10.1109/ISCC58397.2023.10218228
3. Nawaz A, Khan SS, Ahmad A (2024) Ensemble of autoencoders for anomaly detection in biomedical data: a narrative review. IEEE Access 12:17273–17289. https://doi.org/10.1109/ACCESS.2024.3360691
4. Chan HP, Samala RK, Hadjiiski LM, Zhou C (2020) Deep learning in medical image analysis. In: Suzuki K (eds) Advances in experimental medicine and biology, vol 1213. Springer, Cham, pp 3–21. https://doi.org/10.1007/978-3-030-33128-3_1
5. Zhou H-Y., Lu C, Yang S, Yu Y (2021) Preservational learning improves self-supervised medical image models by reconstructing diverse contexts. In: Proceedings of the IEEE/CVF international conference on computer vision (ICCV), pp 3479–3489. https://doi.org/10.1109/ICCV48922.2021.00348

6. Li M, Jiang Y, Zhang Y, Zhu H (2023) Medical image analysis using deep learning algorithms. Front Public Health 11:Article 1273253. https://doi.org/10.3389/fpubh.2023.1273253
7. Vannier MW, Butterfield RL, Jordan D, Murphy WA, Levitt RG, Gado M (1985) Multispectral analysis of magnetic resonance images. Radiology 154(1):221–224. https://doi.org/10.1148/radiology.154.1.3964938
8. Litjens G, Kooi T, Bejnordi BE, Setio AAA, Ciompi F, Ghafoorian M et al (2017) A survey on deep learning in medical image analysis. Med Image Anal 42:60–88. https://doi.org/10.1016/j.media.2017.07.005
9. Huang SC, Pareek A, Seyyedi S, Banerjee I, Lungren MP (2020) Fusion of medical imaging and electronic health records using deep learning: a systematic review and implementation guidelines. npj Digital Med 3:Article 136. https://doi.org/10.1038/s41746-020-00341-z
10. Isensee F, Jaeger PF, Kohl SAA, Petersen J, Maier-Hein KH (2021) nnU-Net: a self-configuring method for deep learning-based biomedical image segmentation. Nature Methods 18(2):203–211. https://doi.org/10.1038/s41592-020-01008-z
11. Mobadersany P, Yousefi S, Amgad M, Gutman DA, Barnholtz-Sloan JS, Velázquez Vega JE, Brat DJ, Cooper LAD (2018) Predicting cancer outcomes from histology and genomics using convolutional networks. J Am Med Inf Assoc 25(6):641–647. https://doi.org/10.1073/pnas.1717139115
12. Chen Z, Song Y, Chang TH, Wan X (2020) Generating radiology reports via memory-driven transformer. Preprint, arXiv:2010.16056. https://arxiv.org/abs/2010.16056
13. Krizhevsky A, Sutskever I, Hinton GE (2012) Imagenet classification with deep convolutional neural networks. In: Advances in neural information processing systems (NeurIPS). https://papers.nips.cc/paper_files/paper/2012/hash/c399862d3b9d6b76c8436e924a68c45b-Abstract.html
14. Cireşan DC, Giusti A, Gambardella LM, Schmidhuber J (2013) Mitosis detection in breast cancer histology images with deep neural networks. In: Medical image computing and computer-assisted intervention (MICCAI), pp 411–418. https://doi.org/10.1007/978-3-642-40763-5_51
15. Esteva A, Kuprel B, Novoa RA, Ko J, Swetter SM, Blau HM, Thrun S (2017) Dermatologist-level classification of skin cancer with deep neural networks. Nature, 542(7639), 115–118. https://doi.org/10.1038/nature21056
16. Codella NCF, Nguyen QB, Pankanti S et al (2015) Deep learning, sparse coding, and SVM for melanoma recognition in dermoscopy images. In: International Workshop on Machine Learning in Medical Imaging (MLMI), pp 118–126. https://doi.org/10.1007/978-3-319-24888-2_15
17. Ronneberger O, Fischer P, Brox T (2015) U-Net: convolutional networks for biomedical image segmentation. In: Medical image computing and computer-assisted intervention (MICCAI), pp 234–241. https://doi.org/10.1007/978-3-319-24574-4_28
18. Gulshan V, Peng L, Coram M et al (2016) Development and validation of a deep learning algorithm for detection of diabetic retinopathy in retinal fundus photographs. JAMA 316(22):2402–2410. https://doi.org/10.1001/jama.2016.17216
19. Abràmoff MD, Lavin PT, Birch M, Shah N, Folk JC (2018) Pivotal trial of an autonomous AI-based diagnostic system for detection of diabetic retinopathy in primary care offices. NPJ Digital Med 1(1):39. https://doi.org/10.1038/s41746-018-0040-6
20. Dosovitskiy A, Beyer L, Kolesnikov A et al (2020) An image is worth 16x16 words: transformers for image recognition at scale. In: International conference on learning representations (ICLR). https://arxiv.org/abs/2010.11929
21. Hatamizadeh A, Nath V, Tang Y et al (2022) UNETR: Transformers for 3D medical image segmentation. In: Proceedings of the IEEE/CVF winter conference on applications of computer vision (WACV), pp 574–584. https://doi.org/10.1109/WACV51458.2022.00181
22. Zhang, Y, Imoto S (2024) Genome analysis through image processing with deep learning models. J Human Genet 69:519–525. https://doi.org/10.1038/s10038-024-01275-0

23. Chen T, Kornblith S, Norouzi M, Hinton G (2020) A simple framework for contrastive learning of visual representations. In: International conference on machine learning (ICML), pp 1597–1607. https://doi.org/10.48550/arXiv.2002.05709
24. Grill JB, Strub F, Altché F et al (2020) Bootstrap your own latent: a new approach to self-supervised learning. In: Advances in neural information processing systems (NeurIPS). https://doi.org/10.48550/arXiv.2006.07733
25. Azizi S, Mustafa B, Ryan F et al (2021) Big self-supervised models advance medical image classification. In: Proceedings of the IEEE/CVF international conference on computer vision (ICCV), pp 3478–3488. https://doi.org/10.48550/arXiv.2101.05224
26. ElBedoui K, Barhoumi W, Cho J (2025) SoK: federated learning and unlearning for medical image analysis. Expert Syst 42:e70063. https://doi.org/10.1111/exsy.70063
27. Ho J, Jain A, Abbeel P (2020) Denoising diffusion probabilistic models. In: Advances in neural information processing systems (NeurIPS). https://doi.org/10.48550/arXiv.2006.11239
28. Pinaya WHL, Tudosiu P, Portela A et al (2022) Brain imaging generation with latent diffusion models. Preprint, arXiv:2209.07162. https://doi.org/10.48550/arXiv.2209.07162
29. Li X, Zhang Z, Zhao H, Lin H, Liu Y, Zhang J, Zhou J, Zhang Y (2023) BiomedGPT: a unified and generalist biomedical generative pre-trained transformer for vision, language, and multimodal tasks. https://doi.org/10.48550/arXiv.2305.17100
30. Van der Velden BHM, Kuijf HJ, Gilhuijs KGA, Viergever MA (2022) Explainable artificial intelligence (XAI) in deep learning-based medical image analysis. Med Image Anal 79:102470. https://doi.org/10.1016/j.media.2022.102470
31. Sanchez P, Voisey JP, Xia T, Watson HI, ONeil AQ, Tsaftaris SA (2022) Causal machine learning for healthcare and precision medicine. https://doi.org/10.48550/arXiv.2205.11402
32. Ronneberger O, Fischer P, Brox T (2015) U-Net: convolutional networks for biomedical image segmentation. In: Navab N, Hornegger J, Wells WM, Frangi AF (eds) Medical image computing and computer-assisted intervention – MICCAI 2015. Lecture notes in computer science, vol 9351. Springer, Cham, pp 234–241. https://doi.org/10.1007/978-3-319-24574-4_28
33. Wang Z, Zou Y, Liu PX (2021) Hybrid dilation and attention residual U-Net for medical image segmentation. Comput Biol Med 134:Article 104449. https://doi.org/10.1016/j.compbiomed.2021.104449
34. Chen J, Lu Y, Yu Q, Luo X, Adeli E, Wang Y et al (2021) TransUNet: transformers make strong encoders for medical image segmentation. Preprint, arXiv:2102.04306. https://doi.org/10.48550/arXiv.2102.04306
35. Wang Z, Zou N, Shen D, Ji S (2020) Non-local U-Nets for biomedical image segmentation. Proc AAAI Conf Artif Intell 34(04):6315–6322. https://doi.org/10.1609/aaai.v34i04.6100
36. Krishnan R, Rajpurkar P, Topol EJ (2022) Self-supervised learning in medicine and healthcare. Nature Biomed Eng 6(12):1346–1352. https://doi.org/10.1038/s41551-022-00914-1
37. Menze BH et al (2015) The multimodal brain tumor image segmentation benchmark (BRATS) IEEE Trans Med Imaging 34(10), 1993–2024. https://doi.org/10.1109/TMI.2014.2377694
38. Oktay O, Schlemper J, Folgoc LL et al (2018) Attention U-Net: learning where to look for the pancreas. In: Medical imaging with deep learning (MIDL). https://arxiv.org/abs/1804.03999
39. Lin J, Huang X, Zhou H, Wang Y, Zhang Q (2023) Stimulus-guided adaptive transformer network for retinal blood vessel segmentation in fundus images. Med Image Anal 89:102929. https://doi.org/10.1016/j.media.2023.102929
40. Milletari F, Navab N, Ahmadi S-A. (2016) V-Net: fully convolutional neural networks for volumetric medical image segmentation. In: Fourth international conference on 3D vision (3DV), pp 565–571. https://doi.org/10.1109/3DV.2016.79
41. Çiçek Ö, Abdulkadir A, Lienkamp SS et al (2016) 3D U-Net: learning dense volumetric segmentation from sparse annotation. In: Medical image computing and computer-assisted intervention (MICCAI), pp 424–432. https://doi.org/10.1007/978-3-319-46723-8_49
42. Zhou Z, Sodha V, Pang J et al (2021) Models genesis. Med Image Anal 67:101840. https://doi.org/10.1016/j.media.2020.101840

43. Kalusivalingam AK, Singh R, Bose M, Chopra R, Bose A (2024) Enhancing anomaly detection in histopathological images using convolutional neural networks and variational autoencoders. Eur Adv AI J 13(3). https://www.eaaij.com/index.php/eaaij/article/view/52
44. Showrov AA, Aziz MT, Nabil HR, Jim JR, Kabir MM, Mridha MF et al (2024) Generative adversarial networks (GANs) in medical imaging: advancements, applications and challenges. IEEE Access 12:35728–35753. https://doi.org/10.1109/ACCESS.2024.3370848
45. Tian Y, Pang G, Liu F, Chen Y, Shin SH, Verjans JW et al (2021) Constrained contrastive distribution learning for unsupervised anomaly detection and localisation in medical images. In: de Bruijne M et al. (eds) Medical image computing and computer-assisted intervention – MICCAI 2021. Lecture notes in computer science, vol 12904. Springer, Cham, pp 128–140. https://doi.org/10.48550/arXiv.2103.03423
46. Nazih W, Aseeri AO, Atallah OY, El-Sappagh S (2023) Vision transformer model for predicting the severity of diabetic retinopathy in fundus photography-based retina images. IEEE Access 11:117546–117561. https://doi.org/10.1109/ACCESS.2023.3326528
47. Shin H-C, Roth HR, Gao M et al (2016) Deep convolutional neural networks for computer-aided detection: CNN architectures, dataset characteristics and transfer learning. IEEE Trans Med Imaging 35(5):1285–1298. https://doi.org/10.1109/TMI.2016.2528162
48. Tajbakhsh N, Shin JY, Gurudu SR et al (2016) Convolutional neural networks for medical image analysis: Full training or fine tuning? IEEE Trans Med Imaging 35(5):1299–1312. https://doi.org/10.1109/TMI.2016.2535302
49. Raghu M, Unterthiner T, Kornblith S et al (2021) Do vision transformers see like convolutional neural networks? In: Advances in neural information processing systems (NeurIPS). https://doi.org/10.48550/arXiv.2108.08810
50. Xie Y, Zhang J, Shen C, Xia Y (2021) CoTr: efficiently bridging CNN and transformer for 3D medical image segmentation. In: de Bruijne M et al. (eds) Medical image computing and computer assisted intervention – MICCAI 2021. MICCAI 2021. Lecture notes in computer science, vol 12903. Springer, Berlin. https://doi.org/10.1007/978-3-030-87199-4_16
51. Li X, Yu L, Fu C-W, Fang M, Heng P-A (2020) Revisiting metric learning for few-shot image classification. Neurocomputing 406:49–58. https://doi.org/10.1016/j.neucom.2020.04.040
52. Perre AC, Alexandre LA, Freire LC (2019) Lesion classification in mammograms using convolutional neural networks and transfer learning. In: Computer methods in biomechanics and biomedical engineering: imaging & visualization. https://doi.org/10.1080/21681163.2018.1498392
53. Bhandary A, Prabhu GA, Rajinikanth V, Thanaraj KP, Satapathy SC, Robbins DE et al (2020) Deep-learning framework to detect lung abnormality–a study with chest X-Ray and lung CT scan images. Pattern Recogn Lett 129:271–278. https://doi.org/10.1016/j.patrec.2019.11.013
54. Davri A, Birbas E, Kanavos T, Ntritsos G, Giannakeas N, Tzallas AT, Batistatou A (2022) Deep learning on histopathological images for colorectal cancer diagnosis: a systematic review. Diagnostics 12(4):Article 837. https://doi.org/10.3390/diagnostics12040837
55. Ramani R, Ganesh SS, Rao SPV, Aggarwal N (2024) Integrated multi-modal 3D-CNN and RNN approach with transfer learning for early detection of Alzheimer's disease. Iranian J Sci Technol Trans Electr Eng 1–25. https://doi.org/10.1007/s40998-024-00769-z
56. Acharya UR, Oh SL, Hagiwara Y, Tan JH, Adeli H (2018) Deep convolutional neural network for the automated detection and diagnosis of seizure using EEG signals. Comput Biol Med 100:270–278. https://doi.org/10.1016/j.compbiomed.2017.09.017
57. Yin W, Mostafa S, Wu FX (2021) Diagnosis of autism spectrum disorder based on functional brain networks with deep learning. J Comput Biol 28(2):146–165. https://doi.org/10.1089/cmb.2020.0252
58. Paul JF, Rohnean A, Giroussens H, Pressat-Laffouilhere T, Wong T (2022) Evaluation of a deep learning model on coronary CT angiography for automatic stenosis detection. Diagn Interv Imaging 103(6):316–323. https://doi.org/10.1016/j.diii.2022.01.004
59. Gao Y, Zhou Z, Zhang B, Guo S, Bo K, Li S et al (2023) Deep learning-based prognostic model using non-enhanced cardiac cine MRI for outcome prediction in patients with heart failure. Eur Radiol 33(11):8203–8213. https://doi.org/10.1007/s00330-023-09785-9

60. Anjum N, Sathi KA, Hossain MA, Dewan MAA (2023) A temporal transformer-based fusion framework for morphological arrhythmia classification. Computers 12(3):Article 68. https://doi.org/10.3390/computers12030068
61. Johnson JM, Khoshgoftaar TM (2019) Survey on deep learning with class imbalance. J Big Data 6(1):Article 27. https://doi.org/10.1186/s40537-019-0192-5
62. Zech JR, Badgeley MA, Liu M, Costa AB, Titano JJ, Oermann EK (2018) Variable generalization performance of a deep learning model to detect pneumonia in chest radiographs: a cross-sectional study. In: PLOS Med 15(11):e1002683. https://doi.org/10.1371/journal.pmed.1002683
63. Haibe-Kains B, Adam GA, Hosny A, Khodakarami F, Waldron L, Wang B et al (2020) Transparency and reproducibility in artificial intelligence. Nature 586(7829):E14–E16. https://doi.org/10.1038/s41586-020-2766-y
64. Frid-Adar M, Klang E, Amitai M, Goldberger J, Greenspan H (2018) Synthetic data augmentation using GAN for improved liver lesion classification. In: 2018 IEEE 15th international symposium on biomedical imaging (ISBI). IEEE, pp 289–293. https://doi.org/10.1109/ISBI.2018.8363576
65. Chen W-Y, Liu Y-C, Kira Z, Wang Y-CF, Huang J-B. (2019) A closer look at few-shot classification. In: International conference on learning representations (ICLR). https://openreview.net/forum?id=HkxLXnAcFQ
66. Sheller MJ, Edwards B, Reina GA, Martin J, Pati S, Kotrotsou A et al (2020) Federated learning in medicine: facilitating multi-institutional collaborations without sharing patient data. Sci Rep 10(1):Article 12598. https://doi.org/10.1038/s41598-020-69250-1
67. Thummerer A, van der Bijl E, Galapon A, Verhoeff JJC, Langendijk JA, Both S, van den Berg CAT, Maspero M (2023) SynthRAD2023 grand challenge dataset: generating synthetic CT for radiotherapy. Med Phys 50(7):4664–4674. https://doi.org/10.1002/mp.16529
68. Selvaraju RR, Cogswell M, Das A, Vedantam R, Parikh D, Batra D (2017) Grad-CAM: visual explanations from deep networks via gradient-based localization. Proceedings of the IEEE international conference on computer vision (ICCV), pp 618–626. https://doi.org/10.1109/ICCV.2017.74
69. Rajpurkar P, Joshi A, Pareek A, Chen P, Kiani A, Irvin J et al (2020) CheXpedition: investigating generalization challenges for translation of chest x-ray algorithms to the clinical setting. J Med Imaging 7(4):045504. https://doi.org/10.48550/arXiv.2002.11379
70. European Commission (2021) Regulation (EU) 2021/2282 on medical devices: amendments to Annex II (Technical documentation) for AI-based products. Official J Eur Union L:456/1
71. Arrieta AB, Díaz-Rodríguez N, Del Ser J, Bennetot A, Tabik S, Barbado A et al (2020) Explainable artificial intelligence (XAI): concepts, taxonomies, opportunities and challenges toward responsible AI. Inf Fusion 58:82–115. https://doi.org/10.1016/j.inffus.2019.12.012
72. Amershi S, Weld D, Vorvoreanu M, Fourney A, Nushi B, Collisson P et al (2019) Guidelines for human-AI interaction. In: Proceedings of the 2019 CHI conference on human factors in computing systems, pp 1–13. https://doi.org/10.1145/3290605.3300233
73. Obermeyer Z, Powers B, Vogeli C, Mullainathan S (2019) Dissecting racial bias in an algorithm used to manage the health of populations. Science 366(6464):447–453. https://doi.org/10.1126/science.aax2342
74. Cheplygina V, de Bruijne M, Pluim JP W. (2019) Not-so-supervised: a survey of semi-supervised, multi-instance, and transfer learning in medical image analysis. Med Image Anal 54:280–296. https://doi.org/10.1016/j.media.2019.03.009
75. Ganin Y, Ustinova E, Ajakan H, Germain P, Larochelle H, Laviolette F et al (2016) Domain-adversarial training of neural networks. J Mach Learn Res 17(59):1–35. http://jmlr.org/papers/v17/15-239.html
76. Mei X, Wang R, Yang W, Qian B, Mulcahey MK, Samet H et al (2022) RadImageNet: an open radiologic deep learning research dataset for effective transfer learning. J Digital Imaging 35(4):851–861. https://doi.org/10.1148/ryai.210315
77. The Medical Imaging and Data Resource Center (MIDRC) (2021) Open-access repositories for medical imaging research data. https://www.midrc.org

78. Pierson E, Cutler DM, Leskovec J, Mullainathan S, Obermeyer Z (2021) An algorithmic approach to reducing unexplained pain disparities in underserved populations. Nature Med 27(1):136–140. https://doi.org/10.1038/s41591-020-01192-7
79. Grari V, Ruf B, Lamprier S, Detyniecki M (2019) Fair adversarial gradient tree boosting. Preprint, arXiv:1911.05369. https://doi.org/10.48550/arXiv.1911.05369
80. Bellamy RKE, Dey K, Hind M, Hoffman SC, Houde S, Kannan K et al (2018) AI Fairness 360: an extensible toolkit for detecting and mitigating algorithmic bias. IBM J Res Dev 63(4/5):4:1–4:15. https://doi.org/10.1147/JRD.2019.2942287

AI-Enhanced Tumour Detection and Segmentation

Muhammad Zunnurain Hussain, Muhammad Zulkifl Hasan, Khadeeja Anjum, and Arha Anwar

1 Introduction to AI in Medical Imaging

Nonetheless, early detection and diagnosis of disease has always been part of medical imaging. When identifying, segmenting and analysing tumours with Artificial Intelligence (AI), this is really the most powerful tool, and especially when it is used to bypass error and save time. It is from this perspective that the existence of various deep learning (DL) and machine learning (ML) models with the role, limit, benefits and ethical considerations of AI on its role in the tumour detection and segmentation were brought in this chapter.

1.1 Evolution of AI in Medical Imaging

Computer assisted detection (CAD) machines, born in 1990s to 2010s, were the early use of AI in medical imaging. Discovered abnormalities of medical image by using the rule based algorithms and hand crafted feature extraction methods.

M. Z. Hussain (✉)
Lahore Campus, Bahria University, Islamabad, Pakistan
e-mail: Zunnurain.bulc@bahria.edu.pk

M. Z. Hasan
Faculty of Information Technology, Department of Computer Science, University of Central Punjab, Lahore, Pakistan
e-mail: zulkifl.hasan@ucp.edu.pk

K. Anjum
Senior Demonstrator, CMH Medical & Dental College, Lahore, Pakistan

A. Anwar
Registrar at Rashid Latif Medical & Dental College, Lahore, Pakistan

N. Ben Aoun et al. (eds.), *AI for Medical Image Analysis*,
https://doi.org/10.1007/978-3-032-02963-8_6

Machine learning classifiers are also introduced to increase pattern recognition in Support Vector Machines, Decision Trees and Bayesian Networks. However, these are less efficient methods as they became lacking in adaptability and required tuning for each imaging modality, making them not so useful and one could expect a high false positive rate. This paved the way to further development with these challenges [1].

1.2 *Role of AI in Oncology and Tumour Detection*

As the use of the technology of the use of AI has grown in the field of oncology, this has completely changed the field of work by it; from high detection, accurate segmentation, classification, to better prognosis outcome forecast. Artificial Intelligence has already been applied to the oncology and tumor detection especially the Artificial intelligence techniques based on tumor segmentation, fusion of Artificial Intelligence in the various modalities, then Artificial intelligence based on prognosis and risk assessment [2]. Early tumor detection is the main uses of the AI in oncology. For instance, in detecting tumours, imagine, for example, at very early stages when the tumours are being detected with imaging modalities or scanning (such as MRI, CT or PET), AI can significantly aid in detecting abnormalities often overlooked by radiologists at the first glance. This in turn reduces the many errors in the medical diagnostics and makes diagnostic procedures more reliable. That's where AI comes in when it comes to microcalcifications of breast cancer or small nodule lung cancer, which are not detectable using regular imaging alone. These functions of the AI made it necessary for prevention, though these functions render the AI necessary for early and accurate detection timely intervention to improve patient's outcome [3].

AI also has a role in oncology in that it plays a role in tumor segmentation. They belong in the series of many models, such as U-Net and Mask R-CNN and Deep Lab, which are specially designed to do accurate segmentation of tumor. Furthermore, with the assistance of the easily doable AI driven segmentation models, radiologists have the means to characterize their tumor boundaries with the aptitude of distinguishing true tumor from normal tissue. In oncology, especially the correct segmentation, is important and it is due to the fact that an understanding of the tumor is needed, for example tumor shape, tumor size, for diagnosis or in order to prepare a treatment plan. Automatic estimation of volume of tumors also helps doctors to know how much the tumors grow and how much it will respond to treatment. By using AI driven segmentation, manual measurements are eliminated, and the human error is decreased and ultimately improve oncology workflow efficiency. The other field that has great promise for AI is that of multi modal image analysis where disparate forms of images are being explored (MRI, CT, PET scans etc.) to create a complete diagnostic picture. Traditionally, a single imaging modality is used for the diagnosis and typically offers a low view depth. For example, AI analyses several imaging sources to obtain a more detailed, more accurate measurement of the tumor while AI does not. The multi modal fusion of the malignant tumors and benign tumor together is a good point were combining morphologic and metabolic features. AI is helping oncologists to solve a harder clinical problem for which they are trying to more accurately identify the tumor characteristics and therefore diagnose and plan the treatment more accurately, by processing data that is collected using multiple imaging modalities [4].

AI has already changed detection and segmentation in oncology and is now more about prognosis and risk assessment. We are analysing large amount of each record (or 'instance') in historical medical data to predict the tumor aggressiveness, how fast their tumor is growing and their survival rate as a patient. By learning on huge patient record datasets, imaging scan sets and the confounding endpoints; clinical outcomes, these models learn to predict very accurately patient disease progression rates. In some sense, AI also is used at some point in the process to generate a personalized treatment plan, usually based on predictive analytics. Oncologists use AI to examine patient specific characteristics such as genetic markers, tumor characteristics and to foresee past response history to oncology and so select a most effective treatment approach each patient. It effectively increases treatment efficacy, is not traumatic, and improves the quality of patient care in general. By its incorporation, AI radically transforms the way oncology is conducted for detection, measurement and treatment. Currently, AI helps with the early detection, segmentation accuracy, small, but growing multi modal image analysis, and strong prognostic insights to improve while enables more precise and effective cancer management. Since the advancing of AI, AI will do much more work on the optimization of the treatment of cancer, diagnostic errors of the cancer patients and their survival rate [5].

1.3 Advantages of AI Over Traditional Diagnostic Methods

The limitations of such traditional methodology are such that an effective solution to well detect and discriminate the tumor has been recorded with the use of AI. Accuracy, speed, image quality, barrier to cost are serious disadvantages for traditional approaches. Several shortcomings are tackled with an AI driven approach that improves diagnostic precision and analysis speed, improves image processing, provides automated segmentation for the treatment planning and provides scalable and cost effective solutions. Apart from that, AI models are better accurate and sensitive than typical radiological assessments. However, some cases, studies show that ai systems can have a sensitivity and specificity higher that human radiologist, therefore, it is generally considered to be accurate. Advanced pattern recognition capabilities of AI can identify tumors; the size and appearance of which may be low, allowing identification that could otherwise be overlooked. Along these lines, AI also lessens inter-observer variability by making standardizing and increasing the reliability radiologists to make the same diagnosis. As opposed to subjectivity of human interpretation affected by fatigue, previous knowledge, or subjective judgement, AI is claimed to objectively and reproducibly make the measurements and hence minimize differences between the medical evaluations [6]. A good part of the use of AI for detecting tumor is the speed. Manual interpretation of medical images is used in current methods that have long time and extend a delay in the diagnosis and treatment. AI means image analysis and processing take seconds or minutes, not hours, with a huge amount of time cut from the process. Drivers of action: These accelerations seamlessly in lines with clinical workflows and drives real time oncologist insights after a simple click. Faster decision means IE faster diagnosis means we can intervene earlier and save lives as well. In the field image processing, AI is very crucial and such as when having a medical image, medical images would be improved in quality. More importantly, this noise, poor contrast, and image artifacts are likely to mask the important details in the tumor of interest. Enhancing image enables us to see the image with the look of the image itself clearer and the tumors are therefore more distinguishable; in doing so, these advanced image techniques denoising, contrast adjustment, and normalization are borrowed from the AI models. It therefore allows for a more accurate diagnosis when the original images are of poor quality. By high pass filtering image data, it enables compensation of the image technology vulnerabilities that can lead to diagnostic errors due to poor scan quality [7].

Another important breakthrough in the field of tumor segmentation, which uses AI, is in the sense of treatment planning. It is this accuracy of delineation of tumor boundaries using AI driven segmentation technique which is possible for radiotherapy and surgical planning. In radiotherapy, knowing precisely where a tumor is in the body and its exact shape, radiation can be precisely targeted directly to the tumor and avoided completely healthy tissues and organs behind it as well as next to it. The third generation of AI transforms tumors reconstructions from 3D, which further improve the strategies of treatment creating a more personal one for each patient based on the architecture of his tumor. At this or lower level of precision, we lessen complications and can have more effective interventions. The real value in AI lies in its ability to be cost efficient and scalable for tumor detection and treatment, even though it is important to know that the technical capabilities of AI are available. The AI automates the work processes surrounding diagnostic procedure, cutting down tons to deal with doctors and radiologists in oncologists, saving the time to deal with the more complicated cases. This means such an automated testing provides availability of high quality diagnostics even in a low resource setting and is of value in low resource setting where specific professionals are not that common [8]. Using remote diagnosis based on AI driven cloud platforms, the experts do a scan review and provide second opinions even they are not nearby. It is critical to fill the gap between equity of access to healthcare and application of cutting edge cancer detection and treatment to underserved populations using this technological advancement. Overall, AI improves the tumor detection and segmentation by increasing accuracy and sensitivity, speeding up the diagnosis, improving image processing, auto and precise segmentation, optimizing time in it, and cost effective and cheaper larger solutions. AI will generate more reliable, more efficient and more universal cancer diagnosis and treatment, leading to better patients' care and better rate of patients' survival.

1.4 Current State of AI-Driven Imaging Techniques

Medical imaging by AI has made significant progress, and today there are many models approved clinically for the cancer tumor detection, segmentation and cancer planning. The state of the art of AI driven tumor imaging is currently the combination of various types of deep learning for tumor segmentation, the AI integrated multi modal imaging, up to explainable AI (XAI) for tumor detection and real time AI integration into clinical practice.

The tumor segmentation became the core of deep learning as recently deep learning models outperformed U-Net and its variants in that task and generated the standard for precise segmentation of MRI, CT, and PET scans. These are encoder decoder architectures, which are suited to pixel wise tumor boundary detection, hence making these models very fit for identifying non regular growths in medical images. Unlike the other deep learning methods, Mask R-CNN is the most convenient for the instance segmentation in the brain and in lung tumor imaging. Traditional segmentation techniques don't always provide accurate results and fine details because tumors have irregular shapes and there are different contrasts in the images; however, Mask R-CNN extracts the image of each tumor instance from the image and creates an accurate as well as fine segmentation. The level of precision gained by radiologists improves their ability to evaluate not only tumor size, shape and spinal relationships to surrounding tissues for management planning, but also for subsequent follow ups [9].

The other major advance in AI driven tumor imaging is integration of multimodal imaging. At the same time, as an individual modality, each of MRI, CT and PET scans provides unique information about tumors that is not captured by their study alone. Using multiple modals fell data in combination, AI derives a superior and more accurate tumor assessment. A fusion allows you to go much deeper because it means that the models learned by fusion are more effective and could make deeper insights. Radiomics belongs to the strongest AI issues, and it is one of the strongest applications of AI, involving imaging data with tumor features such as texture, shape and pattern of image intensities. The predicted tumor behaviour using these features are used in diagnosis, prognosis, or selection with respect to treatment. In place of multiple modal abrasion, AI can be applied to the multi-modal fusion, allowing the clinicians to make a better decision, thereby reducing the uncertainty in the tumor classification and improve the patient outcome [10].

Thus, in the case of tumor detection, explainable AI (XAI) is of great interest, as AI models are black boxes, i.e. decision making processes are not explainable. But until AI is properly adopted in clinical practice, it must be able to give transparent reasons for its diagnoses. These XAI techniques such as SHAP (Shapley additive explanations) and Grad-CAM (Gradient weighted Class Activation Mapping) are developed to handle this problem. In the AI model's decision making process, SHAP assigns a importance value to each feature used by the AI model to help in the diagnosis of tumor. Unlike Grad-CAM which gives heatmaps that reflects where the AI model looked at while making a prediction, tableau vis' goals are to find what our AI model did not focus on when it made a prediction. What makes these techniques important to clinician trust in AI recommendations (and key to getting healthcare authorities to approve AI)[11]. However, when XAI is combined with artificial intelligence-based tumor imaging, these systems become more transparent, and radiologists and oncologists can check AI-based diagnoses and have confidence in using AI insights in clinical decision making.

Integration of AI into real-time clinical practice represents the next such milestone in modern tumor imaging. In recent progress to AI to real-time diagnostic systems, AI was assisted by radiologists in live screening Tumors, which was able to assist in analysis time-reducing and accuracies in diagnostic. They are applied in these radiology workflows and deliver automatic notification and instant feedback of suspicious regions in images. AI has also been used in robot-aided surgery to screen the surgery in the form of tumor resection procedures, where AI speaks the surgery [12]. Similarly, AI, expressed in the form of real-time imaging overlays and predictive models that help a surgeon to distinguish between cancerous and healthy tissues, is used in complex tumor removal surgeries to complement them. So, this real-time support gives you more accurate information that is used in surgery, which decreases the probability of missing the tumor and causing damage to the surrounding organs.

Similarly to the current era, AI-based tumor imaging has realized a transformational advancement in medical diagnostics and treatment planning. Deep learning has been proven highly accurate for performing tumor segmentation, as has comprehensive tumor assessment by multimodal imaging integration with the use of AI. Explainable AI guarantees that such AI-based diagnoses are interpretable and trustworthy, resulting in an approach to present an exact picture to clinicians to be compliant with regulations. Now, the process of integration with real time AI is helping to diagnose workflows and other complex surgical procedures. Together these advances enhance early detection of tumor, increase accuracy of treatment, and improve patient outcomes. On its way of evolution, AI will continue to contribute more value in oncology, making cancer detection and treatment therapeutically more effective, precise, and accessible all around the world [13].

1.5 Ethical and Regulatory Considerations in AI-Based Tumour Detection

AI offers great potential to medical imaging that can be practised ethically and regulated so that AI medical imaging adoption does not happen haphazardly nor unfettered. While all the above is rarely addressed, in the future, AI development will be based on these steps. In the field of AI based medical imaging one of the most urgent tasks is medical electronic information security and medical electronic information privacy [14]. The massive amounts of high-quality medical data that have been used to train training AI models have been causing concern on how to use

Table 1 Common datasets for brain tumor detection

Dataset name	Source/Link	Features	Usage in literature
BraTS (2014–2023)	BraTS challenge [15]	Multimodal MRI, annotated tumors	Widely used for CNN-based segmentation
Figshare dataset	Figshare MRI dataset[16]	3 tumor types, grayscale MRIs	Classification studies
TCGA-GBM/LGG	TCGA via GDC [17]	Genomic + MRI data	Segmentation & survival analysis
Kaggle MRI dataset	Kaggle (https://www.kaggle.com)	Labeled glioma and non-tumor scans	Federated learning research

the collection and storage of such patient information to train training AI models. Generally, most of the AI training methods are based on centralized data storage that is open to outsiders' access, via breaching etc and the public of patients' privacy. Federated learning allows for the training of AI models across different institutions without requiring the data from any of the institutions to leave the institutional boundaries. The model learns from such a decentralized data source, that is instead of transferring sensitive information, patient's records are not compromised. This helps with data protection laws such as HIPAA on the US side or GDPR on the EU side for innovation in AI as shown in Table 1.

Numerous publicly available datasets such as BraTS, TCGA-GBM/LGG, Figshare, and Kaggle MRI datasets have been employed in recent years to develop automated detection frameworks. These datasets typically include multimodal MRI sequences (T1, T1ce, T2, FLAIR) and come with expert annotations of tumor subregions, making them suitable for supervised deep learning approaches. Preprocessing pipelines generally involve normalization, resizing, and augmentation techniques like flipping and rotation to improve model generalization.

- BraTS is widely adopted in segmentation challenges from 2014-2023.
- Kaggle datasets offer pre-classified tumor images, used in federated learning experiments.
- TCGA provides genomic + imaging data, valuable for survival prediction.

Bias is another great ethical issue pertaining to AI models. An AI system learns from the data an AI system was trained on and will reflect that data in terms of the amount of bias in the data, which will be as fair as the data that an AI system looks at. Training the model on the data, that Favors one group and makes it biased for the other too, will also be biased as the model may be biased in a way in which the prediction is skewed against the racial, gender or economic groups. If the AI model the tumor detecting AI model uses is later trained on data from the patients of a certain ethnic group in which the model does not perform that well in predicting patients that are not from the ethnicity. It could mean that people receive less accurate medical care or that they have a difference in medical care.

To avoid the bias in the dataset there should be each of the datasets in two different sources. This helps make AI models trained higher in term of generalizability and fairness, as the population is being trained in wide and fair fashion. In addition, constructions of bias correction technologies like adversarial debiasing algorithms, and fairness aware learning frameworks are pursued as well to allow for equitable use of AI in healthcare. Secondly, AI in medical imaging faces regulatory approvals. However, if models are to be practically usable in the real world, born with the strict regulations like FDA in USA, CE in Europe and any other health authorities worldwide. Because of booming demand in trustworthy AI models, the amount of required dependable accuracy and the reliability, the safety, and transparency of the AI models has been high. Many of the AI models are a black box, thing which is not clear to how the clinician can put trust in how the AI model came to that decision—it is a major hurdle to regulatory approval. In fact, once explainability and model transparency are critical factors of regulatory processes, they become critical factors of regulatory processes.

Interpretability of AI predictions is done using techniques like SHAP (Shapley Additive explanations) and Grad-CAM (gradient weighted class activation mapping) which again builds the trust with the healthcare professional as well as the regulatory bodies. Unfortunately, there are also regulatory requirements for safe use and safe integration to the clinical workflow, that are not fulfilled. There is also the issue regarding the legal and liability issues through the adoption of AI in medical imaging. There is no easy way to hold AI to responsibility for misdiagnosis, or for issuing a wrong treatment recommendation. When at fault in an AI model that is unable to find a tumor like a human radiologist would be, is the AI developer or the health care institution or the individual practitioner using the AI tool? While current guidelines say that AI is not supposed to replace human judgment, it should rather be seen as an extra support in the hands of clinician expertise formed by AI. Of course, the medical community (and the legal folk) are forging ahead to determine who gets pinned for the baggage caused by AIs taking their inopportune holidays.

Future AI development is still being worked upon by the researchers as well as the policymakers. A lot of work is done to bias correct and explain AI models to make the models paint unfairly or transparent. As the AI systems are getting used, people are developing ethical AI frameworks with monitoring on the performance of the AI systems continuously and fine tuning their predictions so as to eliminate any bias in the AI systems as it operates and auditing the same regularly. Also, the legal norms of governance rule of AI have been becoming more formalizes in formulating the regulatory bodies. Moreover, they wish to demonstrate that AI is being deployed in a proper way, and for monitoring and continuous evaluation of the deployment. As AI advances, there will be arrival of ethical and regulatory standards for how AI can be responsibly used for medical imaging. These ethical and regulatory challenges need to be addressed in order to make AI in medical imaging safe and effective. However, apart from this it can serve in such areas of the healthcare space as it can be protecting data privacy, reducing the bias, complying to regulatory requirements, define the rights of patients and their obligations, going further even in ethics of the

AI development. The point being that: There should be best use of AI to prevent risk inflicted to the healthcare system, otherwise open to a just and efficient one.

2 Machine Learning Algorithms for Tumour Detection

Since it realized that the milling of the past few weeks in both machine learning (ML) and its use to discover the cancer, it fell into the hands of the doctors to do the same. Nevertheless, it is important to note that the usage of ml has come to a positive side for oncology, in terms of neural network. They are statistical learning models that take the imaging data and try to learn the most relevant features for discriminating between one type of tumor and another using it. The manual work was eliminated by ML, the speed up of early diagnosis has been made, and ML has become an integral part of the oncology of modern times [18].

The essence of basic concepts of ML in medical imaging resolution is the ability to learn complex patterns on large sets of data by means of mathematical models and algorithms. In this field, it feeds the medical scans such as MRI, CT, PET, and ultrasound to the ML to classify and segment a tumor. Since the datasets for the ML models training requires to be high quality, we need to start collecting and annotating. Shape, texture and intensity feature from tumor are analysed. Estimation of tumor patterns in new imaging data are made once features are extracted and the model is trained and trained on to find patterns indicative of tumors. These tumors are trained on these models to identify malignant and benign tumors and figure the values with metrics like accuracy, sensitivity and sensitivity to verify the correctness of the results. The proportion of tumor classes in the dataset is shown in below Fig. 1.

Tumor detection can be expressed in the supervised and unsupervised learning paradigms using machine learning. The other thing to note is that supervised learning is used as it trains the models on tumor datasets that are capable to differentiate benign and malign from tumor, for instance, to differentiate tumor type of glioblastoma and meningioma in MRI scans from brain. k nearest neighbours (k NN), Decision Trees, Random Forests, Support Vector Machines, Neural Networks are all supervised learning algorithms. However, as opposed to unsupervised learning, the supervised learning makes use of the labelled datasets that are very different from the ones used by the unsupervised learning that is identifying the tumor patterns in the data and training the model using the dataset that is labelled. This method may be applied to organize tumors based on their imaging features, and identify new types of cancers, for such application. In unsupervised learning, techniques based upon unsupervised learning are widely used for discovering the hidden tumor patterns such as Keans Clustering, Gaussian Mixture Models (GMM) and Autoencoders respectively [19].

Yet, deep learning is time and data consuming, and therefore, although they are a major player for tumor detection, classical ML models still play a role. While Decision Trees do not predict well out of sample one of their reasons for both popularity and interpreting them is that they can code tumors as linear combinations

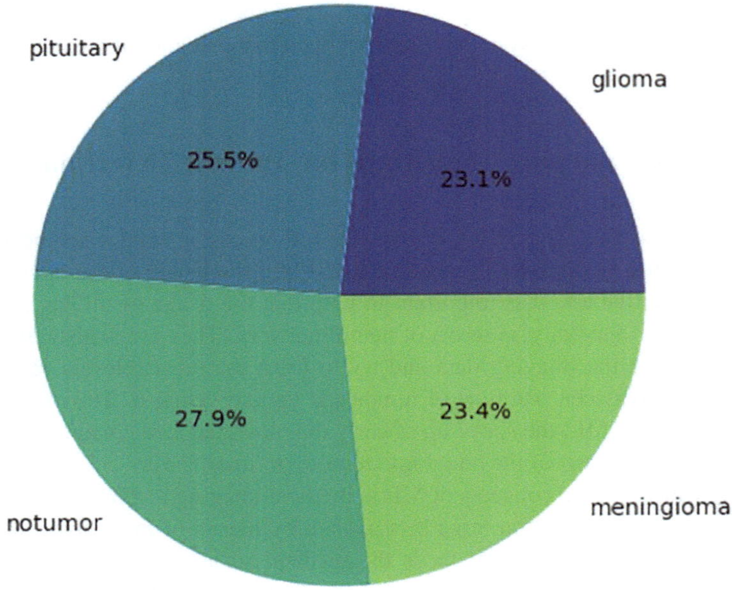

Fig. 1 Proportion of tumor classes in dataset (Kaggle.com, from https://www.kaggle.com/datasets/navoneel/brain-mri-images-for-brain-tumor-detection)

of yes/no splits and features. If the data such as discriminating whether the tumors of a breast cancer mammography is malignant or benign is high dimensional, then random forest, a concatenation of many decision trees, complemented and very powerful, is useful. If dataset size is small, then SVMs are employed to solve such a problem over the tumor where they seek the most efficient hyperplane in a huge dimensional feature space. The lack of being able to use nonlinear data makes it difficult for SVMs to work, but with the use of kernel tricks, they are able to do so in the cases of being able to recognize the lung cancer from CT and segmenting a human brain tumor. For cases of when the underlying distribution (for which the data belong) is unknown, the k nearest neighbour (k-NN) algorithm uses the next neighbour data in feature space for predicting the tumor. We demonstrate that k-NN is useful by histopathology slide in early stage tumor detection but comes with computational cost when there is large volume of data set. The Bayesian Networks help with probability of malignancy with probabilistic graphical models where data scarcity or high uncertainty is present. In addition, they are also employed to predict ontologically the malignancy of tumors from MRI and CT scan features and to see if a tumor is predisposed to progress. As feature engineering is necessary for tumor classification, it can find meaning characteristics in medical image, which increases the model accuracy. On the morphological features including the shape and size as well as border irregularity, they can differentiate the tumor. Pixel intensity, entropy and texture contrast are fed into as into into insights as regards the tumor's internal structure. High order statistics attributes from imaging data, that is, radiomics features, improve model fit [20]. And further improving classification accuracy, features from convolutional neural network (CNN) layers have also been used with the help of deep learning. PCA based feature selection improved the SVM accuracy by 12% in the breast cancer diagnosis. The need for performance evaluation metrics is clearly put forward in order to ensure reliability of the ML model in detecting tumor. In general, the accuracy is the whole correctness of the model and the precision, that is the so-called positive predictive value (PPV), subsequently represents how many of those detected tumors are malignant. Specificity and recall tell us what is the fraction of tumors we have correctly called and the fraction of non tumors we have correctly called. This is because the harmonic mean between precision and recall is convenient to use, when there are many more samples from one class, than from another. After this ROC curve is used to see at any stages of classification threshold the model performs, and the AUC between cases of Tumor and non tumor can be said. In fact, a model of an AUC of 0.97 (Random Forest).

Revolutionary machine learning in the automation of tumor detection and classification analysis in medical imaging has reduced the burden of workload, helped in quick diagnosis and early detection and further improved treatment planning. In classification task cases we are using Supervised learning models like SVM, Decision Trees, Random Forest, Neural Networks etc whereas Unsupervised learning models like k means cluster or Auto encoders are used to find new tumor patterns. Computational resource means that classical ML models are still very valuable. Machine Learning is modelling based, feature engineering is the key part of machine learning based on which model will be built in order to increase the accuracy and to evaluate the performance of the model in respective metrics. In oncology, ML will have even more in its role because it will use ML to enhance diagnostic precision for the patient as shown in Fig. 2 [21].

This study aims to describe the importance of sample MRIs of notumor, meningioma, pituitary, and glioma in AI assisted tumor detection and segmentation. Each MRI scan is labelled, we show the characteristic of tumor, notumor is the control, the rest is tumor with different shape, different size. Labelled images are needed for training AI models for the segmentation and for automated classification to improve the diagnostic accuracy and to detect tumors at an earlier stage. AI methods in this approach are able to determine exactly what tumor is there, and so it can ultimately improve the treatment plan, and the patient's outcome.

The image shows use of AI to detect and segmentation of tumor over a grid of pre-processed MRI scans of brain with different classes of tumor types. The grayscale conversion, contrast enhancement and normalization were applied to the input data so that it can be used as input to the machine learning models. It shows these tumor location and structures in the axial, coronal, and sagittal views. Most important thing in this setup is that it shows us how much the quality of medical image is important for any AI based diagnostics tool, which in this setup can achieve high accuracy for tumor identification as well as segmentation and will return an accurate clinical decision. This implies that the data is organized in a manner in which individual units of the information aren't on most outstanding distinction

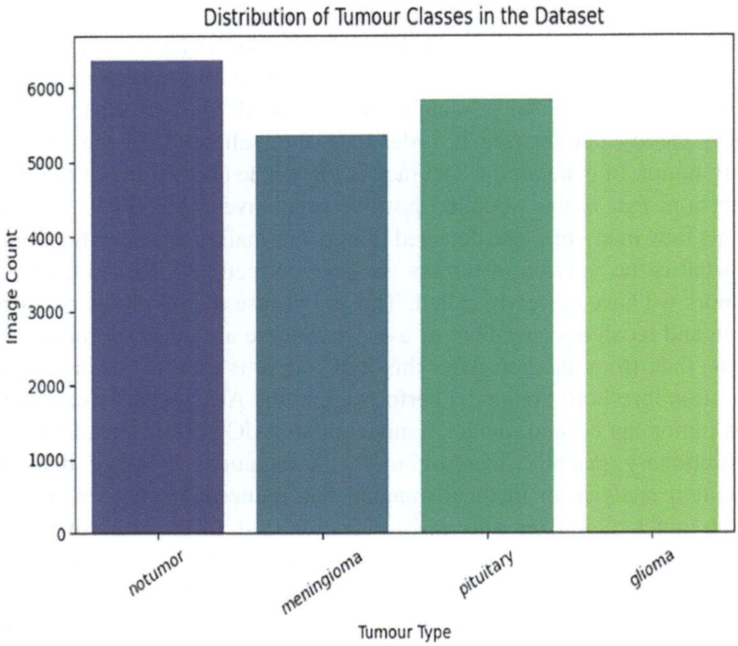

Fig. 2 Distribution of tumor classes in brain MRI dataset (Kaggle.com, from https://www.kaggle.com/datasets/navoneel/brain-mri-images-for-brain-tumor-detection)

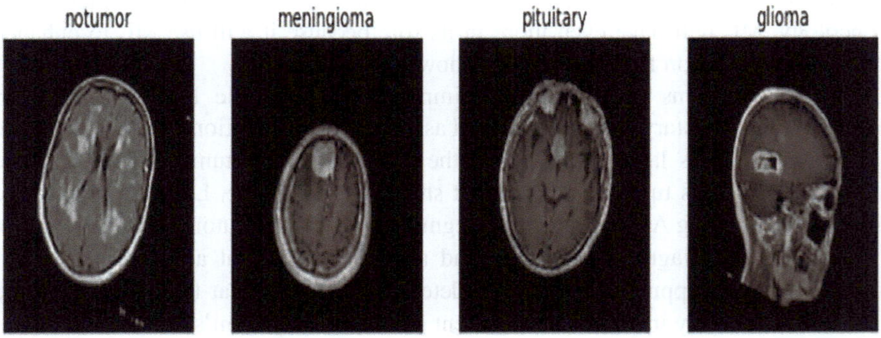

Fig. 3 Sample images from each tumor class of brain MRI dataset (Kaggle.com, from https://www.kaggle.com/datasets/navoneel/brain-mri-images-for-brain-tumor-detection)

contrasted with other portions of the information since these matters when preparing protected AI models in clinical picture investigation as shown in Fig. 3.

The tumour detection using machine learning as a tool has been a success, yet there are more challenges such as the development of an efficient and reliable method of tumour detection that need to be met for it to be brought into practice in clinic. The problem with the problems is that these are the most challenging aspect: data imbalance and of course not enough high quality and large datasets.

In the case that there are countably fewer malignant samples than benign, in tumor datasets for instance, the models bias and perform well in the majority class (benign) but not in the minority, important, class of malignant samples. To resolve this problem, researchers use a data augmentation techniques and synthetic data generation methods such as Generative Adversarial Networks (GANs) and Synthetic Minority Over-sampling Technique (SMOTE). It creates new synthetic samples to create system handles for the datasets and help classify tumour as a malignant case with high accuracy.

The other challenge stems from the variability of different types of image modalities, that is, each modality is treated differently in different modalities of image modalities, while each modality of image modalities has its own image characteristics that make it hard to train a universal ML model. This is because tumors can manifest in other ways, according to different imaging technique, and they must, at least, adopt to a shift in contrast, resolution and noise level. Transfer learning to fine tune these pre trained models on a gigantic medical image dataset with respect to the application is utilized broadly to take care of this issue. In addition, multi modal fusion models that incorporate information of multiple imaging modalities can be built to construct more holistic and universal ML systems with greater diagnostic potentials across imaging modalities as shown in Fig. 4.

However, the explanation of ML based tumor detection results—variations on explaining the system (explainability)– presents a major hindrance for the clinical adoption of the system. And all too often, a lot of ML models and nearly all deep learning algorithms will operate in their black box form, where clinicians can't investigate how decisions are made. Since medical professionals are supposed to prove their cases, they do not accept, and trust AI generated diagnosis if there no transparency. SHAP (Shapley Additive Explanations) and Grad CAM (Gradient weighted Class Activation Mapping) are used for explaining the decisions of this model and derived and implemented using Explainable AI (XAI) methods. Nevertheless, these methods help clinicians to see visual or statistical reasoning from AI predictions to help understand how a prediction is made and to increase the possibility of AI application in routine medical practice because they provide clinicians with explanations.

Besides the challenges in employing ML for tumor detection, there are other challenges that come with it, such as overfitting and generalization. Training these ML models late on small single centre datasets can cause it to learn patterns that do not relate to the data from other hospitals or different imaging devices. In worst case overfitting causes the model to have high accuracy on training set but poor accuracy on unseen cases, which makes the model not reliable for application in real world. Methods that you can use to solve this problem are using cross calibration methods to put dropout normalization in your neural networks or use ensemble learning methodologies at least aggregate several models to make your predictions stronger. It can moreover give readiness on more assorted multi focus datasets, which are all the more regularly recognized to lead to superior generalization, or uniformity, in practice over various patient populaces and clinical offices. Another major challenge of adopting ML based tumor detection systems is comprised of

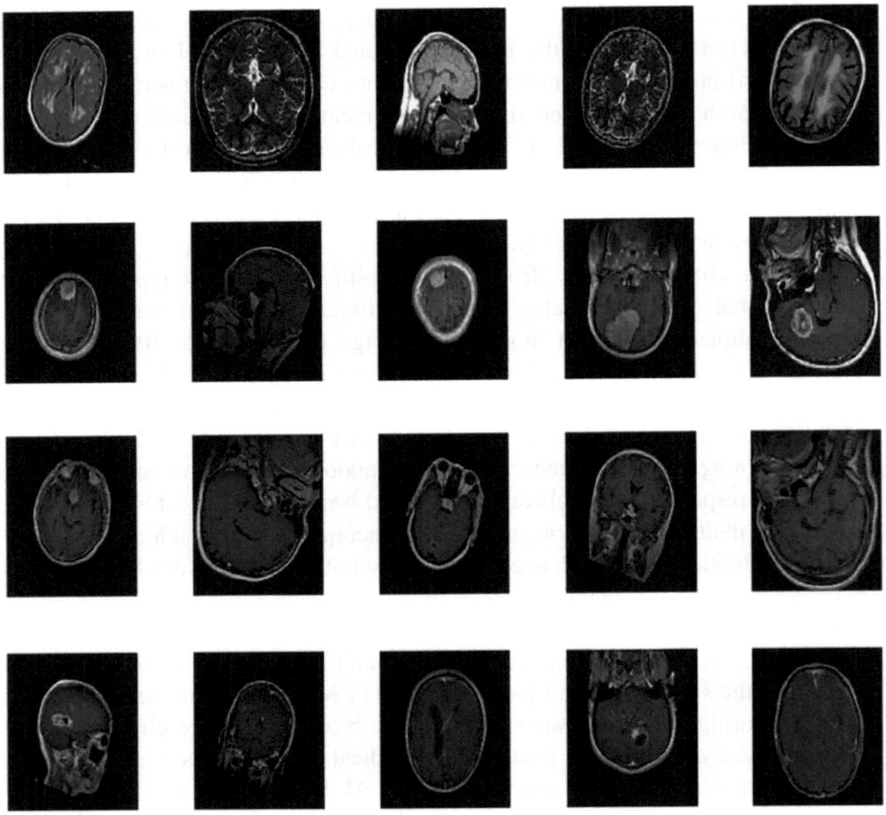

Fig. 4 Processed images from each class of brain MRI dataset (Kaggle.com, from https://www.kaggle.com/datasets/navoneel/brain-mri-images-for-brain-tumor-detection)

ethical and regulatory challenges. Before they can approve their models for use, they have to be subjected to an extremely strict regulatory framework for approvability through several entities—the food and drug administration of the US and the CE marking system of EU, to name a few. Those systems that are powered with AI issues of safety, accuracy, and ethical behaviour have been as good as validated if one after the other has to go through exhaustive trials in various centres continuously including trials with multiple AI regulatory bodies. This also brings other ethical concerns cantered on key issues including data privacy, consent, and AI fairness that are to be handled with utmost care to avoid any probability of harm and disparity on patients' healthcare outcomes. In order for these challenges to be addressed, it will need rigorous testing of their AI models, transparency in the performance of their AI models, and dialog between AI researchers, regulators, and healthcare professionals. Other important issues such as imbalanced data, variability in the imaging quality, interpretability of the model, overfitting, and regulatory requirements have to be tackled for ML to succeed in clinical implementation. In addition, more reliable, accurate, secure and regulatory compliance, cross validation methods, explainable AI techniques, and more ethical AI tumor detection systems can be built using additional advanced data augmentation, transfer learning, rigorous compliance, and advanced ML techniques [22]. By doing this, we are able to come up with useable ML models that are very far along the scale of clinically viable and actually used and accepted within the medical field.

3 Deep Learning Frameworks for Precise Segmentation

Deep learning has revolutionized the detection and segmentation of tumor with the aim of performing an automatic, highly accurate and efficient analysis of the medical images. Traditional machine learning approaches are based on handcrafting of feature extraction and are, therefore, very sensitive to domain changes and hard to apply to complex segmentation tasks but unlike these, deep learning models learn hierarchical features directly from the raw imaging data and therefore are very powerful for such complex tasks. However, intensifying effort has been used recently towards improving the accuracy and efficiency of tumor analysis, which may have been paved with convolutional neural networks (CNNs), more complex

Table 2 Comparison of machine learning methods

Algorithm	Key features	Strengths	Limitations
SVM [23]	Max-margin hyperplanes	Works well on small datasets	Sensitive to kernel & noise
KNN [24]	Lazy learning, distance-based	Simple & interpretable	Struggles with high dimensions
Random forest [25]	Ensemble of decision trees	High accuracy, handles overfitting	Black-box nature, slower inference
CNN [26]	Deep feature extraction	High performance on image data	Needs large data and compute
Decision tree [27]	Rule-based structure	Easy to interpret, fast training	Prone to overfitting
Logistic regression[28]	Linear classification	Simple, interpretable	Not suitable for complex decision boundaries
Naive Bayes [29]	Probabilistic model	Fast, good for text or categorical data	Strong independence assumption
Gradient boosting [30]	Sequential tree boosting	High accuracy on structured data	Can overfit, long training time
XGBoost [31]	Optimized boosting framework	Regularization + speed	Requires tuning, may not scale for huge images
MobileNet (DL) [32]	Lightweight CNN	Good accuracy with less compute	Lower accuracy than heavy CNNs

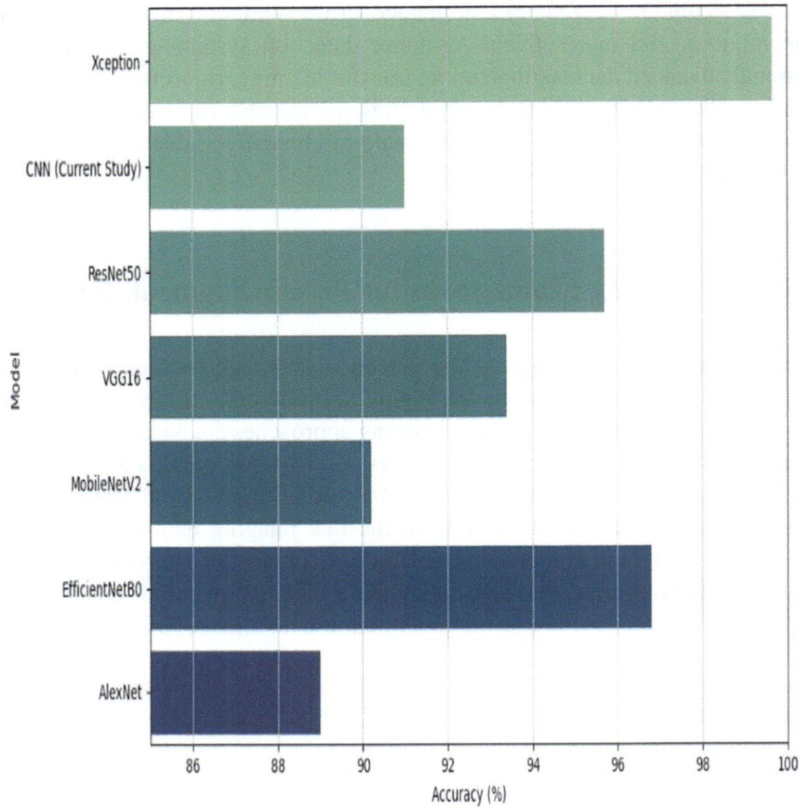

Fig. 5 Accuracy comparison of deep learning models using brain MRI dataset (Kaggle.com, from https://www.kaggle.com/datasets/navoneel/brain-mri-images-for-brain-tumor-detection)

neural architectures like U-net, Mask R-CNN and Vision Transformers, multi-modal fusion, better optimized training schemes, and sophisticated validation metrics to assess results as shown in Table 2.

Using deep learning technology, the technology of analysing medical images involves using multi-layered artificial neural networks. These models perform sub–mm accurate segmentation between malignant and healthy tissue on tumor segmentation problems. Deep learning has also one of the best advantages, which is that it can extract the features automatically while traditional machine learning models required the selection of features manually. In addition, deep learning models are sensitive and specific at their state of the art, making them ideal for tumor segmentation. In addition, such probes are common across various imaging modalities, including MRI, CT, PET, sonography, and are readily useful for flexible diagnostic purposes as shown in Fig. 5.

Furthermore, these models are extremely scalable and transferable given that they are capable of fine-tuning printed pre-trained architectures to different cancer

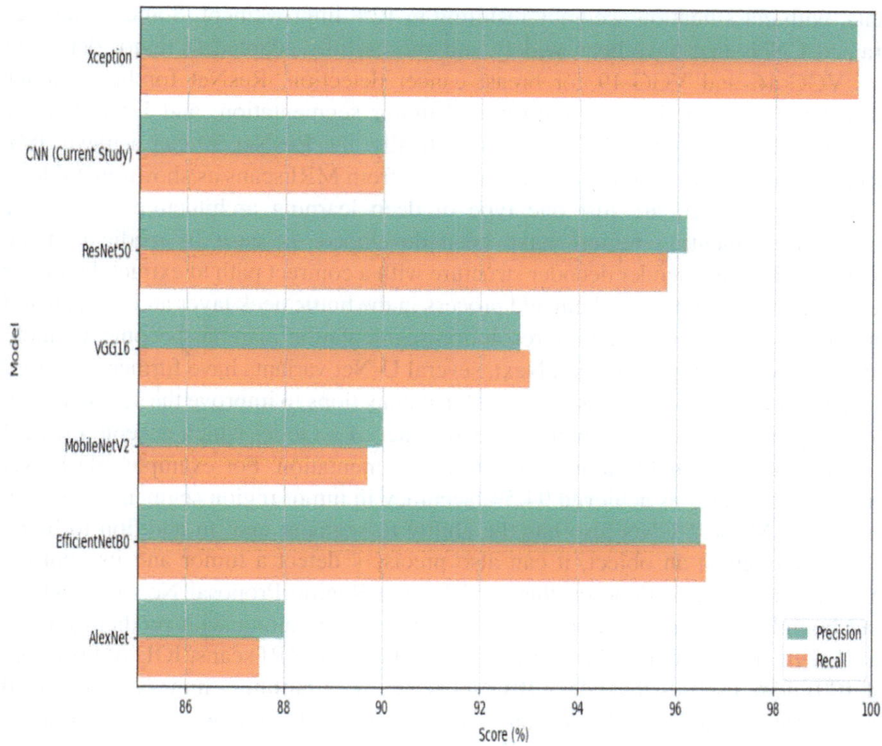

Fig. 6 Precision and recall comparison of deep learning models using brain MRI dataset (Kaggle.com, from https://www.kaggle.com/datasets/navoneel/brain-mri-images-for-brain-tumor-detection)

types. For example, with brain MRI, the accuracy of glioblastoma segmentation with the model trained with the CNN is over 96%. CNNs form the main constituent of medical image segmentation, and because CNNs are very good at feature extraction of tumor, they have strong ability of learning spatial hierarchy in medical scans. Images are fed into convolution layers that learn to extract features like edges, shapes, textures, etc. Fully connected layers classify the extracted features for tumor whereas pooling layers reduce dimensionality to improve computational efficiency as shown in Fig. 6.

Unfortunately, CNNs have widely been used for the task of lung cancer detection where it has achieved the performance of an excellent and at the same time a significantly reduced number of false positives in early stage lung cancer screening. Besides that, transfer learning improves CNN performance by reusing the pre-trained models in new medical imaging tasks. In the medical domain, for which the training data set is limited, it is advantageous with reduced training time, used fewer number of labelled images and better generalization. In the example, image data of ResNet-50 was trained to ImageNet and fine-tuned to perform MRI tumor data, with classification accuracy resulting in 12% improvement. Some of the pre-trained CNNs that have been widely and successfully adapted to tumor detection are VGG-16 and VGG-19 for breast cancer detection, ResNet for brain tumor classification, Inception for multi-modal tumor segmentation, and DenseNet for lung nodule detection in CT scans. Specifically, the ResNet 50 can achieve 98% accuracy for classification of glioma subtypes from MRI scans as shown in Table 3.

CNNs, however, are just one type of deep learning architecture; others for precisely segmenting tumors have been developed. In case of medical image segmentation, an encoder decoder structure with a contract path to extract the tumor related features, compress them and process in the bottle neck layer and a expansion path for reconstructing the high resolution segmentation map has become a widely adopted model called as U-Net. Next, several U-Net variants have further increased the performance. U-Net++ uses dense skip connections to improve the segmentation accuracy; and 3D U-Net, when extended to act as a model which accepts medical volume data such as brain and lung tumor segmentation. For example, 3D U-Net on lung CT scans has achieved 94.5% accuracy in tumor region segmentation from the scans. Mask R-CNN also has the ability to segment and, in addition to being able to recognize an object, it can also precisely detect a tumor and its contour. A region proposal is done on this model using Region Proposal Network (RPN), and bounding box regression used to refine detection along with predicting pixel level segmentation mask. At the time of breast cancer MRI scans, IOU of 96% (out of 100) demonstrates that Mask R-CNN accuracy in outlining tumors is perceived to be great. In 2021, 2020, Vision Transformers (ViTs) yielded a new paradigm within tumour detection, using self-attention over the entire image. Additionally, just as with ViT, ViBe does not use overlapping pooling or any unspooling layers, thus global receptive fields are available to it, which finally results in the ViBe's incredible decomposition performance even in the case of limited training data. Yet, it is shown that for that kind of limited dataset, ViT models work better than CNNs for brain tumor segmentation. More importantly, multi-modal AI models are linked with various imaging techniques, such as MRI, PET, CT, to understand the tumor better. The developed approach integrates morphological and metabolic tumor characteristics into the feature representation which allows to improve feature representation and to make detection more robust. Though sometimes, they occur as a result of limits of contrast or resolution on single modality imaging, multi modal AI nullifies that by cross comparing information from multiple scans. For instance, deep learning is used to enhance accuracy of brain tumor segmentation selection by 18%, for instance, by combining deep learning with MRI and PET scan. To ensure effective performance of deep learning models used for training and optimization of medical imaging, it is essential to have the models. For example, rotation, contrast adjustment and flipping are the data augmentation techniques, as a strategy to improve training that actually increases the training dataset size to improve the model generalization. The second main application for transfer learning is to fine tune pre-trained model on specific medical imaging dataset. There is no hyperparameter tuning and that is one of the most important reasons for hyperparameter tuning so that one can optimize how the model performs with

Table 3 Performance metrics of deep learning models

Study/Model	Accuracy	Precision	Recall	Dice score	IoU	Dataset used
Xception + Adam [33]	99.66%	99.66%	99.68%	~0.996	~0.994	Internet benchmarked dataset
CNN [34]	94% (train), 91% (*val*)	High	High	Not reported	Not reported	Not specified
ResNet50 [35]	95.7%	96.2%	95.8%	~0.95	~0.93	Figshare brain MRI dataset
VGG16 [32]	93.4%	92.8%	93.0%	~0.94	~0.91	Kaggle brain MRI dataset
MobileNetV2 [36]	90.2%	90.0%	89.7%	~0.89	~0.87	Custom dataset (Lightweight)
EfficientNetB0 [37]	96.8%	96.5%	96.6%	~0.97	~0.95	Public benchmark MRI dataset
AlexNet (Baseline DL) [38]	89.0%	88.0%	87.5%	~0.86	~0.85	Internet brain dataset

several factors like the learning rate, the batch size and the unrelated models or the dropout rates and so on. While the Adam optimizer is a form of an optimization technique that learns how to adjust the learning rates of the algorithm adaptively to make it converge faster, the gradient clipping helps to avoid the exploding gradients in deep networks. They also ran studies that showed that data augmentation techniques are found to be helpful for improving the accuracy of tumor segmentation considerably (10%) with robust training methods being necessary. Rigorous study of performance for the validation of deep learning models used for medical imaging is quite dependent on whether they are fit for clinical use in real world. The metrics used to evaluate the model are: The Dice Similarity Coefficient (DSC) is the standard overlap measure between predicted and actual tumor regions and, therefore, has been used as one common evaluation metric of segmentation quality. To quantify the accuracy of the predicted tumor boundaries, the most common used metric of Mask R-CNN evaluations is Intersection over Union (IoU). This is especially true when the F1 score only gives an overall balance between precision and recall, and for pure imbalanced datasets the malignant tumors do not represent, but precision and recall are not balanced. Sensitivity (recall) relates the rate at which the model correctly detects true tumors, as well as the early stage cancers are identified, while specificity is concerned with the extent to which the model reduces false positives under the consideration of over diagnosis. The IoU score in the clinical application of glioblastoma segmentation is also reported as high at 0.89 using a U-Neted model [12].

In terms of tumor detection and segmentation, feature extraction in an automatic fashion has been revolutionized by deep learning, which is highly accurate and can be done quickly, in multiple modalities. CNNs remain the core of deep learning based medical imaging with some interesting paths, and advanced architectures such as U-Net, Mask R-CNN, and Vision Transformers have helped push segmentations to the level of computational precision. Yet the multi-modal AI models can provide more detection than that by including more evidence from different types of imaging techniques. Data augmentation training strategies such as crop and flip and transfer learning in addition to relying on performance metrics for model validation make the models resilient while performance metrics are useful in validating the reliability of the models in the clinical settings. However, since deep learning will continue to advance, it will also bring more benefits to the oncology field, allowing early detection, precise delineation, and accurate treatment planning, and more.

4 Data Challenges and Solutions in Oncology Imaging

To obtain the success of tumor detection and segmentation there with AI, high quality medical imaging data is required. The issue: imaging data is far from consistent, dataset labels don't agree, there is noise and moreover the data is protected and so private. There are two ways to accomplish that: using a combination data sources, data preprocessing for various data sources, data annotation, a balanced dataset, generated synthetic data and a privacy preserving AI. In our case, we currently had three types of the main source of medical imaging datasets of tumors detection and segmentation: MRI, CT, PET, and ultrasound. Due to its high soft tissue contrast, MRI qualifies as one of the best methods for segmentation of brain tumour, detection of prostate cancer and detection of breast tumour. For the analysis of lung nodule and liver tumor analysis, CT scans are usually introduced based on the principle of X-ray based cross sectional imaging and can potentially achieve relatively high spatial resolution. On the other hand, as the information obtained out of PET scans depends highly on the metabolism in tissues, and the finding out malignant tumors, and, consequently, the stage of cancer. That is because an ultrasound imaging uses sound waves featured by real time images and the technology is valuable for breast cancer screening, and even for detecting thyroid nodule. For example, combining PET and MRI scans, an AI system fuses PET and MRI scans to achieve higher glioblastoma tumor segmentation accuracy of 22% than being able to see just one modality alone. Some of these imaging modalities are in existence, but the main problem of imaging data variability is that there are no ways or means to amalgamate or compare imaging data over imaging modalities. This work contributes to the variability by considering different scanner hardware, patient populations and image artifacts, which makes the challenge that needs to be overcome by the performance of the AI model. For instance, one can see those two scanners with different Tesla strength, for example, 1.5T vs. 3T, could carry different resolutions and contrast of an MRI scan. Furthermore, it is not possible to standardize as different hospitals use different acquisition protocol such as different contrast agents and image resolutions. In addition, tumor morphology is based on demographics such as age, gender or ethnicity, prohibiting models trained for one segment of a patient population to be applied to the other segments. Moreover, image quality can be degraded such as due to the presence of noise, image artifacts, motion artifacts connected to patient movement or metal artifacts from implants that could result in the misguidance of the AI models. The problem with addressing these challenges is that the different datasets need to be adapted to by the AI models, fine-tuned across the different institutions. Since these models are trained on multi centre datasets, scanning imaging data from different scanners is harmonized, and likewise training on such multi centre datasets and the trained models help generalizability. Consistency of the data is used to keep the performance of MRI tumor segmentation similar between different manufacturer scanners using a GAN based domain adaptation model. The data in imaging datasets need to be pre-processed, making it is an essential process prior to feeding the imaging data to AI models so that they can learn from the datasets. Image normalization or standardization techniques are used to reduce the scanning induced variability by rescaling pixel values to some pre-defined scale or zero mean and unit variance. The CNN segmentation accuracy improves by 18% in comparison to standard brain MRI scans. Second, the noise reduction and artifact removal are needed as the medical image is mostly affected by unwanted distortions. Image stabilization and other motion artifact reduction techniques can be used to reduce motion artifacts due to patient movement while artifact reduction software can be used to reduce metal artifacts acquired in CT and MRI images.

Gaussian Noise (which might be coupled with other medical imaging problem), can be removed from the input by using wavelet based filtering and anisotropic diffusion and tangibly, result in 11% improvement in tumor detection in lung CT scanners image. Besides, also artificially using image augmentation, extend the training data, which adds more examples of dataset diversity. Simulation of different scanning conditions such as rotation flipping, contrast adjustment and elastic deformations help to improve the model robustness. Applying data augmentation to deep learning algorithms on brain tumor MRI datasets was another first for us in this work and led to a 15% increase in segmentation for U-Nets [14]. The annotations needed are of good quality, and the ground truth labels are noted manually, which constitutes multiple challenges and is the reasons for the high quality tumor segmentation and classification. There is a highly strenuous task in medical imaging and is immensely time consuming that it may take an hour or so of a radiologist for the annotation of a single scan which in turn demands huge expertise from that radiologist. Additionally, since it is well known that annotation of tumor varies widely among radiologists, the training data will be inconsistent if each tumor gets annotated by different radiologists independently. Along with high cost of creating large well labelled datasets that are produced through expert annotations. One of the ways to try and overcome these challenges would be semi supervised learning, techniques that use the help of an AI models in annotation without drastically burdening manual work. Some of these AI assistances labelling tool has features of these crowdsourced annotation platforms, which aims to help with speeding up the annotation process. However, there is consensus labelling aggregation of expert inputs to label the same scan to mitigate biases in annotations and make them more reliable. With active learning for AI augmented annotation helps us achieve 60% time saving in human segmentation—AI to accelerate dataset prep. However, there is paucity of large, diverse medical datasets, such that synthetic data generation is an important technique to train AI models. Global provides the power to generate actual realistic MRI, CT, and PET scans and propagate the current dataset without even having to obtain more from the real world. Variational Autoencoders (VAEs) learn to pick out the subtle morphological differences in tumor using, which can then be generated into tumor samples. It also has the capacity to produce data generation simulation (e.g., generate more phantom tumor images for an augmented set of training data for the model training). The CNN models trained to segment MRI scans generated by GAN were 12% more accurate. With the way the approaches that are used in this work, Data Scarcity issues are overcome and the performance of the AI model used in the detection and classification of tumor is improved. Furthermore, there is another major challenge of Privacy in AI driven medical imaging as HIPAA in the U.S and GDPR in Europe do not allow us to share the data. Federated learning allows AI models to be created that learn from data residing in different hospitals, without the data needing to reside in one central point. The decentralized approach guarantees patient privacy and utilizes the benefit of multi institutional dataset that can help AI. However, federated learning suffers from very high communication overheads as the updates during model update consumption significant band width, and heterogeneity in data since each hospital may use different imaging protocol.

Table 4 MRI modalities used for tumor detection

MRI modality	Purpose	Tumor insight
T1-weighted [39]	Anatomical structure	Baseline shape
T1 with contrast (T1ce) [40]	Highlights blood-brain barrier breakdown	Enhancing tumor
T2-weighted [41]	Fluid-sensitive regions	Edema detection
FLAIR [42]	Suppresses CSF signals, highlights lesions	Peritumoral edema

Other ways to achieve it is homomorphic encryption of training of encrypted patient data, differential privacy where noise is added to sensitive data in a controlled manner while maintaining the model, and secure multi-party computation that allows collaborative model training between hospitals without disclosing raw data. Classifying tumor based upon MRI scans across 5 hospitals with less accurate results, they relied on the federated learning method without violating the privacy regulations as shown in Table 4.

To develop robust AI models to detect and segment tumors on high quality medical imaging sources, resolving data related challenges in terms of preprocessing, improving the annotation, dataset balancing, synthetic data generation as well as privacy preserving AI framework is necessary. Harmonization and domain adaptation techniques for model generalizability and noise reduction and artifact removal techniques for data quality enhance this. So, the learning process is coupled with AI annotations, which eases the manual labelling process thus making them easier to deal with. Since the data are imbalanced, SMOTE and ensemble learning are applied; in solving the problem and making good the design of the AI model in detecting or predicting the malignant tumor. Meanwhile, some methods to expand these training datasets are by utilizing data generation and federated learning and privacy preserving techniques so that machine learning can learn from samples from multi-centre while not compromising confidentiality of the patient. As AI continues to progress, such solutions must be part of it to build reliable and clinically deployable models of tumor detection [19].

5 Clinical Implementation and Future Perspectives

Early tumor detection, personalization of treatment and, eventually, AI knows what to do with your tumor: that's what will radically change oncology workflows. However, aspects such as explainability, the ethical issues, obtaining regulatory approval, and the deployment itself in a practical real time context have to be dealt with fully for such integrations into a clinical setting.The integration of AI in oncology assists radiologists, oncologists, and pathologists in tumor diagnosis, segmentation, and treatment planning. A commonplace use of image analysis in AI for MRI, CT or PET scans is to detect, differentiate between benign or

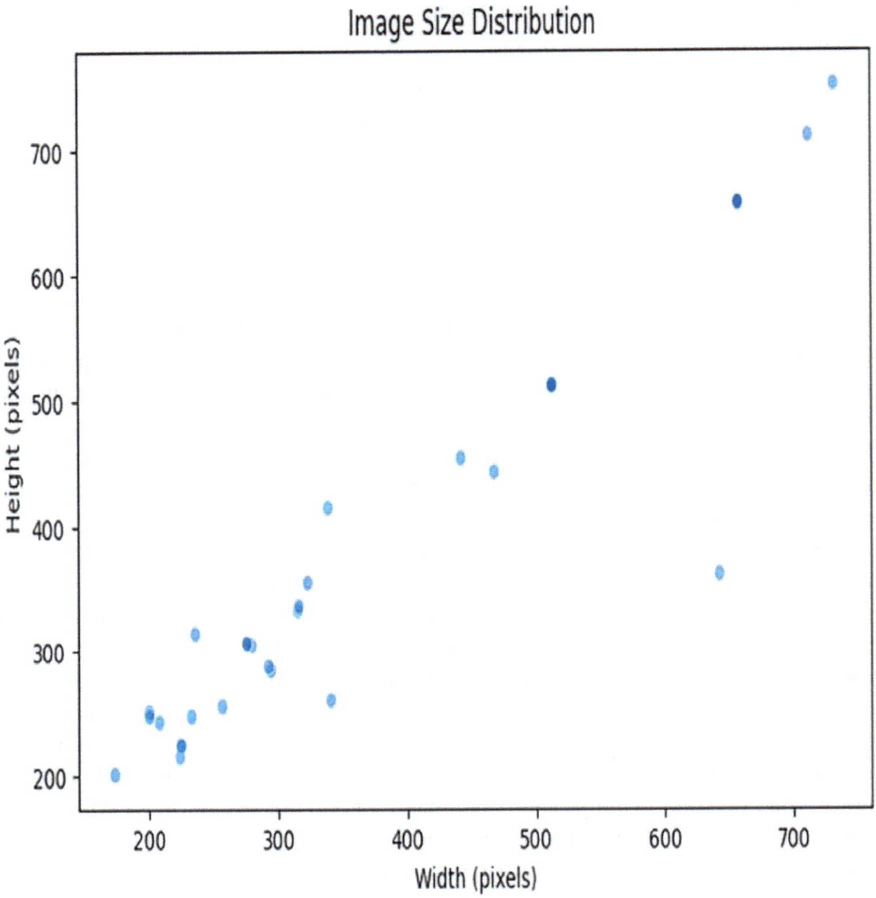

Fig. 7 Image size distribution of brain MRI dataset (Kaggle.com, from https://www.kaggle.com/datasets/navoneel/brain-mri-images-for-brain-tumor-detection)

malignant, or predict the chemotherapy response of tumors. In the context of AI powered clinical decision support systems we use the patient records to support personalized treatment planning by offering evidence based recommendations to them. Nevertheless, there are several reasons why AI cannot be used in clinical areas. There is no protocol in hospitals, and as PACS and EHR systems in hospitals are existing infrastructure for the hospitals energy and are not talking to the new developments, such as the AI, as no one wants the AI to take the place of the clinical expertise. For example, it assists radiologists with breast cancer screening, which substantially reduced the false positives for 37%, and sped up a radiologists' time to do it. With the use of AI, clinical decision support systems (CDSS) are of aid to oncologists with real-time insights about patient's data and imaging as shown in Fig. 7.

Cancer progression is estimated, radiology reports are auto generated, response of tumors to treatment options (chemotherapy and immunotherapy) is predicted and potential malignancies are flagged for further review. For example, IBM Watson for Oncology helps lessen diagnostic errors in oncology by evaluating patient records to suggest patient specific cancer treatment consistent with matching the patient's data with clinical guidelines. The problem of further strengthening the roles of black models in ensuring AI adoption by patients, clients, and medical staff, however, stems from the fact that they at the same time are a significant barrier and a substantial obstacle to the requirement of explainability, which is essential for establishing clinical trust. The techniques of explainable AI (XAI) are used to attempt to aid in the interpretability and capitalization of the same for tumor detection. However, Grad-CAM finds out the regions of the image which AI looks into when diagnosing tumor, SHAP helps explain the calculated risk to dig into why such AI decision-making is done and LIME offers local interpretability, particularly, to identify reasons in predicting a specific patient. These increase clinician trust, are transparent, obey regulations and facilitate model debugging. The AI system we know as Grad-CAM helped radiologists verify their lung nodule detections by cutting down the false positives by 29%. AI will also alter personalized treatment strategies that are biology driven and based on tumor characteristics for individual patients in personalized oncology. With that being said, the combination of the genomic data enables the AI to check the genetic mutations in tumors to determine which algorithm to use to make a decision on which targeted therapy options are available, to develop predictive oncology models to predict the likelihood of tumor progression and metastasis, as well as for the forecasting of drug response for the determination of the best possible chemotherapy regimen. Additionally, they are able to predict the targeted therapy with Tristeza based on a prediction of the HER2 gene expression thus achieving an 18% better rate of survival and fewer accompanying side effects. Similarly, cancer treatments have also started using AI to give personalized treatments in which the risk of chemotherapy side effects has been reduced by 35% [43].

AI in oncology, regulatory compliance and ethical checking, both are the prerequisites. Consequently, in this report, AI based medical imaging tools had to get approval for the patient safety and efficacy from FDA in the USA, CE certification in Europe, and MHRA in the UK. In addition, AI models must follow data privacy rules like HIPAA law in the U.S.A and EU GDPR law in Europe. The related ethical issues of the study were bias in the models to be trained on diverse dataset, protecting patient privacy and responsibility associated with AI misdiagnosis when it comes to jurisdiction. While such rigorous regulatory validation is a necessity for clinical use, on clinical trials with 95% sensitivity, FDA then approved an AI lung cancer detection system. AI is now using multi modal data such as genomic, imaging, and clinical in its effort to understand tumors diagnosis better. To augment precision medicine, AI models combine PET, CT and MRI scans to give a genetic biomarker and imaging features to give a more complete tumour analysis. The two models are more reliable than the two models in diagnosis, they are also more accurate than two models in tumour staging. By multi modal AI

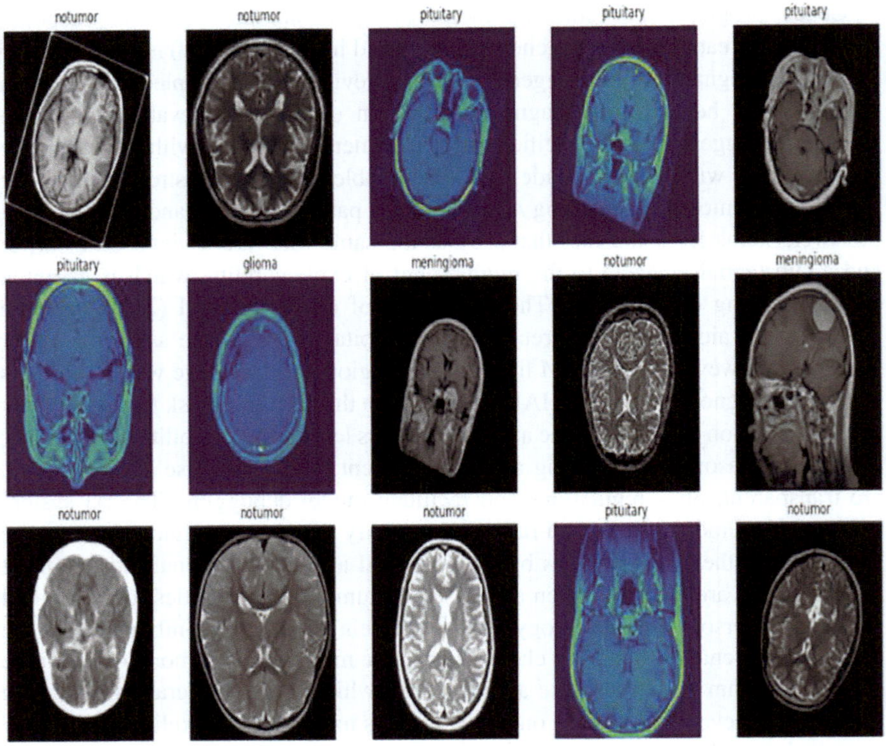

Fig. 8 Random sample images from tumor classes from brain MRI dataset (Kaggle.com, from https://www.kaggle.com/datasets/navoneel/brain-mri-images-for-brain-tumor-detection)

merging MRI and CT scans from many sources of data, it raises the accuracy of brain tumor diagnosis by 21% [44].

Real time AI applications: Being created in oncology to help oncologists to use it in consultation as well as in surgeries [45]. AI aided biopsy helps making real time optimal biopsy site selection, AI directed surgical navigation provides real time visualisation of the tumor inner boundary and point of care AI models mostly rule out the time aspects and enable quick diagnostic insightful almost seconds with the addition of the ultrasound images alone. Real time it is possible to detect 40% fewer lung nodule biopsy errors, so in the case of using AI you can assist clinical decision making during the procedure. Further research on AI based tumor segmentation is then conducted for use in fast application and with more advanced learning techniques. AI models are trained in self-supervised learning that helps the ML models learn the tumor features without labelling large amounts of data, in federated learning where training of AI models is distributed across several hospitals without compromising on patient's privacy and in real time AI adaptation that permits the AI models to auto update with latest imaging protocols as shown in Fig. 8.

With only 3 contexts, it's possible for AI to learn liver tumor segmentation, with an improvement over that of a baseline of 19%. AI guided immunotherapy is among potential future AI applications in cancer prognosis and treatment: AI models predicting the patient response to immunotherapy drugs from the genetic and clinical data. Tumor growth prediction models powered by AI, based on the models, can predict the tumor growth over time. Finally, the tool is also speeding up the process of drug discovery in particular, the discovery of anti-cancer compounds, faster than the conventional means. One such case involved a new lung cancer drug discovered using AI based drug discovery, which drug discovery was accomplished in 1/10th the time as would have with traditional methods, thus proving that AI can advance the development of new treatments. Dice Score and Intersection over Union (IoU) are not just mathematical constructs–they carry significant clinical relevance. A higher Dice score reflects better overlap between the predicted tumor region and the ground truth, crucial in surgical planning and radiation therapy. For instance, accurate delineation of tumor margins ensures complete resection, reducing recurrence risk. Similarly, IoU helps quantify segmentation performance, guiding dosage planning in radiotherapy. Consequently, AI segmentation not only improves diagnostic accuracy but also informs personalized treatment strategies, thereby improving survival rates and quality of life where:

- Random Forest + CNN feature extraction correlated tumor segmentation with survival prediction.
- U-Net-based segmentations are often used for guiding surgical interventions.

The artificial intelligence revolution is fundamentally reshaping the map of oncology by helping with early tumor detection, new personalized treatment prescriptions, assisting with the clinical decision and is already in the pipeline to be implemented in real time in the medical practice. Yet, to make such systems more widely adopted in a clinical setting, explainability, ethical considerations, regulatory compliance, and similar systems deployment would also need to be addressed. Over time, more of the uses of AI in oncology will be more embedded in workflows to help with more precise diagnoses, more effective treatment, and better outcomes in patients.

6 Conclusion

Artificial Intelligence (AI) in oncology image has revolutionized and improved greatly with the help of AI for tumour detection, segmentation and classification. Yet, the capability of making this real-time decision cannot be ignored as a strong, or especially, important factor, and ways in which current diagnostic approaches will still need subjectivity, diversity, timeliness, expertise, inaccuracy and automation must not be. All this happens in many ways in oncology as there are classifications, using machine, or segmentation like U-Net and Mask R CNN etc. Finally, AI integration with multi modal data and predictive analytics as well as explainable

AI (XAI) further improve diagnostic precision, in such a way that the AI models meet clinical requirements to produce the patient outcome. Still, there are several issues: inconsistency of data, bias in the AI models, privacy issues; and regulation ones, no less. It has been found that the medical imaging data in combination of several modalities (including MRI, CT, PET, Ultrasound and etc) is suffering from the interinstitutional discrepancy that restricts the capability of generalizing the AI model.

The two main problems with deep learning being currently adopted for the clinic are in the area of availability of large, well annotated datasets, and black box nature of deep learning models . To solve the problems of this thesis, I will use federated learning, synthetic data generation and domain adaptation, taking advantage of them to train more transparent and ethically safe AI systems. AI reality for oncology is a real time detection of tumour, AI drug discovery, AI personalized treatment recommendation. Following the AI driven innovation, the immunotherapy, skin cancer detection, biopsy guidance and self-supervised driving are a few examples. However, indeed, growingly there are such medical devices approved for AI use in a clinical workflow. In fact, we are already downstream of human surgeons, and the AI will no longer be downstream of surgeons, the oncologist will interact with the AI to make the decision of whether to respect the tumour at the millimetre scale.

The future of AI for oncology is precision and efficiency of cancer diagnosis. Similar comments are also applicable for cancer treatment planning scale and efficiency. Hence, one doctor does not have to stifle the technological advancement of AI or how it's used for medical imaging by any other party working on such technology, but rather cooperate with each other, collaborate with other parties such as AI researchers as well as clinicians, and complementary bodies working to create safe regulation in the field of medical imaging. Solving the problems will switch on the inter disciplinary research in AI oncology that will generate an amazing surge in survival rates of patients along with overall quality of the entire healthcare outcome.

References

1. Amin J, Sharif M, Haldorai A, Yasmin M, Nayak RS (2021) Brain tumor detection and classification using machine learning: a comprehensive survey. Complex Intell Syst 8(4):3161–3183. https://doi.org/10.1007/s40747-021-00563-y
2. Nazir M, Shakil S, Khurshid (2021) Role of deep learning in brain tumor detection and classification (2015 to 2020): a review. Comput Med Imaging Graph 91:101940. https://doi.org/10.1016/j.compmedimag.2021.101940
3. Image segmentation for MR brain tumor detection using machine learning: a review. https://ieeexplore.ieee.org/document/9804867
4. Saeedi S, Rezayi S, Keshavarz H, Kalhori SRN (2023) MRI-based brain tumor detection using convolutional deep learning methods and chosen machine learning techniques. BMC Med Inf Decision Making 23(1). https://doi.org/10.1186/s12911-023-02114-6
5. Abunasser BS, Al-Hiealy MRJ, Zaqout IS, Abu-Naser SS (2022) Breast cancer detection and classification using deep learning xception algorithm. Int J Adv Comput Sci Appl 13(7). https://doi.org/10.14569/ijacsa.2022.0130729

6. Talukder MA, Islam MM, Uddin MA, Akhter A, Hasan KF, Moni MA (2022) Machine learning-based lung and colon cancer detection using deep feature extraction and ensemble learning. Exp Syst Appl 205:117695. https://doi.org/10.1016/j.eswa.2022.117695
7. Amethiya Y, Pipariya P, Patel S, Shah M (2021) Comparative analysis of breast cancer detection using machine learning and biosensors. Intell Med 2(2):69–81. https://doi.org/10.1016/j.imed.2021.08.004
8. Sadad T et al (2021) Brain tumor detection and multi?classification using advanced deep learning techniques. Microscopy Res Tech 84(6):1296–1308. https://doi.org/10.1002/jemt.23688
9. Dipu NM et al (2021) Deep learning based brain tumor detection and classification | request PDF. ResearchGate. https://www.researchgate.net/publication/353695989_Deep_Learning_Based_Brain_Tumor_Detection_and_Classification
10. Dildar M et al (2021) Skin cancer detection: a review using deep learning techniques. Int J Environ Res Public Health 18(10):5479. https://doi.org/10.3390/ijerph18105479
11. Iqbal S et al (2021) Prostate cancer detection using deep learning and traditional techniques. IEEE Access 9:27085–27100. https://doi.org/10.1109/ACCESS.2021.3057654
12. Din NMU, Dar RA, Rasool M, Assad A (2022) Breast cancer detection using deep learning: datasets, methods, and challenges ahead. Comput Biol Med 149:106073. https://doi.org/10.1016/j.compbiomed.2022.106073
13. Mahmud MI, Mamun M, Abdelgawad A (2023) A deep analysis of brain tumor detection from MR images using deep learning networks. Algorithms 16(4):176. https://doi.org/10.3390/a16040176
14. Vankdothu R, Hameed MA, Fatima H (2022) A brain tumor identification and classification using deep learning based on CNN-LSTM method. Comput Electr Eng 101:107960. https://doi.org/10.1016/j.compeleceng.2022.107960
15. Multimodal Brain Tumor Segmentation Challenge 2020: Data | CBICA | Perelman School of Medicine at the University of Pennsylvania. https://www.med.upenn.edu/cbica/brats2020/data.html
16. Cheng J (2015) Brain tumor dataset [Data set]. https://figshare.com/articles/dataset/MRIdataset/1512427
17. Khan MSI et al (2022) Accurate brain tumor detection using deep convolutional neural network. Computat Structural Biotechnol J 20:4733–4745. https://doi.org/10.1016/j.csbj.2022.08.039
18. Nassif AB, Talib MA, Nasir Q, Afadar Y, Elgendy O (2022) Breast cancer detection using artificial intelligence techniques: a systematic literature review. Artif Intell Med 127:102276. https://doi.org/10.1016/j.artmed.2022.102276
19. Ramkumar G, Prabu RT, Singh NP, Maheswaran U (2021) WITHDRAWN: experimental analysis of brain tumor detection system using machine learning approach. Materials today proceedings. https://doi.org/10.1016/j.matpr.2021.01.246
20. Sanjay S, Anjali G (2020) Performance analysis of machine learning algorithms for cervical cancer detection. Int J Healthcare Inf Syst Inf 15:1–21. https://doi.org/10.4018/IJHISI.2020040101
21. Das A, Mohanty MN, Mallick PK, Tiwari P, Muhammad K, Zhu H (2021) Breast cancer detection using an ensemble deep learning method. Biomed Signal Process Control 70:103009. https://doi.org/10.1016/j.bspc.2021.103009
22. Kousis I, Perikos I, Hatzilygeroudis I, Virvou M (2022) Deep learning methods for accurate skin cancer recognition and mobile application. Electronics 11(9):1294. https://doi.org/10.3390/electronics11091294
23. Huang S, Cai N, Pacheco PP, Narrandes S, Wang Y, Xu W (2018) Applications of support vector machine (SVM) learning in cancer genomics. Cancer Genom Proteom 15(1):41–51
24. Ayyad SM, Saleh AI, Labib LM (2019) Gene expression cancer classification using modified K-Nearest Neighbors technique. Biosystems 176:41–51
25. Divya S, Vignesh R, Revathy R (2019) A distincitve model to classify tumor using random forest classifier. In: 2019 third international conference on inventive systems and control (ICISC). IEEE, pp 44–47

26. Bnouni N, Rekik I, Rhim MS, Amara NEB (2018) Dynamic multi-scale CNN forest learning for automatic cervical cancer segmentation. In: International workshop on machine learning in medical imaging. Springer International Publishing, Cham, pp 19–27
27. Sankar M, Baiju BV, Preethi D, Ananda Kumar S, Mathivanan SK, Shah MA (2024) Efficient brain tumor grade classification using ensemble deep learning models. BMC Med Imaging 24:297. https://doi.org/10.1186/s12880-024-01476-1
28. Gajula S, Rajesh V (2024) An MRI brain tumour detection using logistic regression-based machine learning model. Int J Syst Assurance Eng Manag 15(1):124–134
29. Zaw HT, Maneerat N, Win KY (2019) Brain tumor detection based on Naïve Bayes classification. In: 2019 5th international conference on engineering, applied sciences and technology (ICEAST). IEEE, pp 1–4
30. Selvapandian A, Manivannan K (2018) Performance analysis of meningioma brain tumor classifications based on gradient boosting classifier. Int J Imaging Syst Technol 28(4):295–301
31. Tseng CJ, Tang C (2023) An optimized XGBoost technique for accurate brain tumor detection using feature selection and image segmentation. Healthcare Anal 4:100217
32. Kia M, Sadeghi S, Safarpour H, Kamsari M, Jafarzadeh Ghoushchi S, Ranjbarzadeh R (2025) Innovative fusion of VGG16, MobileNet, EfficientNet, AlexNet, and ResNet50 for MRI-based brain tumor identification. Iran J Comput Sci 8(1):185–215
33. Verma G (2024) Xception-based deep learning model for precise brain tumour classification. In: 2024 8th international conference on I-SMAC (IoT in social, mobile, analytics and cloud) (I-SMAC). IEEE, pp 1481–1485
34. Chattopadhyay, 2022, MRI-based brain tumour image detection using CNN based deep learning method. Neuroscience Informatics, 2(4), p. 100060. Available at: https://doi.org/10.1016/j.neuri.2022.100060.
35. Kumar K, Jyoti K, Kumar K (2024) Machine learning for brain tumor classification: evaluating feature extraction and algorithm efficiency. Discov Artif Intell 4:112. https://doi.org/10.1007/s44163-024-00214-4
36. Xu L, Mohammadi M (2024) Brain tumor diagnosis from MRI based on Mobilenetv2 optimized by contracted fox optimization algorithm. Heliyon 10(1)
37. Mahesh TR, Gupta M, Anupama TA, Geman O (2024) An XAI-enhanced efficientNetB0 framework for precision brain tumor detection in MRI imaging. J Neurosci Methods 410:110227
38. Sarkar A, Maniruzzaman M, Alahe MA, Ahmad M (2023) An effective and novel approach for brain tumor classification using AlexNet CNN feature extractor and multiple eminent machine learning classifiers in MRIs. J Sensors 2023(1):1224619.
39. Gasmi K, Ben Aoun N, Alsalem K, Ltaifa IB, Alrashdi I, Ammar LB, Mrabet M, Shehab A (2024) Enhanced brain tumor diagnosis using combined deep learning models and weight selection technique. Front Neuroinf 18. https://doi.org/10.3389/fninf.2024.1444650
40. Dhandapani A, Gunasekaran M, Palanisamy B, Velusamy M, Krishnakumar G (2025) Revolutionizing intracranial tumour detection: a significant convolutional neural network approach to MRI analysis. In: Hybrid and advanced technologies. CRC Press, Boca Raton, pp 180–185
41. Miao H, Fukatsu H, Ishigaki T (2007) Prostate cancer detection with 3-T MRI: comparison of diffusion-weighted and T2-weighted imaging. Eur J Radiol 61(2):297–302
42. Soltaninejad M, Yang G, Lambrou T, Allinson N, Jones TL, Barrick TR, Howe FA, Ye X (2017). Automated brain tumour detection and segmentation using superpixel-based extremely randomized trees in FLAIR MRI. Int J Comput Assisted Radiol Surgery 12:183–203
43. Sahoo PK, Mishra S, Panigrahi R, Bhoi AK, Barsocchi P (2022) An improvised deep-learning-based mask R-CNN model for laryngeal cancer detection using CT images. Sensors 22(22):8834. https://doi.org/10.3390/s22228834
44. Qureshi SA et al (2022) Intelligent ultra-light deep learning model for multi-class brain tumor detection. Appl Sci 12(8):3715. https://doi.org/10.3390/app12083715
45. Majib MS, Rahman MM, Sazzad TMS, Khan NI, Dey SK (2021) VGG-SCNet: a VGG net-based deep learning framework for brain tumor detection on MRI images. IEEE Access 9:116942–116952. https://doi.org/10.1109/ACCESS.2021.3105874

Personalized Medicine Through AI-Driven Imaging

Rohit Doke, Jeevan Rajguru, and Kuldeep Vinchurkar

1 Introduction to Personalized Medicine in Imaging

Recently personalized medicines have gained much more attention as it made transformative shift in the healthcare from traditional one -size -fits -all approach to specific, more customized and individualized model of patient care. Personalized medicines can be defined as a medical model that offers customization of healthcare facilities including diagnosis, analysis and treatment options based on the unique genetic, biological, and lifestyle characteristics of each patient. The concept of personalized medicines though it started from the genetics, it has now covered the various areas including imaging, therapeutic and disease management [1].

Over the last few years, AI has emerged as one of the key enablers of personalized medicine, particularly in medical imaging. AI has been described as the imitation of human thought processes by machines such that computers can perform complex processes such as perception of visual stimuli, decision-making, and linguistic processing [2]. Through techniques such as machine learning (ML), deep learning (DL), and natural language processing (NLP), AI is able to process large volumes of data efficiently, identify subtle patterns, and generate correct therapeutic and diagnostic suggestions that might be beyond the human brain's capability to understand [3]. In healthcare imaging, artificial intelligence (AI) has transformed the methods employed by clinicians when interpreting medical images and developing tailored treatment strategies. AI technologies enhance every

R. Doke
Jaihind College of Pharmacy, Pune, Maharashtra, India

J. Rajguru
Delight Institute of Pharmacy, Pune, Maharashtra, India

K. Vinchurkar (✉)
Sandip Institute of Pharmaceutical Sciences (SIPS), Nashik, Maharashtra, India

N. Ben Aoun et al. (eds.), *AI for Medical Image Analysis*,
https://doi.org/10.1007/978-3-032-02963-8_7

stage of the medical imaging pipeline—from preprocessing and segmentation to disease detection, diagnosis, and treatment planning—offering unprecedented levels of accuracy and efficiency. These developments can analyze imaging data to the minutest detail, identifying intensity, texture, and shape-related features—factors that are at the heart of radiomics, a field dedicated to the quantitative extraction of data from images in order to facilitate decision-making processes [4].

The AI techniques such as ML when specifically integrated with imaging tools including radiomics and texture analysis, have shown immense results in identification of disease-specific biomarkers and therapeutic outcome prediction [5]. however, another AI technique named DL has provide much more excellent performance in image classification and feature extraction, conventional ML methods remain significant in certain applications. For instance, ML has been proven to be more accurate in predicting patient age from computed tomography scans using vertebral texture analysis compared to certain DL algorithms [6].

The use of AI in medical imaging is applied to more than a single organ system and imaging modality, such as MRI, CT, ultrasound, radiography, and even microscopic imaging. These applications are intended to enhance image quality, facilitate pathology detection and classification, deliver simulations of anatomical models, and predict disease development. The potential of AI in the improvement of therapeutic results and diagnostic accuracy is enormous, as observed from its diagnostic performance ranging from varied to 65% to almost 100% depending on the application [7, 8].

In summary, the most sophisticated among the personalized medicine technologies is the application of AI to medical imaging. Technology enables medical professionals to transition from generic diagnostic methods to more specialist and sophisticated ones. AI-supported imaging is a precision medicine milestone because it delivers personalized imaging analysis and treatment planning depending on patient profiles.

AI models have been found to be highly effective in the interpretation of medical images in a wide variety of fields, such as dermatology, electrocardiography, pathology, and ophthalmology. In radiology, AI has been found to be useful in detecting and classifying abnormalities in radiographs, CT scans, and MRI scans, resulting in enhanced diagnostic accuracy and improved treatment plans [8]. More than 200 radiology AI products have been FDA cleared, but challenges are still faced before their extensive clinical application. The use of AI in radiology is of great value but also poses challenges that need to be overcome by the medical and AI communities [9].

AI is extremely useful in radiology because it reads images from multiple modalities like radiography, CT, ultrasonography, and MRI. Such sophisticated algorithms enable functions such as quantification, workflow triage, and image enhancement. Quantification models enable anatomical structure segmentation and measurements of abnormalities, while workflow triage enables marking and reporting potential positive findings [8]. AI enables detection, localization, and classification of diseases such as pulmonary nodules and breast lesions too. Apart from human experience, AI is capable of aiding diagnostic interpretation. For example, AI algorithms can predict clinical outcome from CT imaging in traumatic brain injury and cancer. Imaging biomarkers based on AI offer important information on body composition and disease processes, enabling early screening of health conditions. Recent research emphasizes the potential of radiologic AI to measure coronary artery calcium scores through cardiac ultrasonography, thus demonstrating its clinic value [10]. The availability of commercially developed AI algorithms from over 20 countries indicates increased interest in radiologic AI worldwide. The majority of hospitals and point-of-care sites have initiated the implementation of AI solutions, and major health organizations have been at the forefront [11].

While promising, AI uptake in radiology is hindered by concerns such as radiologists' fears of knowledge gaps, trust in AI-driven diagnoses, and its impact on professional roles and autonomy. Tackling these fears demands committed local champions, training, education, and support. Most radiologists and trainees expect radical change in their job in the coming decade, and they see AI as a "co-pilot" that makes workflow more efficient and not as a substitute for human skill. While AI uptake in the U.S. radiology market is presently at a paltry 2%, increasing radiologist preparedness and the evolving capabilities of AI point to its broader integration into clinical practice in the near term. Global use of medical imaging AI by non-radiologist physicians is on the rise and is a promising opportunity to deliver greater access to imaging services and reduce diagnostic errors, especially in resource-poor environments and emergency departments [12]. AI-powered systems designed for chest radiograph interpretation and the detection of large-vessel occlusions in the central nervous system have demonstrated performance levels comparable to those of board-certified radiologists. Additionally, AI has streamlined medical imaging acquisition beyond conventional referral pathways through clinician-oriented mobile applications that provide real-time notifications of AI-generated results. This transformation makes technical image interpretation less complex so that clinicians who are not radiologists can use imaging equipment without only depending on radiology experts [13].

Moreover, AI has enabled the seamless integration of low-cost and portable imaging devices, including the Swoop mobile MRI scanner and handheld ultrasound probes, and hence expanding the availability of medical imaging across varied clinical environments. By overcoming technological bottlenecks, AI is driving the widespread application of medical imaging outside of hospitals, hence improving diagnostic efficacy across a broader spectrum of clinical settings.

2 Role of AI in Precision Diagnostics

The application of AI in precision diagnosis is transforming medical imaging by improving accuracy, minimizing diagnostic errors, and allowing patient-specific evaluation (Table 1). In personalized medicine, the diagnostic process is becoming more personalized not just to the clinical condition of the patient but also to his or her own characteristics, in an effort to choose the most suitable imaging modality,

Table 1 Key pillars of AI in precision diagnostics and medical imaging [8]

Pillar	Description	Applications/examples	Key benefits
Precision image analysis	AI detects complex patterns in images, ensuring consistent and accurate diagnoses	• AI detects rectal cancer margins • Outperforms radiologists in lung nodule detection • Improves cervical myelopathy diagnosis	• Reduces errors • Consistent, high-accuracy results
Operational efficiency	AI speeds up image processing, reducing turnaround times and optimizing workflows	• AI detects lung nodules • Enhances CT for lumbar disc herniation • Cuts unnecessary scans	• Reduces waiting times and costs • Boosts speed and efficiency
Predictive and personalized healthcare	AI predicts disease risks and tailors care to individual profiles	• AI predicts prostate cancer survival • Cardiovascular MRI for infarction risk • AI monitors diabetic nephropathy	• Enables early intervention • Personalizes diagnostics
Clinical decision support	AI aids clinicians in complex decision-making by integrating imaging and patient data	• AI in stress echocardiography • Integrated with EHRs for comprehensive health views • Guides surgery in real-time	• Enhances decision-making • Improves accuracy and confidence

maximize image quality, and reduce possible risks or side effects. These concepts fit well within the personalized medicine approach [14].

Radiological societies have developed modality-specific imaging protocols to cover a broad range of clinical situations. These protocols differ in a number of technical parameters such as contrast dosage, rate of injection, method of image reconstruction, and slice thickness— ach optimized based on the patient's status and type [15]. For instance, low-dose CT for kidney stone detection, CT angiography for arterial stenosis, and MRI protocols for spinal cord disorders are examples of targeted approaches. Furthermore, patient-based adjustments, such as weight-based contrast dosing, bolus tracking for optimized scan delays, and radiation-avoidance strategies for sensitive populations (e.g., children, pregnant women), exemplify how diagnostics are increasingly personalized. In this framework, AI really boosts precision diagnosis by operating under four broad pillars: image diagnostics, operational excellence, predictive/individualized care, and decision support.

2.1 *Precision Image Analysis and Interpretation*

AI has an unparalleled ability to detect very fine, complex patterns within medical images that would not be noticeable by the naked eye. Such a center is especially valuable in the case of highly complex illnesses such as cancer and neuro illnesses. Moreover, AI eliminates human error as it attains incessant diagnostic accuracy regardless of exhaustion or personal discretion—succumbing to reliable and consistent opinions [16].

For example, AI-powered systems such as Faster R-CNN achieved very high accuracy in detecting positive circumferential resection margins in rectal cancer with high-resolution MRI. In the same way, in pulmonary imaging, AI was found to perform better than experienced radiologists in spotting lung nodules in chest CT scans. The ability of AI to reduce human mistake and provide consistent picture interpretation independent of clinical heterogeneity or weariness is noteworthy [8]. Studies have shown that AI improves the diagnosis of cervical spondylotic myelopathy using cervical radiographs and the distinction of breast lesions using contrast-enhanced MRI to produce extremely accurate and repeatable results. By lowering interpretation mistakes, AI-enabled quantitative CT angiography enhances the assessment of atherosclerosis in coronary artery diagnosis. The importance of AI in enhancing diagnostic precision and supporting well-informed clinical decision-making is highlighted by all of these characteristics [17].

2.2 *Operational Efficiency*

With the integration of AI in medical imaging, AI greatly accelerates image processing and interpretation, which is crucial during emergency or time-sensitive situations. Efficiency is also achieved through workflow optimization, reduction of waiting times, and allowing medical practitioners to give quicker clinical judgments. Apart from that, AI helps to reduce costs by reducing unnecessary scans and decreasing rates of misdiagnosis, hence reducing overall healthcare costs.

With precision, AI also significantly boosts procedural effectiveness in diagnostic procedures. Its capacity for rapid processing of large amounts of medical imaging information results in lower diagnostic turnaround times and increased cost savings. Not only have AI algorithms equaled sensitivity rates with experienced radiologists, but also, they have picked up ancillary findings—such as lung nodules—that might otherwise have remained undetected, thus accelerating diagnostic procedures for pulmonary-related ailments [18].

Additionally, spinal diagnostic research shows that computed tomography analysis with AI greatly enhances the assessment of lumbar disc herniation. By reducing diagnostic mistakes and the frequency of unnecessary interventions, these technologies help reduce overall healthcare costs. This cumulative evidence supports that AI not only saves time but also promotes resource-effective diagnostic processes within modern healthcare systems.

2.3 Predictive and Personalized Healthcare

Using historical data and real-time information, AI can predict the chances of disease occurrence and development, hence enabling early intervention and prevention measures. The predictive analytics drive proactive health condition management. With AI-powered imaging, too, it is possible to tailor this to a patient's individualized profile—thus making more accurate diagnostic evaluations possible and helping the cause of personal medicine. For example, DL models have been employed to predict survival in prostate cancer by examining bone scintigraphy and enabling clinicians to identify high-risk patients. In cardiology, AI-powered cardiovascular MRI enables myocardial strain imaging to risk stratify after infarction. Likewise, light-weight AI models have enhanced patient monitoring in diabetic nephropathy by examining MRI images [19].

AI has also demonstrated diagnostic superiority in coronary artery disease and skin cancer detection over traditional methods, such as smartphone-based AI systems that were on par with specialist-level accuracy. In oncology, AI has facilitated the distinction between malignant and benign breast tumors using multiparametric MRI, and enhanced patient selection for soft tissue sarcoma treatment using radiomics and deep learning. Moreover, AI has enabled quantification of macular degeneration disease progression and breast mass differentiation, improving longitudinal disease tracking. CNN-based diagnostic systems evaluating rectal cancer resection margins are an example of the promise of personalized diagnostics, allowing surgical procedure planning based on patient-specific tumor and anatomical characteristics. Such observations underscore AI's transformative role in revolutionizing diagnostics towards individualized care.

2.4 *Clinical Decision Support and Integration*

Clinical Decision assistance Systems (CDSS) with AI assistance improve healthcare delivery by assisting physicians in making challenging choices. AI has enabled automated image processing in complex procedures like stress echocardiography, improving diagnostic precision and physician confidence.

AI supports clinicians during challenging diagnostic and surgical procedures with comprehensive, real-time imaging guidance, improving accuracy and confidence in decision-making. Integrated with electronic health records (EHRs) and other technologies, AI provides a more comprehensive picture of the patient's health, and clinicians make better-informed decisions. Quantitative research identifies AI's greatest contributions in predictive analysis, assistance in complex processes, speed and efficiency, enhanced image interpretation, and error reduction. Although its contributions to cost reduction, compatibility with digital technology, and customized diagnostics have been debated less often, ongoing innovation should expand AI's contribution in every aspect of precision diagnostics [20].

3 AI-Driven Radiomics and Imaging

Radiomics, a new field in the realm of medical imaging, represents an important intersection of radiology and AI. Radiomics has its origins in the vast body of work over several decades of computer-aided diagnosis, prognosis, and treatment planning through quantitative imaging analysis of large image feature datasets acquired from standard medical modalities, such as CT, MRI, and PET scans. The central tenet of radiomics is that biomedical images harbor much non-humanly interpretable information. Leverage by the power of advanced ML algorithms and high-throughput computational architectures, AI systems can derive hundreds to thousands of quantitative imaging biomarkers—such as intensity, shape, texture, and wavelet features—that provide a window into disease phenotypes and the tumor microenvironment in a non-invasive manner. These features are often employed as complementary features to standard clinical, histopathological, and genomic data, thus enhancing the predictive performance of clinical decision-support systems (CDSS).

The radiomics pipeline is generally divided into five broad stages: data selection, image acquisition, feature extraction, exploratory analysis, and modeling. The first step is to define an optimal imaging protocol and to define the volume of interest (VOI), usually the main tumor or region of abnormality. Delineation of this region is done using manual, semi-automatic, or automatic techniques, and segmentation is critical as it affects the reliability of the extracted features. Variability of segmentation, particularly between various clinicians or imaging protocols, has the potential to introduce large bias. To fight such biases, processes such as carrying out several segmentation tests, introducing noise perturbation, and using several segmentation algorithms are used. Phantom studies are also carried out in order to establish inter-scanner and inter-vendor variability and therefore ensuring uniformity in multiple imaging modalities and institutions [21].

Radiomics is particularly useful for imaging-based disease characterization and prediction modeling. After segmentation, features are extracted using specialized algorithms that quantify aspects of image patterns not detectable by human vision. However, feature extraction is highly sensitive to image pre-processing methods such as filtering, intensity discretization, and reconstruction techniques. Hence, standardization of imaging protocols and feature nomenclature is required to enable interoperability and consistency across studies. After feature extraction, exploratory analysis is performed where radiomic and non-radiomic features are combined and contrasted with regard to clinical endpoints like overall survival or disease recurrence. Dimension reduction is obtained through clustering techniques by determining redundant or unstable features, keeping only features with high predictability and robustness across various imaging conditions.

The modeling process involves the phases of feature selection, ML algorithm selection, and thorough validation. Feature selection is an integral part, since the inclusion of too many features may result in overfitting and decreased generalizability. Dimensionality reduction methods such as principal component analysis or hierarchical clustering are employed to preserve only the most representative features. The selection of the modeling method often relates to the expertise of the research team and can vary from logistic regression to DL models. Individual algorithms have their limitations; for example, logistic regression takes the independence of features for granted, and Bayesian networks necessitate feature discretization [22]. Therefore, comparison and use of several modeling approaches could provide more reproducible and stable results. Of particular interest, model validation is a significant part of the radiomics pipeline. Internal validation methods (e.g., cross-validation) in combination with external validation based on independent data play a critical role to ensure generalizability of the model and its applicability to the clinic. Model performance is typically evaluated using discrimination metrics such as the area under the receiver operating characteristic (ROC) curve (AUC), which reflects the model's sensitivity and specificity.

The application of AI-driven radiomics has unmatched potential to enable precision medicine by improving personalized diagnosis, risk assessment, and treatment planning. Radiomic information-based decision-support systems are increasingly recognized as valuable assets in modern medical practice, especially in oncology. However, there are still a number of challenges that must be overcome, such as the need for standardized imaging protocols, uniform reporting standards, and efficient data-sharing systems. The integration of radiomics with other data types—genomics, pathology, and EHRs into a federated database system can facilitate the development of rapid learning healthcare (RLHC) systems. Such systems can have the potential to learn continuously and improve their functionality using large, multimodal datasets across institutions and geographic locations. However, processing such large volumes of data present logistical and computational challenges that must be overcome using advanced data infrastructure and privacy-preserving technologies.

In summary, although radiomics is not a standalone solution to clinical decision-making, its capacity to non-invasively acquire complex imaging biomarkers renders it a useful complement to current diagnostic and prognostic methods. The field is undergoing radical transformation with the help of improvements in ML and AI and the ability to transform radiology from being largely a descriptive science to one that is quantitatively robust, data-based science. Further improvements will be dependent on collaborative multidisciplinary effort among radiology, oncology, computer science, and bioinformatics to break current barriers, cross-validate models in multiple clinical settings, and make possible their broad incorporation into standard clinical practice.

4 Integration with Genomics and Multi-Omics Data

The intersection of AI and genomics as well as multi-omics data is transforming the landscape of precision medicine and biomedical research (Table 2). Multi-omics can be described as the combined analysis of two or more types of biological data such as genomics, transcriptomics, proteomics, metabolomics, and epigenomics. Each of these dimensions gives individual perspectives of molecular mechanisms; yet, when examined collectively, they provide systems and holistic insight into health, disease progression, and therapeutic responses. The combination of AI-enhanced imaging data with multi-omics analysis is full of potential to reveal hidden patterns of biology and facilitate highly individualized treatment plans [23].

The multi-omics approach has come to be the main methodology of modern biomedical science due primarily to the increasing access to high-throughput sequencing and molecular profiling technology. In genomics, genomics sequencing technology makes it possible to identify disease-associated genetic mutations. Proteomics and metabolomics, by contrast, enable one to decipher patterns of protein expression and metabolic profiles, respectively, that signal functional and phenotypic changes within the organism. In addition, epigenomics illuminates inheritable gene expression changes that are not dependent on DNA sequence changes, thus providing additional context for disease regulation [24].

By combining these types of data, clinicians and researchers can achieve high-dimensional perspectives of disease processes. This global consideration is particularly enlightening in precision medicine—particularly oncology and cardio-vascular disease—where patients will be stratified by molecular means to inform targeted, individualized therapies. In the treatment of cancer, for instance, multi-omics enables stratification of tumors by molecular patterns, not by tissue of origin, opening the way to more targeted therapy. Similarly, in neurodegenerative diseases, where multiple interacting pathophysiologic processes dominate, multi-omics will enable the detection of primary molecular drivers of disease onset and progression.

Table 2 Role of genomics and transcriptomics in personalized medicine and imaging integration through AI [27, 28]

Omics type	Focus	Tools/technologies	Key applications in personalized medicine	AI role in imaging integration
Genomics	DNA sequence, mutations, SNPs	Whole Genome/Exome Sequencing (WGS/WES)	Genetic risk assessment, tumor classification, pharmacogenomics	AI links imaging phenotypes with genomic alterations (radio genomics); predicts mutation-driven imaging biomarkers
Transcriptomics	RNA expression profiling	RNA-seq, microarrays	Identifying active pathways, disease subtyping	AI detects expression-based imaging signatures; assists in radio transcriptomics for treatment stratification
Proteomics	Protein levels, modifications (PTMs)	Mass spectrometry, protein arrays	Drug target validation, response prediction	DL connects proteomic markers with lesion features in imaging (e.g., MRI, PET)
Metabolomics	Small molecule metabolite profiling	NMR spectroscopy, LC-MS	Metabolic phenotyping, disease monitoring	AI correlates metabolic shifts with imaging features in cancer, diabetes, neurodegeneration
Epigenomics	DNA methylatio, histone modification	ChIP-seq, bisulfite sequencing	Cancer diagnostics, immune profiling	AI integrates epigenetic patterns with image-based tissue classification; supports early detection

Although promising, multi-omics data integration is a formidable analytical and computational task. The inherent heterogeneity, high dimensionality, sparsity, and incompleteness of multi-omics data render conventional statistical methods insufficient. Each platform of omics possesses unique data distributions, scales, and noise characteristics, complicating direct comparison and fusion. Normalization, dimensionality reduction, and missing data imputation preprocessing steps are required but problematic in the case of various data types. Furthermore, informative biological knowledge is buried in vast amounts of data, necessitating the use of sophisticated computational frameworks to identify salient patterns. Integration is also plagued by scalability, particularly when handling thousands of features in various omics platforms. This has prompted increased reliance on ML and AI software, which are capable of revealing buried patterns, modeling nonlinearity, and ranking biologically informative variables for interpretation.

AI, and in particular deep learning, has emerged as a potential solution to the limitations of conventional multi-omics analysis. The capacity of AI to handle large-scale, unstructured, and complex data makes it appropriately suited for multi-omics integration. Techniques such as autoencoders—design of neural network architecture for unsupervised learning—have been used to map high-dimensional omics information into low-dimensional informative representations with considerable biological information captured. These resulting representations can then be used to make predictions regarding therapeutic targets, patient outcomes, or disease subtypes. In cancer research, for instance, autoencoders have been able to detect underlying molecular signatures related to patient outcomes. Such models remove noise and redundancy from the data, hence enabling researchers to analyze the most informative biological signals. Supervised AI methods like support vector machines (SVMs), random forests, and neural networks have also been extensively employed in biomarker discovery, patient stratification, and prediction of outcomes. Another very important field where AI enjoys a considerable advantage is feature selection. Methods like recursive feature elimination (RFE) and LASSO regression are applied routinely to select subsets of variables that substantially enhance the predictive capacity of models Not only does this improve model interpretability but also provides clinical utility by removing non-informative features.

Apart from feature selection and classification, AI has also progressed significantly in multi-omics network analysis. Graph-based methods, including graph neural networks (GNNs), demonstrate excellent performance in capturing intricate biological interactions between genes, proteins, and metabolites. GNNs enable scientists to construct interaction networks that correspond to disease-specific molecular pathways, thus providing new opportunities for the discovery of therapeutic targets [25]. These models can combine prior knowledge of biology with empirical evidence to further clarify functional modules and signaling cascades in disease. In addition, NLP tools powered by AI further enable multi-omics analysis by reading biomedical literature and databases to infer implicit relationships between biological entities. NLP-created knowledge graphs have been employed to place omics data within the framework of existing scientific knowledge, thereby facilitating hypothesis generation and testing.

AI multi-omics integration is at the core of precision medicine. Through the integration of genomics, transcriptomics, proteomics, and metabolomics data with clinical data and imaging data, AI algorithms can produce personalized disease models for every individual. These models can potentially provide more accurate predictions of disease trajectories, drug response, and side effects [26]. In oncology, it involves stratification of patients based on their molecular profile to personalize therapy to maximize effectiveness and reduce the toxicity. In cardiology, AI algorithms combining genetic risk, proteomics, and metabolomics are able to predict cardiovascular risk better than the current models.

These methods are being applied to create personalized treatment protocols for hypertension, atrial fibrillation, and heart failure. AI drug repurposing platforms are also employing multi-omics data to discover new drug-disease interactions. Methods such as generative adversarial networks (GANs) and variational autoencoders (VAEs) are being applied to simulate biological systems and generate candidate drug molecules or combination therapies, especially for treatment-resistant diseases.

With continued developments in AI technologies, their uses with multi-omics data will be even more important. XAI, digital twins, and reinforcement learning are also on the horizon to render multi-omics models more interpretable and reliable in clinical application. Despite challenges of data standardization, privacy, and computational resource requirements, the synergistic marriage of AI and multi-omics is the answer to realizing the maximum potential of personalized medicine.

5 Real-Time AI Applications in Personalized Medicine

AI has come forward as a strong enabler in the field of personalized medicine, particularly by way of real-time applications with continuous monitoring, rapid diagnostics, and instantaneous clinical decision-making support. AI's real-time applications involve the use of information from different imaging modalities, like MRI, CT, X-ray, PET, and ultrasound, by virtue of sophisticated algorithms with convolutional neural networks (CNNs), restricted Boltzmann machines (RBMs), and fully convolutional networks (FCNs) to offer individualized medical intelligence (Fig. 1). These developments are transforming the methods used by doctors for detecting diseases, monitoring, and treatment, thus turning the visions of personalized and precision healthcare into a reality.

Figure 1 illustrates the integration of AI into the medical imaging process, from patient consultation to improved health outcomes. AI-powered imaging methods significantly accelerate data processing faster than traditional methods), assisting radiologists in diagnosis and report generation. By enhancing image interpretation speed and accuracy, AI supports faster clinical decisions and better patient care, ultimately transforming the traditional workflow in diagnostic Imaging.

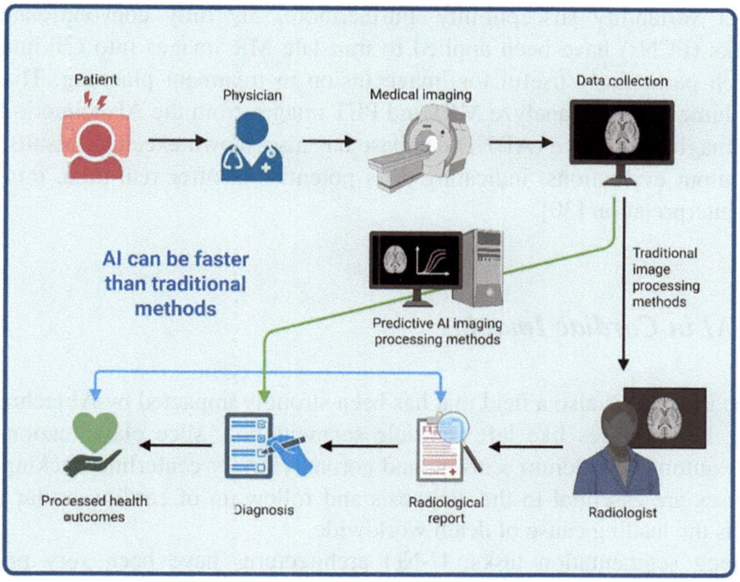

Fig. 1 Applications of artificial intelligence in medical imaging

5.1 AI in Brain Imaging

One of the most promising uses of real-time AI in personalized medicine is neuroimaging, particularly for neurological diseases like Alzheimer's disease (AD), mild cognitive impairment (MCI), and brain neoplasms. Traditional diagnostic methods in neuroimaging are usually limited because they are based on manual interpretation, which is time-consuming and prone to human errors. AI is useful because it allows automation of classification and segmentation processes.

AI models, like the Gaussian Restricted Boltzmann Machine (RBM), have been applied with high degree of success to learn features from patches of 3D volumes of MRI and PET scans for the classification of AD, MCI, and HC. Early and proper diagnosis is essential for early intervention. Moreover, 3D CNNs have been reported to perform better than traditional classifiers by learning complex features and patterns in imaging data automatically. The networks are able to segment magnetic resonance (MR) images properly. AI-based methods, like the proposed ensemble model that integrates Vision Transformers (ViT) and EfficientNet-V2, greatly improve medical imaging tasks such as brain tumor classification. By optimizing model weights with genetic algorithms, AI enhances classification accuracy and precision, ultimately supporting better diagnostic decisions [29].

In addition to segmentation, newer deep-learning models such as VoxResNet, with its 25-layer architecture setup, have been created to aid in the automation of the delineation of complex brain structures. These models can overcome the limitations of manual segmentation, which is not only time-consuming but also observer variability susceptibility. Furthermore, 3D fully convolutional neural networks (FCNs) have been applied to translate MR images into CT images, an approach particularly useful for image fusion in treatment planning. The use of two-volume CNNs to analyze MRI and PET images from the Alzheimer's Disease Neuroimaging Initiative (ADNI) database has also shown excellent results in both input/output evaluations, indicating AI's potential to offer real-time, multimodal image interpretation [30].

5.2 AI in Cardiac Imaging

Cardiac imaging is also a field that has been strongly impacted by AI technologies, namely for purposes like left ventricle segmentation, slice classification, image quality, automatic calcium scoring, and coronary artery centerline tracking. All of these uses are essential to the diagnosis and follow-up of cardiovascular disease, which is the leading cause of death worldwide.

Among segmentation tasks, U-Net architectures have been very promising because of their ability for localization and segmenting regions with great efficacy even in cases of working with quite small datasets. Both three-dimensional and two-dimensional convolutional neural networks (CNNs) have also been employed for slice classification and motion tracking. Notably, a very advanced image super-resolution (SR) method based on DL has been employed for enhancing the resolution of two-dimensional stacks of images to high-quality three-dimensional volumes. Such development has greatly improved the visibility of cardiac structures and the accuracy of follow-up analysis [31].

Moreover, real-time detection of coronary artery calcification (a key predictor of cardiovascular risk) has been achieved using multi-stream CNNs, which analyze low-dose chest CT images. These models provide intensity thresholding (for instance, > 130 Hounsfield Units) to identify calcium deposits. AI models have been utilized in coronary CT angiography (CCTA) with the aid of both 3D CNNs and multi-stream 2D CNNs and have performed extremely well to detect and measure coronary plaque burden—thus benefiting cardiologists by making rapid decision-making possible in real time during the procedure [32].

5.3 AI in Chest Imaging

Chest imaging is widely used for the diagnosis of a range of medical conditions, such as pneumonia, tuberculosis, interstitial lung disease (ILD), and lung cancer. In this use, AI is at the forefront of the automation of detection, classification, and segmentation tasks in real-time application scenarios. One specific methodology employs the multiple-instance learning (MIL) framework, where deconvolutional neural networks generate heat maps that mark areas of interest on chest radiographs.

Convolutional neural network (CNN)-based methods have been trained on large public datasets to identify up to 17 different pathological patterns in chest X-rays, thus serving as a useful assistive tool for radiologists. A segmentation-oriented label propagation method has been applied to interstitial lung disease datasets, identifying abnormal interstitial patterns that are typically hard to identify with naked eyes. Similarly, CNNs have been used to classify lung texture patterns, thus enhancing the granularity of disease description. Furthermore, methods that identify frontal and lateral chest X-rays using DL methods have automated the process of metadata annotation, thus saving precious time in large-scale screening programs [33, 34]. AI models, such as those using Vision Transformers (ViT) and EfficientNet-V2, significantly enhance medical image analysis, including lung disease diagnosis. Their ability to optimize feature extraction and classification accuracy ensures precise identification of diseases like COVID-19, pneumonia, and pulmonary opacity, leading to better patient outcomes [35].

Among the notable advancements in real-time diagnosis is the application of 3D CNNs to identify pulmonary nodules from volumetric CT scans. The models are able to decrease false positives and increase sensitivity by considering spatial context across slices. The algorithm has been validated on the LUNA16 Challenge with high Competition Performance Metric (CPM) values and extended to 3D PET images for wider application.

5.4 *AI in Breast Imaging*

Breast imaging is important for early diagnosis of breast cancer and associated disorders. AI, and more so deep learning, has been extremely useful in this regard owing to the large amount and two-dimensional character of mammographic data. CNNs and RBMs have been extensively used for lesion detection and tumor lesion and micro-calcification classification, and risk estimation. For instance, breast density, which is a known risk factor for breast cancer, can be measured using CNNs for feature extraction. An R-CNN has also been used for lesion localization to make it more accurate and less subjective to interpretation [36].

Advanced segmentation techniques such as U-Net have been applied to breast and fibro-glandular tissue (FGT) in MR images, yielding high-accuracy density calculations. Furthermore, a short-term breast cancer risk assessment model has been created using mammographic images and a multiple layer perceptron (MLP) classifier, achieving a predictive accuracy of 71.4%. This model enables clinicians to assign personalized risk scores and develop individualized screening and prevention strategies [37].

5.5 AI in Musculoskeletal Imaging

AI has also made substantial contributions to musculoskeletal imaging, which is used to assess bones, joints, and soft tissues. Real-time analysis is particularly helpful for diagnosing fractures, degenerative disorders, and evaluating skeletal maturity. 3D CNN architecture has been developed to automatically segment vertebral bodies (VBs) from MR spine images, achieving a Dice similarity coefficient of 93.4%, indicating a high level of agreement with expert manual segmentation. This not only conserves time and money invested in diagnosis but also enhances reproducibility [38, 39].

Difficult tasks like spine posture correction and vertebra localization have been solved using the assistance of the Transformed Deep Convolution Network (TDCN), which automatically corrects spinal curvature discrepancies and aligns images. Real-time registration techniques in 2D/3D have also been improved, with CNN regressions now being capable of working well over wider capture ranges. Deep-learning models have also been used for skeletal age estimation from X-ray imaging [40]. These models have demonstrated an average discrepancy of only 0.8 years from chronological age and are a valuable tool for pediatric assessments and growth monitoring.

6 Challenges in Implementing AI for Personalized Imaging

AI has demonstrated revolutionary potential in individualized medical imaging, particularly in the diagnosis of diseases such as breast cancer, colon cancer, brain tumors, and neurodegenerative diseases like Alzheimer's disease. Yet, even with these developments, the deployment of AI in clinical practice continues to be hampered by a number of key challenges. These include algorithmic bias, data privacy issues, regulatory and legal constraints, restricted clinical uptake, and stakeholder trust. Solving these issues is crucial to maximizing the potential of AI in customized imaging [41].

One of the most prominent challenges is the potential for bias in AI algorithms. As good as AI systems are, they are so only through the data that they are trained upon. When training sets are unrepresentative—failure to represent ethnic, racial, or socio-economic diversity—models can mirror and even enhance disparities in healthcare. Predictive models based on genomic data, for instance, typically underrepresent minority groups, producing inaccuracies in diagnosis and treatment for these groups [42]. This issue extends to medical imaging, where AI can preferentially choose for certain demographic trends due to biased training inputs. Ethnic and gender bias in AI has already been a source of issues in numerous fields and raises ethical issues in medicine. In imaging, these biases could result in misinterpretation of radiographs or MRIs, or erroneous risk prediction for conditions such as breast cancer or cardiovascular disease. Mitigating this involves

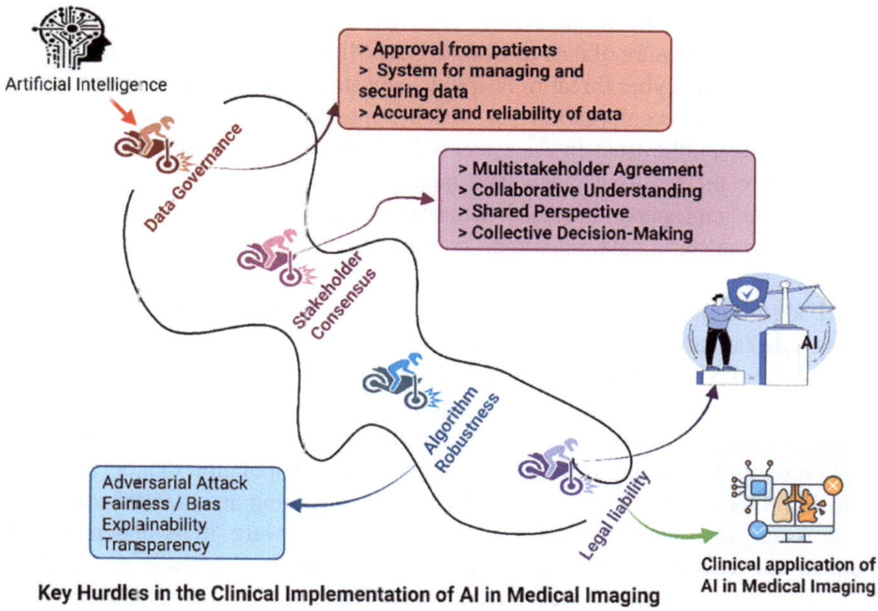

Fig. 2 Key hurdles in the clinical implementation of AI in medical imaging

concerted efforts in training models from large, representative datasets and using fairness-aware algorithms in model development [43].

The objective of AI design is a serious issue. Although numerous AI technologies exist to support diagnosis and clinical efficacy, economic imperatives can distort development goals (Fig. 2). Some commercial developers may design AI algorithms for the purpose of driving unnecessary imaging studies, spending more money without necessarily enhancing the result [44]. Furthermore, when AI systems are optimized or trained to favor specific diagnoses for profit (e.g., prescribing high-cost interventions), patient trust and safety may be compromised extensively. Proprietary AI models also hinder transparent ethical review because their lack of transparency makes them opaque to the clinicians and the patients themselves. Most AI algorithms are "black boxes" wherein clinicians and even patients cannot understand the logic for certain decisions. Such lack of transparency makes auditing model behavior, measuring accountability, or checking decisions in high-stakes critical care situations hard. To secure patient-centered innovation, developers and regulators need to give topmost priority to transparency, explainability, and ethical alignment in AI models [45].

Medical imaging and tailored diagnostics require considerable reliance on access to high-fidelity patient data such as genomic, radiographic, and clinical data. Data privacy, however, is still a huge impediment. Strict rules like GDPR (General Data Protection Regulation) and CCPA (California Consumer Privacy Act) are necessary for upholding patient rights but also restrict open data sharing for model learning and research [46]. Historical events, such as the Royal Free NHS Foundation Trust's illegal disclosure of data to Google DeepMind, have drawn attention to these risks. Besides, the cyber threat to hospitals persists, and healthcare cyber breaches have exploded in recent years. Data breaches may uncover sensitive information, again eroding public trust in AI systems [47]. Strong data governance is thus a priority—not merely to manage data quality and access but to ensure it is not misused and improperly disclosed. Governance needs to also have clear policies for data ownership, data retention, consent mechanisms, and interinstitutional interoperability [48].

AI algorithms, especially DL models, are susceptible to respond to minor distortions or variations in input data. Adversarial attacks, for example, where images are slightly tampered with to mislead AI systems, can potentially lead to diagnostic errors of immense scale. Moreover, the ability of models to generalize is still limited; AI tools trained from data in one hospital can fare badly when applied to another owing to variations in equipment, population demographics, or clinical protocols [49]. Explainable AI (XAI) is becoming an essential solution to these issues. In contrast to black-box models, XAI software offers understandable outputs via techniques such as saliency maps or attention mechanisms, enabling clinicians to learn why a model arrived at a specific decision. Interpretability is the foundation of enhancing clinical trust and ensuring proper use of models during diagnosis or treatment planning [50]. The Radiological Society of North America (RSNA) answered these needs with the Checklist for AI in Medical Imaging (CLAIM), a harmonized reporting scheme for AI studies to enhance transparency, reproducibility, and trust in reported research [51].

Notwithstanding technological preparedness, clinical adoption of AI continues to lag behind. Among the key reasons is the disconnection between clinical end-users and technology developers. Most clinicians admit limited exposure to AI systems and are concerned that the use of these tools could erode their decision-making powers [52]. A poll indicated that over 50% of radiologists had insufficient knowledge about AI, calling for professional education and training. Stakeholders are also varied geographically. In China, for instance, IT experts are concerned about misuse of data, but healthcare regulators would like to be able to trust algorithms. Business leaders are optimistic about AI in Europe but believe that masses view it as a threat. Closing this gap will involve establishing collaboration among AI developers, clinicians, hospital administrators, patients, and policy-makers to co-design patient-centered, accountable AI systems [53, 54].

With more and more incorporation of AI technologies into diagnostics, the question of legal liability becomes multifaceted. Presently, the "learned intermediary doctrine" shields device makers by assigning blame to clinicians. But when AI errors injure—via misdiagnosis or the inadvisability of suggested treatment—it is difficult to know where fault lies: with the clinician, software engineer, or hospital. Additionally, the non-explainability of AI decision-making makes it difficult for adjudication in court. Without transparent explanation of supporting reasons for AI conclusions, regulators and judges can't articulate fault in cases of malpractice [55, 56]. In the context of protecting patients and making the patient accountable, governments and institutions must frame legal regulations that can be easily understood by making provision for accountability, ensuring transparency, and oversight in the creation and use of AI in healthcare.

7 Conclusion

AI imaging is a cornerstone in the modern move towards personalization in medicine, with innovative solutions for individualized diagnosis, risk estimation, and tailored treatment planning. Integration of ML and DL into imaging modalities not only enhanced disease detection precision but also enabled earlier intervention, especially in high-stakes conditions like oncology, neurology, and cardiology. By processing rich imaging data and correlating them with clinical and molecular profiles, AI bridges the gap between unusable medical information and actionable knowledge. One of the most groundbreaking subjects covered is radiomics—a discipline enhanced by AI—which allows the derivation of imaging features of high dimensions that are invisible to the human eye. Such features can be matched against genomic, proteomic, and clinical information to give a better overall picture of disease pathophysiology. The combination of multi-omics data with imaging by AI has also enabled an integrative, systems-level perspective on health and disease, and paved the way for truly personalized treatment. Additionally, the real-time applications of AI in imaging for various specialties such as neuro, breast, cardiac, and musculoskeletal radiology show how personalized diagnosis is being made increasingly accessible and efficient. Yet algorithmic bias, explainability of AI models, ethical considerations, and legal accountability remain valid concerns. Bridging the clinician-AI developer gap by way of training, open model development, and standardized frameworks will be essential to enable broad clinical application.

While the journey toward fully personalized, AI-powered healthcare is still unfolding, the advances in AI-driven imaging provide a compelling roadmap. With continued interdisciplinary collaboration, regulatory oversight, and technological refinement, AI will undoubtedly play a central role in delivering precision medicine that is not only effective but also equitable and ethically sound.

References

1. Whitcomb DC (2012) What is personalized medicine and what should it replace? Nat Rev Gastroenterol Hepatol 9:418–424. https://doi.org/10.1038/nrgastro.2012.100
2. Schork NJ (2019) Artificial intelligence and personalized medicine. Cancer Treat Res 178:265–283. https://doi.org/10.1007/978-3-030-16391-4_11
3. Parekh A-DE, Shaikh OA, Simran et al (2023) Artificial intelligence (AI) in personalized medicine: AI-generated personalized therapy regimens based on genetic and medical history: short communication. Ann Med Surg 85:5831–5833. https://doi.org/10.1097/ms9.0000000000001320
4. Diao S, Huang D, Jiang G (2024) The role of artificial intelligence in personalized medicine through advanced imaging. Front Sci Eng 4:92–100. https://doi.org/10.54691/fbpgw554
5. Banegas-Luna AJ, Peña-García J, Iftene A et al (2021) Towards the interpretability of machine learning predictions for medical applications targeting personalised therapies: A cancer case survey. Int J Mol Sci 22:4394. https://doi.org/10.3390/ijms22094394
6. Wang P, Fan E, Wang P (2021) Comparative analysis of image classification algorithms based on traditional machine learning and deep learning. Pattern Recogn Lett 141:61–67. https://doi.org/10.1016/j.patrec.2020.07.042
7. Obuchowicz R, Strzelecki M, Piórkowski A (2024) Clinical applications of artificial intelligence in medical imaging and image processing—a review. Cancer 16:1870. https://doi.org/10.3390/cancers16101870
8. Khalifa M, Albadawy M (2024) AI in diagnostic imaging: Revolutionising accuracy and efficiency. Comput Methods Programs Biomed Update 5:100146. https://doi.org/10.1016/j.cmpbup.2024.100146
9. Zhang K, Khosravi B, Vahdati S, Erickson BJ (2024) FDA review of radiologic AI algorithms: Process and challenges. Radiology 310:e230242. https://doi.org/10.1148/radiol.230242
10. Singh M, Babbarwal A, Pushpakumar S, Tyagi SC (2025) Interoception, cardiac health, and heart failure: The potential for artificial intelligence (AI)—driven diagnosis and treatment. Physiol Rep 13:e70146. https://doi.org/10.14814/phy2.70146
11. Yuan N, Kwan AC, Duffy G et al (2023) Prediction of coronary artery calcium using deep learning of echocardiograms. J Am Soc Echocardiogr 36:474–481.e3. https://doi.org/10.1016/j.echo.2022.12.014
12. Lastrucci A, Giansanti D (2024) Radiological crossroads: Navigating the intersection of virtual reality and digital radiology through a comprehensive narrative review of reviews. Robotics 13:69. https://doi.org/10.3390/robotics13050069
13. Sharma A, Singh A, Verma A et al (2023) Potential of AI in the advancement of the pharmaceutical industry. In: Pharmaceutical Industry 40: Future, Challenges & Application, pp 107–143. https://doi.org/10.1201/9781003442493-5
14. Mesko B (2017) The role of artificial intelligence in precision medicine. Expert Rev Precis Med Drug Dev 2:239–241. https://doi.org/10.1080/23808993.2017.1380516
15. Trattner S, Pearson GDN, Chin C et al (2014) Standardization and optimization of CT protocols to achieve low dose. J Am Coll Radiol 11:271–278. https://doi.org/10.1016/j.jacr.2013.10.016
16. Streba CT, Ionescu M, Vere CC, Rogoveanu I (2017) Artificial intelligence and automatic image interpretation in modern medicine, pp 371–407. https://doi.org/10.1007/978-94-024-1045-7_16
17. Alanazi MMF, Mohammed ASF, Owaydhah AN et al (2024) Advancements in AI-driven diagnostic radiology: Enhancing accuracy and efficiency. Int J Health Sci 8:737–749. https://doi.org/10.53730/ijhs.v8ns1.14928
18. Roy R, Srivastava A (2024) Role of artificial intelligence (Ai) in enhancing operational efficiency in manufacturing medical devices. J Multidiscip Res 4:35–40. https://doi.org/10.37022/tjmdr.v4i1.580

19. Dilsizian SE, Siegel EL (2014) Artificial intelligence in medicine and cardiac imaging: Harnessing big data and advanced computing to provide personalized medical diagnosis and treatment. Curr Cardiol Rep 16:441. https://doi.org/10.1007/s11886-013-0441-8
20. Najjar R (2023) Redefining radiology: A review of artificial intelligence integration in medical imaging. Diagnostics 13:2760. https://doi.org/10.3390/diagnostics13172760
21. Maniaci A, Lavalle S, Gagliano C et al (2024) The integration of radiomics and artificial intelligence in modern medicine. Life 14:1248. https://doi.org/10.3390/life14101248
22. Lambin P, RTH L, Deist TM et al (2017) Radiomics: The bridge between medical imaging and personalized medicine. Nat Rev Clin Oncol 14:749–762
23. Tong L, Shi W, Isgut M et al (2024) Integrating multi-omics data with EHR for precision medicine using advanced artificial intelligence. IEEE Rev Biomed Eng 17:80–97. https://doi.org/10.1109/RBME.2023.3324264
24. Phan NN, Chattopadhyay A, Chuang EY (2019) Role of artificial intelligence in integrated analysis of multi-omics and imaging data in cancer research. Transl Cancer Res 8:E7–E10. https://doi.org/10.21037/tcr.2019.12.17
25. Di VM, Silva W (2024) Review on multi-modal AI models to integrate imaging and omics data, pp 1–19
26. Lin B, Ma Y, Wu S (2022) Multi-omics and artificial intelligence-guided data integration in chronic liver disease: Prospects and challenges for precision medicine. OMICS 26:415–421. https://doi.org/10.1089/omi.2022.0079
27. Barbano CA, Beccuti M, Cordero F et al (2023) Artificial intelligence methods for biomedical imaging and omics data. CEUR Workshop Proc 3486:154–159
28. Olayemi Stephen Bakare (2025) AI-driven multi-omics integration for precision medicine in complex disease diagnosis and treatment. Int J Res Publ Rev 16:5070–5084
29. Gasmi K, Ben Aoun N, Alsalem K et al (2024) Enhanced brain tumor diagnosis using combined deep learning models and weight selection technique. Front Neuroinform 18:1444650. https://doi.org/10.3389/fninf.2024.1444650
30. Segato A, Marzullo A, Calimeri F, De Momi E (2020) Artificial intelligence for brain diseases: A systematic review. APL Bioeng 4:041503. https://doi.org/10.1063/5.0011697
31. Jiang B, Guo N, Ge Y et al (2020) Development and application of artificial intelligence in cardiac imaging. Br J Radiol 93:20190812. https://doi.org/10.1259/bjr.20190812
32. Ahmad IS, Dai J, Xie Y, Liang X (2025) Deep learning models for CT image classification: a comprehensive literature review. Quant Imaging Med Surg 15:962–1011. https://doi.org/10.21037/qims-24-1400
33. Morcos G, Yi PH, Jeudy J (2023) Applying artificial intelligence to pediatric chest imaging: reliability of leveraging adult-based artificial intelligence models. J Am Coll Radiol 20:742–747. https://doi.org/10.1016/j.jacr.2023.07.004
34. Schalekamp S, Klein WM, van Leeuwen KG (2022) Current and emerging artificial intelligence applications in chest imaging: a pediatric perspective. Pediatr Radiol 52:2120–2130. https://doi.org/10.1007/s00247-021-05146-0
35. Bennour A, Ben Aoun N, Khalaf OI et al (2024) Contribution to pulmonary diseases diagnostic from X-ray images using innovative deep learning models. Heliyon 10:e30308. https://doi.org/10.1016/j.heliyon.2024.e30308
36. Wang X, Moriakov N, Gao Y et al (2022) Artificial intelligence in breast imaging. In: Medical radiology, pp 435–453. https://doi.org/10.1007/978-3-030-94918-1_20
37. Danala G (2022) Developing and applying CAD-generated image markers to assist disease diagnosis and prognosis prediction
38. Suri A, Jones BC, Ng G et al (2021) A deep learning system for automated, multi-modality 2D segmentation of vertebral bodies and intervertebral discs. Bone 149:115972. https://doi.org/10.1016/j.bone.2021.115972
39. Gitto S, Serpi F, Albano D et al (2024) AI applications in musculoskeletal imaging: a narrative review. Eur Radiol Exp 8:22. https://doi.org/10.1186/s41747-024-00422-8

40. Cai Y, Landis M, Laidley DT et al (2016) Multi-modal vertebrae recognition using transformed deep convolution network. Comput Med Imaging Graph 51:11–19. https://doi.org/10.1016/j.compmedimag.2016.02.002
41. Arabahmadi M, Farahbakhsh R, Rezazadeh J (2022) Deep learning for smart healthcare—A survey on brain tumor detection from medical imaging. Sensors 22:1960. https://doi.org/10.3390/s22051960
42. Farhud DD, Zokaei S (2021) Ethical issues of artificial intelligence in medicine and healthcare. Iran J Public Health 50:i–v. https://doi.org/10.18502/ijph.v50i11.7600
43. D'antonoli TA (2020) Ethical considerations for artificial intelligence: An overview of the current radiology landscape. Diagn Interv Radiol 26:504–511. https://doi.org/10.5152/dir.2020.19279
44. Obermeyer Z, Powers B, Vogeli C et al (2020) Dissecting racial bias in an algorithm used to manage the health of populations. In: Yearbook of paediatric endocrinology. https://doi.org/10.1530/ey.17.12.7
45. Mongan J, Moy L, Kahn CE (2020) Checklist for artificial intelligence in medical imaging (CLAIM): A guide for authors and reviewers. Radiol Artif Intell 2:e200029. https://doi.org/10.1148/ryai.2020200029
46. Alexander CB (2020) The general data protection regulation and california consumer privacy act: The economic impact and future of data privacy regulations. Loyola Consum Law Rev 32:199–245
47. Aggarwal R, Farag S, Martin G et al (2021) Patient perceptions on data sharing and applying artificial intelligence to health care data: Cross-sectional survey. J Med Internet Res 23:e26162. https://doi.org/10.2196/26162
48. Jutzi TB, Krieghoff-Henning EI, Fröhling S et al (2020) Artificial intelligence in skin cancer diagnostics: The patients' perspective. Front Med 7:233
49. Zhang A, Xing L, Zou J, Wu JC (2022) Shifting machine learning for healthcare from development to deployment and from models to data. Nat Biomed Eng 6:1330–1345. https://doi.org/10.1038/s41551-022-00898-y
50. Borys K, Schmitt YA, Nauta M et al (2023) Explainable AI in medical imaging: An overview for clinical practitioners - Saliency-based XAI approaches. Eur J Radiol 162:110787. https://doi.org/10.1016/j.ejrad.2023.110787
51. Tejani AS, Klontzas ME, Gatti AA et al (2023) Updating the checklist for artificial intelligence in medical imaging (CLAIM) for reporting AI research. Nat Mach Intell 5:950–951. https://doi.org/10.1038/s42256-023-00717-2
52. Elise Almestad M, Datateknologi Veileder M, Krogstie Juni J. Exploring explainable AI adoption in medical diagnosis and the empowering potential of collaboration
53. Qian ST, Rony M (2018) Mapping the challenges of artificial intelligence in the public sector: Evidence from public healthcare. Gov Inf Q 36:368–383
54. Ford EW, Menachemi N, Peterson LT, Huerta TR (2009) Resistance is futile: But it is slowing the pace of EHR adoption nonetheless. J Am Med Inform Assoc 16:274–281. https://doi.org/10.1197/jamia.M3042
55. Contaldo MT, Pasceri G, Vignati G et al (2024) AI in radiology: Navigating medical responsibility. Diagnostics 14:1506. https://doi.org/10.3390/diagnostics14141506
56. Raposo VL (2025) The fifty shades of black: about black box AI and explainability in healthcare. Med Law Rev 33:fwaf005. https://doi.org/10.1093/medlaw/fwaf005

AI-Driven Medical Image Analysis: Challenges and Limitations

Moez Krichen and Najib Ben Aoun

1 Introduction

In recent years, artificial intelligence (AI) has revolutionized medical image analysis as well as many other fields. With the incredible advances in artificial intelligence techniques, both in terms of technology and hardware, the use of AI in the medical field has evolved remarkably, particularly in the field of medical imaging, as illustrated in Fig. 1.

Currently, different AI techniques are used in this field, such as those listed in Fig. 2 [1, 6–8, 14, 15, 20, 39, 44]:

- Supervised learning models uses labeled data to extract valuable data features that will used to learn the relationship between inputs and outputs, which enable the model to give accurate predictions on new, unseen data [1, 8, 10, 15, 21, 24, 25, 33, 44, 51]
- Unsupervised learning models explore unlabeled data to uncover hidden patterns and structures [10, 21, 24, 25, 33, 51]
- Reinforcement learning models adapt through trial and error, making it suitable for dynamic medical contexts [16, 30, 50].

M. Krichen (✉)
Faculty of Computing and Information, Al-Baha University, Alaqiq, Saudi Arabia

ReDCAD Laboratory, University of Sfax, Sfax, Tunisia
e-mail: mkreishan@bu.edu.sa; moez.krichen@redcad.org

N. Ben Aoun
Faculty of Computing and Information, Al-Baha University, Alaqiq, Saudi Arabia

REGIM-Lab: Research Groups in Intelligent Machines, University of Sfax, Sfax, Tunisia
e-mail: najib.benaoun@ieee.org

N. Ben Aoun et al. (eds.), *AI for Medical Image Analysis*,
https://doi.org/10.1007/978-3-032-02963-8_8

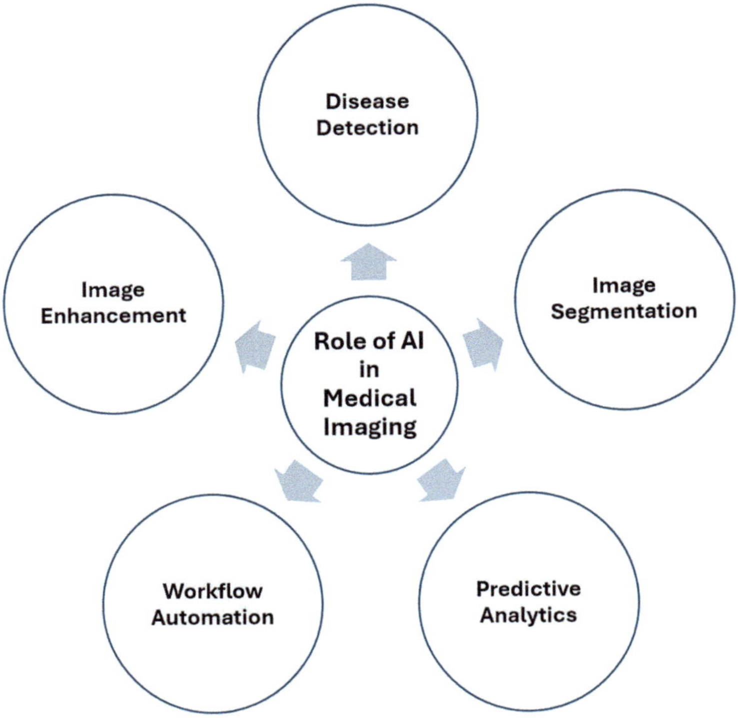

Fig. 1 Role of AI in medical imaging

- Hybrid methods, such as semi-supervised learning [54], self-supervised learning [31], and multi-instance learning [13], combine the strengths of supervised and unsupervised approaches [23, 28, 37].

Despite the increasing use of the AI technique in the field of medical image analysis, things are not as perfect for the moment, and the application of AI for medical imaging still poses significant challenges and difficulties that limit its widespread adoption and effectiveness in real-world healthcare settings. These obstacles are of different types, namely: technical limitations, operational barriers, and systemic issues [2, 11, 18, 26, 47, 53].

In this chapter, our goal is to identify these main obstacles and difficulties by classifying them into different categories [5, 9, 35, 36, 40]. The first category corresponds to data-related challenges, namely the difficulties in accessing medical images and the quality of these images. Another problem in this same category addresses the problem of data imbalance and bias in medical datasets, as well as privacy and security concerns in data sharing [32, 41, 49].

The second category of difficulties corresponds to algorithmic limitations, including, first, issues in model generalization and overfitting [12, 34]. This means that the results obtained may only be acceptable when applied in a specific context

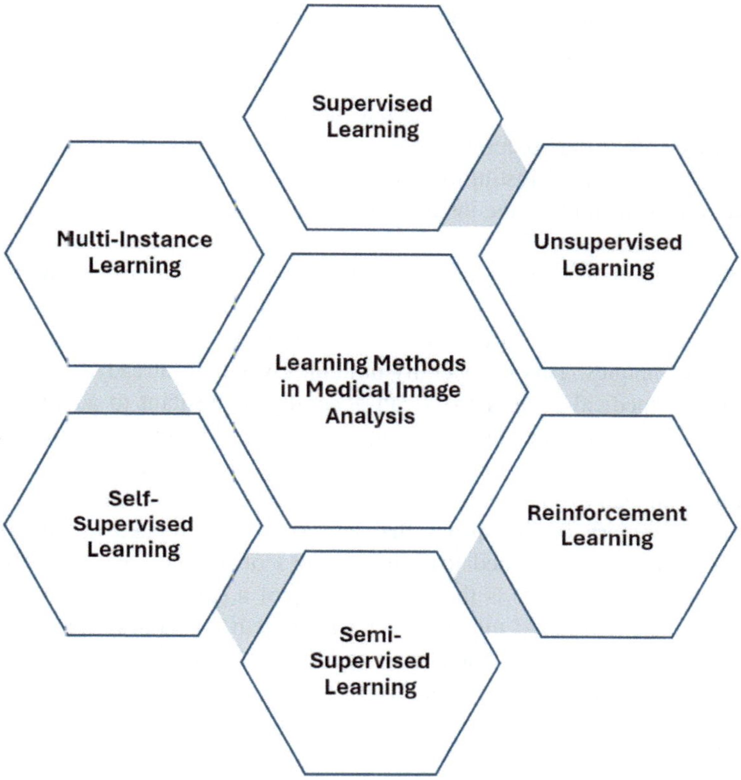

Fig. 2 Learning methods in medical image analysis

that is close to or similar to the learning context used for model development and cannot be generalized to other contexts [42, 43, 48]. Another aspect related to this category corresponds to the problem of explainability and interpretability of AI models, mainly related to the black-box nature of AI models. Indeed, the physician or radiologist will not have sufficient details or arguments justifying the choices and results obtained by the AI model used. Subsequently, it would not be possible to ensure whether the results obtained are truly correct or not, hence the problem of reliability and robustness in clinical settings.

Another category of challenges we cover in this chapter is the integration of these intelligent medical image analysis systems into the general workflow of healthcare institutions [27, 29]. Indeed, when integrating these tools, it is necessary to comply with and take into account the various constraints imposed by existing conventional systems. Among other things, the available resources and calculators are generally not adapted to the requirements of AI techniques, which are most of the time quite demanding in terms of computation and storage memory. The other aspect related to this challenge is the problem of interoperability with existing systems given the use of different storage and data exchange techniques between old and new systems.

We also cover aspects related to legal and legal acceptance issues as well as Liability and Accountability issues for AI Errors. In fact, until now, regulatory systems in the majority countries have not reached a sufficient level of maturity to keep pace with the evolution of AI-based techniques [3, 17, 38, 43, 46]. In particular, if there are errors in the processing of images by intelligent techniques, who will be responsible: the medical institution, or the development company that created the intelligent analysis tool, or the institution that collected and shared the data used to prepare the model, etc.

Another important category of challenges we will cover in this chapter is related to human-AI collaboration. On the one hand, physicians and radiologists must undergo specific training to acquire the minimum knowledge necessary for the use of AI techniques. This is generally difficult given their already high workload. Furthermore, medical professionals can generally be hesitant to adopt or use AI techniques, especially when these techniques go against their beliefs and knowledge [45, 52]. In contrast, another risk related to this category is that excessive use of these techniques can lead to a decrease in medical professionals' knowledge and skills.

Another category of limitations that we consider is related to limitations in addressing edge cases Related to Rare Diseases or unique Patient Profiles. The problem in these situations is the unavailability of a sufficient number of images that can be used to train AI models. Another problem that arises in this case is the different techniques used to obtain, save, and send images. The divergence between these different techniques makes training even more difficult and complicated. Thus, the risks of errors and inaccuracies increase significantly.

The last category we consider relates to significant global and socioeconomic barriers. Indeed, from one institution to another, available resources and technologies can vary significantly. Wealthier regions and countries can obviously afford to spend larger sums than those with limited budgets. Thus, populations in developing countries are disadvantaged, and technologies can be used in an uncontrolled and unregulated manner, leading to the risk of serious medical errors endangering the health or even the life of certain patients.

2 Data-Related Challenges

2.1 Availability, Accessibility, and Quality of the Medical Images

The first challenges encountered in the field of medical image analysis using AI techniques relate to the availability, accessibility, and quality of the medical images themselves [14, 43, 48]. In fact, AI learning algorithms are very data-intensive in order to generate robust and reliable models [43, 48]. Furthermore, the images must be of high quality and high resolution. They must also be properly annotated and standardized so that their use in model training is effective and the results obtained are of good quality and high accuracy [3, 19, 22]. If training databases contain a large number of blurry or low-resolution images, this could negatively impact the quality of the resulting models, resulting in critical errors and inaccuracies.

2.2 Data Imbalance

Another challenge related to training data is the problem of data distribution imbalance. In other words, the majority of data/images correspond to a particular type of patient (or healthy people), while the number of images corresponding to other patients is relatively low. This leads to problems during model training since the learning engine does not have enough samples corresponding to certain anomalies. For example, a model obtained from mammograms of European women might perform less well for African patients due to differences in breast density.

2.3 Confidentiality

Another problem at this level is the confidentiality of medical data, which hinders the construction of databases of acceptable size and good quality [4, 29]. This is mainly due to the different national and international laws governing the storage and sharing of medical images. For example, a project between two institutions located on different continents may be blocked due to possible conflicts in the laws of the two countries. A possible solution to this problem could be based on anonymous data sharing or the use of federated learning techniques, which allow the construction of local models that can then be aggregated into a central model. However, these techniques are still in their preliminary stages and need to be further explored and deepened. Figure 3 summarizes the main data-related challenges.

3 Algorithmic Limitations

3.1 Overfitting

The second category of challenges corresponds to algorithmic problems. First, a difficulty that could be encountered when using AI for medical image analysis is the overfitting problem. The latter corresponds to the fact that the models developed after the training phase can be very accurate and efficient for training data and have very poor quality for other test data or data from real situations. This is mainly due to the great variability of data between different institutions, regions and nations or even between different types of patients in terms of age, sex, origin, etc.

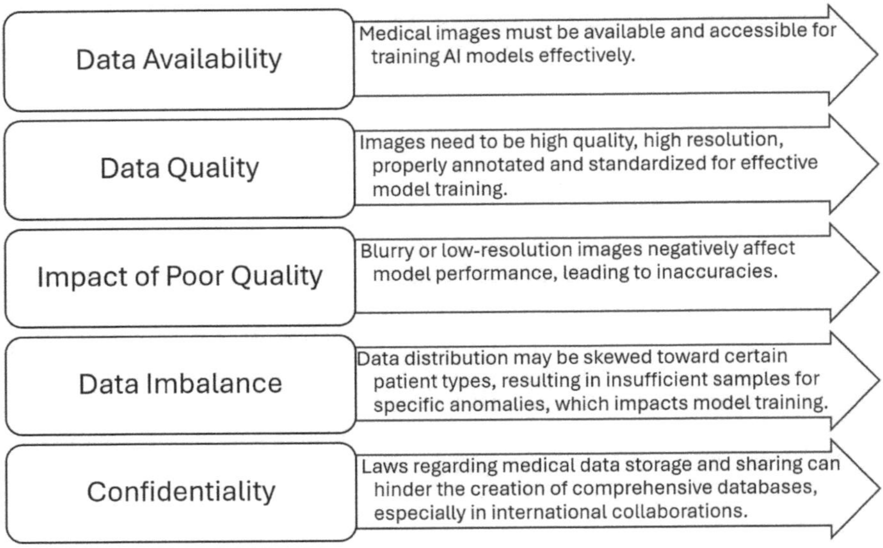

Fig. 3 Summary of data-related challenges in medical image analysis

For example, a model trained to detect brain tumors from MRI scans taken with a specific scanner could fail on images acquired with another device, due to differences in contrast or resolution. Similarly, an algorithm developed using data primarily from adult patients might underperform on pediatric scans, where anatomy and pathological features differ.

3.2 Eexplainability and Interpretability

Another algorithmic challenge relates to issues related to the explainability and interpretability of AI models. More specifically, this is related to the fact that in many cases, AI will provide clinicians with results and decisions but without providing any explanation or justification. In this case, clinicians may remain doubtful and hesitant.

Consider an AI system designed to identify early signs of Alzheimer's disease from brain MRIs. If the model classifies a patient as "high risk" but does not indicate which brain regions influenced this decision, neurologists may hesitate to follow this recommendation. Similarly, in breast cancer screening by mammography, a prediction must be accompanied by a precise location of suspicious lesions to guide the radiologist.

3.3 *Reliability and Robustness*

A third problem related to algorithmic aspects corresponds to the risks of lack of reliability and robustness of the developed intelligent models. This is mainly due to errors that can be contained in the training image databases either due to anomalies in the equipment used, or the divergence between the different technologies for acquiring, storing and transferring images, or due to deliberate attacks targeting the introduction of imperfections in the training data introduced by adversaries to distort the calculations and the results obtained.

For example, an algorithm for detecting pneumothorax on chest X-rays could be fooled by motion artifacts or variations in X-ray exposure, leading to false diagnoses. A more critical case would be an adversarial attack, where an alteration imperceptible to the human eye (such as pixelated noise) could cause a model to ignore a malignant tumor or, conversely, detect one that does not exist. To improve robustness, techniques such as adversarial learning, anomaly detection, and uncertainty calibration are being explored. We provide a summart of these challenges in Fig. 4.

4 Integration into Healthcare Systems

4.1 *Challenges in Workflow Integration*

Integrating AI tools for medical image 'analysis into clinicians workflows poses significant challenges. For example, a physician or radiologist reviewing a patient's X-ray images and using an AI decision-making tool must integrate the results of this tool into their medical report. If the AI model detects an anomaly, the clinician must decide whether it is indeed this anomaly or give a contrary opinion and opt for another decision based on their personal expertise. In all cases, the clinician must provide arguments justifying their choice. In certain critical situations, it may be useful to seek the opinion of other experts or also to compare the current decision with decisions generated by other AI tools. To better master these tools, medical professionals must follow specific and advanced training in the field.

4.2 *Computational Requirements and Infrastructure Constraints*

AI techniques, and deep learning in particular, require significant computing resources, both in terms of computing capacity and storage. This poses a challenge for under-resourced medical institutions, such as medium-sized hospitals in rural areas. Another problem related to infrastructure and resource issues is the rapid

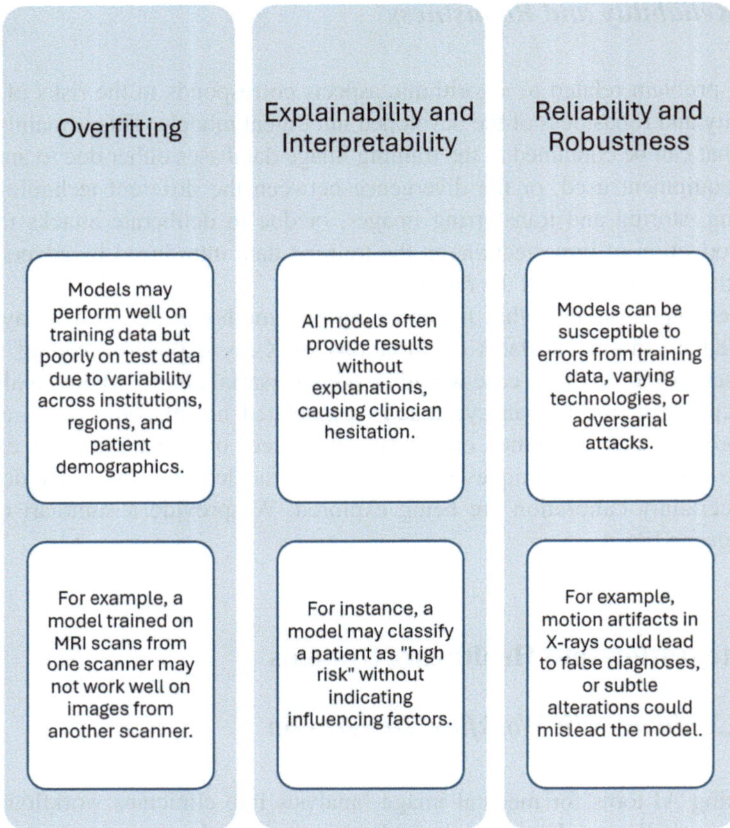

Fig. 4 Summary of algorithmic limitations in AI for medical image analysis

evolution of AI technologies, which necessitates additional budgets for continuous hardware and software updates, as well as training for IT experts in these institutions. Therefore, it is important to consider all these financial aspects from the very beginning of the adoption of AI techniques to avoid any possible delays or procedural bottlenecks.

4.3 Interoperability with Existing Systems

Another challenge related to the integration aspects of AI systems is compatibility and interoperability issues with existing systems. Indeed, existing systems often use specific technologies for storing and sharing electronic data that are not necessarily compatible with the AI technologies and platforms in use. Any incompatibility at this level can lead to calculation errors or at least delays in treatment, resulting in malfunctions that can be critical in the medical sector for certain types of diseases. Therefore, it is important to ensure that new technologies can communicate and exchange data efficiently with existing systems to ensure a smooth flow of information and minimize potential errors. Therefore, it is important to develop common standards and data exchange protocols to overcome these obstacles and promote successful integration. These challenges related to integration issues are summarized in Fig. 5.

5 Regulatory and Legal Challenges

5.1 Regulatory Approval Bottlenecks

Regulatory approval for AI technologies in the healthcare sector can be a lengthy and challenging process. Indeed, if a new AI system is developed for early disease diagnosis, it must necessarily undergo a series of clinical trials to prove its efficacy and safety. These trials can last for unreasonably long periods of time, delaying clinicians' access to potentially beneficial tools. For example, AI devices used for medical image analysis must obtain approval from the relevant authorities to ensure the minimization of the risk of errors and accidents that can be critical and very dangerous. In this way, requirements on compliance with safety and efficacy standards can create bottlenecks, preventing rapid time to market.

5.2 Liability and Accountability for AI Errors

When AI systems make mistakes, it is difficult to know who's truly responsible. If an AI tool makes a diagnosis that could lead to inadequate treatment, the question arises as to whether the responsibility lies with the AI developer, the hospital that used it, or the physician who interpreted the results. These kinds of situations can deter healthcare organizations from adopting AI solutions. As a solution to these kinds of situations, it is essential to clearly define rules of responsibility and accountability to ensure that healthcare professionals understand their obligations when using these technologies. A summary of the regulatory and legal challenges is given in Fig. 6.

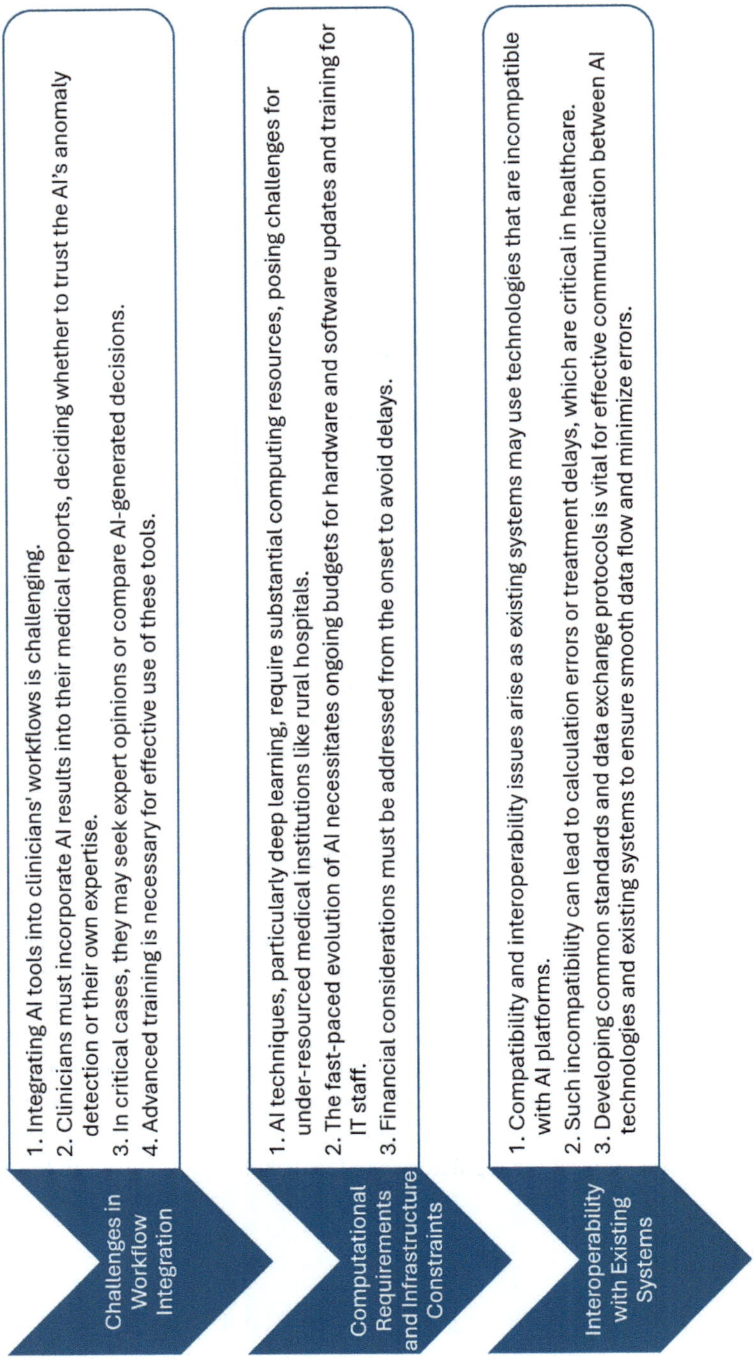

Fig. 5 Summary of integration issues in AI for medical image analysis

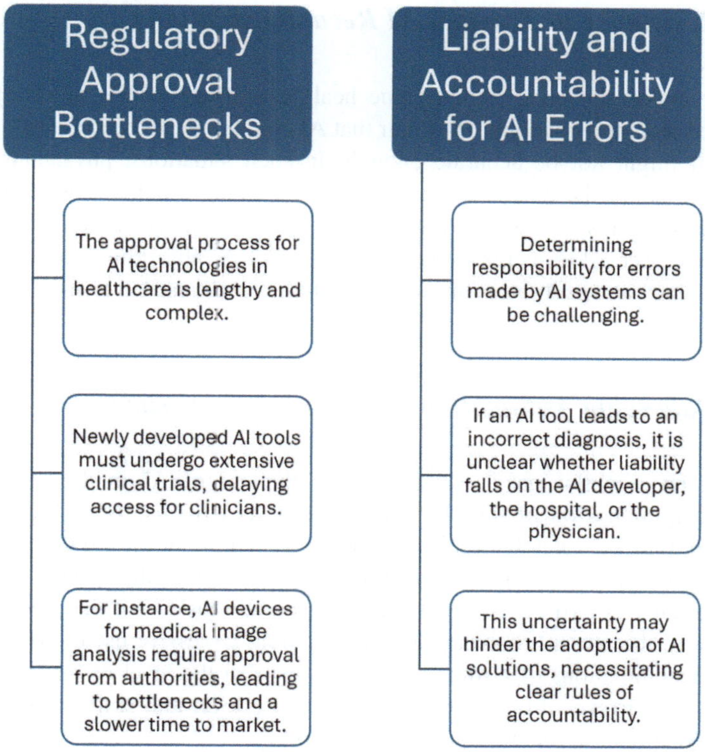

Fig. 6 Summary of regulatory and legal challenges in AI for medical image analysis

6 Human-AI Collaboration Challenges

6.1 Training and Adoption by Healthcare Professionals

One of the major challenges is training healthcare professionals to use AI technologies. For optimal effectiveness, it is extremely important that doctors, nurses, and other practitioners in the medical field understand how to use and interpret the recommendations of AI models. They must also be able to integrate these recommendations into their daily practice. This type of AI tool must be accompanied by appropriate training so that professionals can use it correctly. Without this preparation, there is a risk that users will have difficulty adopting these new technologies, which could limit the potential benefits in patient care or even lead to critical and dangerous accidents.

6.2 Resistance to Trusting AI Recommendations

Another major challenge is that some healthcare professionals are wary of AI-generated recommendations. They fear that AI could replace their clinical judgment or that it might not be accurate enough. In such situations, physicians may be hesitant to adopt the results of an AI tool for treating a patient, especially if the recommendation is not consistent with their expertise or experience. To address this issue, it is essential to increase the transparency of AI algorithms and demonstrate their accuracy and usefulness through case studies and tangible results.

6.3 Balancing Automation with Human Expertise

Among the potential risks associated with the use of AI in the medical field is the marginalization of the clinician's role. Excessive use of AI could lead to the technology completely dominating decision-making at the expense of medical experts. It is necessary to find the optimal balance between the role of AI tools and the clinician's expertise. AI could accelerate certain tasks, but the medical expert must always be present to make the final decision. Excessive use of AI could even lead to accumulations of errors at all levels, even at the level of medical experts' training, thus irreversibly harming their scientific level and skills. A summary of human-AI collaboration challenges is given in Fig. 7.

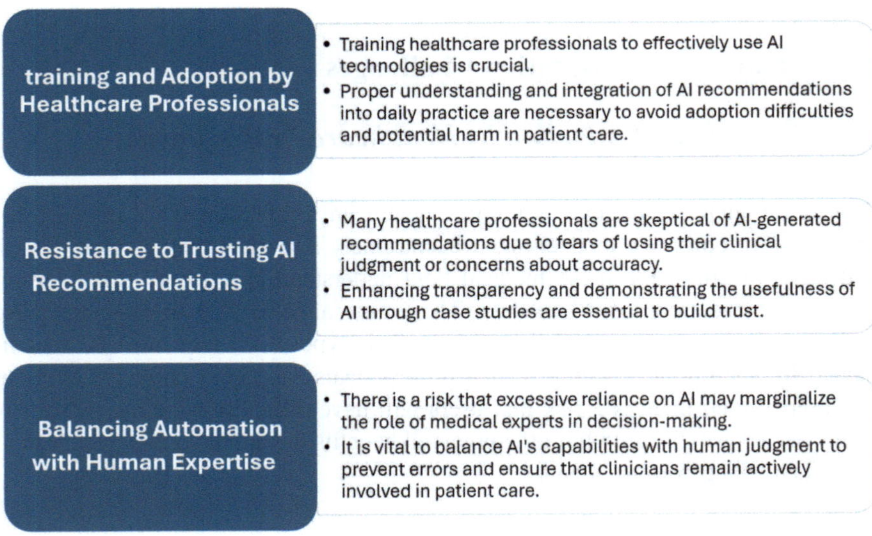

Fig. 7 Summary of human-AI collaboration challenges for medical image analysis

7 Limitations in Addressing Edge Cases

7.1 Rare Diseases and Unique Patient Profiles

Another major challenge facing clinicians who want to take advantage of AI techniques for disease diagnosis and identification is in situations involving very rare diseases or patients with unique profiles. Indeed, the main rule for using AI techniques, and deep learning techniques in particular, is to have a sufficiently large number of images covering the disease in question. However, for rare diseases, the situation is completely opposite. Therefore, the use of these techniques is not appropriate in these cases and could lead to significant diagnostic errors. In these situations, it is therefore necessary to rely on the expertise of medical professionals.

7.2 Limitations of AI in Complex, Multimodal Cases

In some complex situations, the patient may suffer from different simultaneous diseases and several factors and parameters must be taken into account for the medical diagnosis to be made accurately and optimally. In this case, we are talking about a multidimensional situation or multimodal cases for which traditional AI approaches may prove limited and insufficiently appropriate. The solution once again is to have close collaboration between medical experts and available AI systems in order to achieve an optimal decision and a correct evaluation of the patient situation. A summary of the limitations in addressing edge cases is given in Fig. 8.

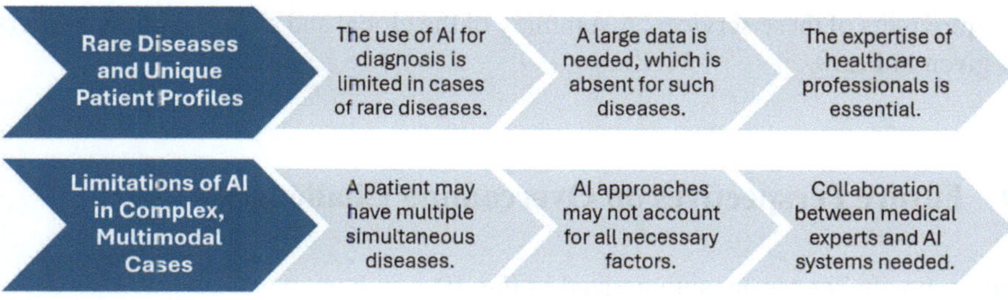

Fig. 8 Summary of limitations in addressing edge cases for medical image analysis

8 Global and Socioeconomic Barriers

8.1 Lack of Access to AI Solutions in Low-Resource Settings

In poor countries or regions, governments generally struggle to provide hospitals and medical institutions with the necessary budgets to properly invest in the adoption of AI solutions. Indeed, these solutions are always quite expensive in terms of necessary equipment (databases, computers, networks, etc.) and also in terms of the salaries of specialized technical staff. Thus, poor populations are less likely to access medical services assisted by AI technologies. Even more dangerous is that some medical institutions in these countries may venture into using the techniques without having the necessary resources, hence the significant risks of errors or even dangerous accidents.

8.2 Disparities in AI Adoption Across Regions

Today, we are witnessing a significant imbalance between rich and poor countries when it comes to the adoption of AI technologies for medical image processing. Poor countries often lack the necessary resources to carry out all the essential steps for developing and implementing AI models. First, the primary challenge is collecting, organizing, storing, and sharing data. In the best-case scenario, data can be stored on foreign clouds. Therefore, rich countries are once again at an advantage, since they have their own data and data from poor countries. Poor countries also lack the computing centers necessary to build AI models. Even in terms of using existing models developed by foreign institutions, the task is not easy and could pose security problems because there is no guarantee how the queries and results will be used by the providers of these services. A summary of the global and socioeconomic barriers is given in Fig. 9.

9 Future Perspectives on Overcoming Challenges

The main challenges are summarized in Fig. 10.

9.1 Collaborative Efforts Across Stakeholders

Fruitful collaboration between various stakeholders working in the healthcare field and AI techniques is the key to solving most of the challenges encountered when applying AI to medical image analysis. This exchange should include governments,

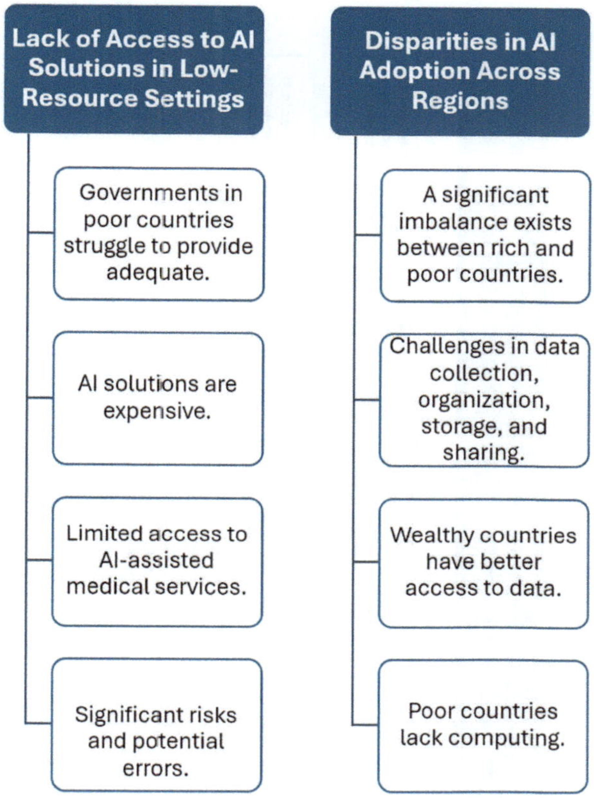

Fig. 9 Summary of global and socioeconomic barriers for medical image analysis

medical institutions, AI technology development companies, associations, etc. This exchange will allow the creation of larger databases with more diverse content. In addition, computing and storage resources will be greater, allowing the creation of more robust, stable, and efficient models. Poor countries and developing populations will have a better chance of benefiting from these technologies for free or at reasonable costs. This would only be possible through the establishment of international laws and multinational non-profit organizations whose primary goal is the interest of patients and human beings, whoever and wherever they are.

9.2 *Preparing for Ethical and Regulatory Evolution*

Another key point to exploit to improve the use of AI in the medical field is the establishment of laws that define the responsibilities of the different actors involved in this field in order to provide guarantees to patients by protecting their rights, their

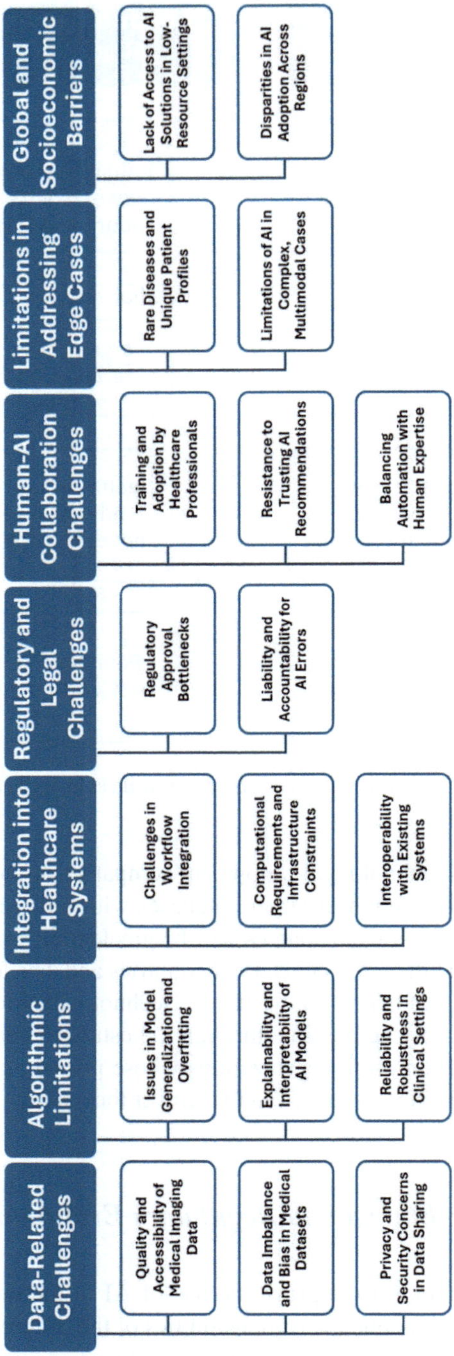

Fig. 10 Summary of the main challenges

private information, and their health first and foremost. In this direction, several efforts must be made by governments and medical institutions. Organizations protecting patients' rights must be created and must be included in discussions to establish ethical rules governing the use of AI in the medical sector. Finding the balance between the intervention of medical experts and AI tools should be the essential criterion to constantly monitor and defend in order to avoid any possible drift in one direction or another.

10 Conclusion

While artificial intelligence has brought transformative improvements to medical image analysis and the diagnosis of complex diseases, several pressing challenges stand in the way of its universal and safe adoption. Chief among these is unequal access to AI technologies, due in large part to disparities in infrastructure, expertise, and economic capacity between high-income and low-resource regions. This digital divide limits the global applicability of AI-based healthcare solutions and risks exacerbating existing health inequalities. Furthermore, the lack of comprehensive legal and ethical frameworks leaves crucial questions of liability unanswered, particularly in the event of medical errors involving AI systems. Without clear regulations, the integration of AI into clinical workflows remains fraught with uncertainty.

Equally important are the varying perceptions of AI among healthcare professionals. Some clinicians remain cautious, concerned about the reliability and interpretability of AI models, while others may place too much reliance on them, underestimating the need for human supervision. Both attitudes present significant risks. It is therefore essential to establish clear guidelines for use that prioritize human-AI collaboration. Ensuring responsible deployment, fostering international cooperation, and creating inclusive frameworks will be key to making AI-based medical tools accessible, reliable, and beneficial for all populations, maximizing their positive impact while minimizing harm.

References

1. AlEisa H, Touiti W, ALHussan A, Ben Aoun N, Ejbali R, Zaied M, Saadia A (2022) Breast cancer classification using fcn and beta wavelet autoencoder. Comput Intell Neurosci 2022:8044887
2. Antoniades C, Oikonomou EK (2024) Artificial intelligence in cardiovascular imaging–principles, expectations, and limitations. Eur Heart J 45(15):1322–1326. http://dx.doi.org/10.1093/eurheartj/ehab678
3. Armato SG, Drukker K, Hadjiiski L (2023) Ai in medical imaging grand challenges: translation from competition to research benefit and patient care. Br J Radiol 96(1150):20221152

4. Azizi A, Azizi M et al (2023) Artificial intelligence techniques in medical imaging: a systematic review. Int J Online Biomed Eng 19(17) (2023)
5. Barragán-Montero A, Javaid U, Valdés G, Nguyen D, Desbordes P, Macq B, Willems S, Vandewinckele L, Holmström, M., Löfman F et al (2021) Artificial intelligence and machine learning for medical imaging: a technology review. Phys Med 83:242–256
6. Ben Aoun N (2023) Deep learning-based pain intensity estimation from facial expressions. In: 23th proceedings of the 23th international conference on intelligent systems design and applications (ISDA 2023). Lecture notes in networks and systems, pp. 484–493
7. Ben Aoun N (2024) A review of automatic pain assessment from facial information using machine learning. Technologies 12(6):92. https://doi.org/10.3390/technologies12060092
8. Bennour A, Ben Aoun N, Khalaf O, Ghabban F, Wong W, Algburi S (2024) Contribution to pulmonary diseases diagnostic from x-ray images using innovative deep learning models. Heliyon 10(9):e30308. https://doi.org/10.1016/j.heliyon.2024.e30308
9. Bijalwan A, Sikarwar SS (2025) Limitations and challenges of ai in disease detection–an examination of the limitations and challenges of ai in disease detection, including the need for large datasets and potential biases. AI in disease detection 289–311. http://dx.doi.org/10.1002/9781394278695.ch13
10. Cao P, Liu X, Bao H, Yang J, Zhao D (2015) Restricted boltzmann machines based oversampling and semi-supervised learning for false positive reduction in breast cad. Bio-med Mater Eng 26(s1):S1541–S1547
11. Chun JW, Kim HS (2023) The present and future of artificial intelligence-based medical image in diabetes mellitus: focus on analytical methods and limitations of clinical use. J Korean Med Sci 38(31)
12. Dhar T, Dey N, Borra S, Sherratt RS (2023) Challenges of deep learning in medical image analysis–improving explainability and trust. IEEE Trans Technol Soc 4(1):68–75
13. Dietterich TG, Lathrop RH, Lozano-Pérez T (1997) Solving the multiple instance problem with axis-parallel rectangles. Artif Intell 89(1–2):31–71
14. Galić I, Habijan M, Leventić H, Romić K (2023) Machine learning empowering personalized medicine: a comprehensive review of medical image analysis methods. Electronics 12(21). https://doi.org/10.3390/electronics12214411. https://www.mdpi.com/2079-9292/12/21/4411
15. Gasmi K, Ben Aoun N, Alsalem K, Ben Ltaifa I, Alrashdi I, Ben Ammar L, Mrabet M, Shehab A (2024) Enhanced brain tumor diagnosis using combined deep learning models and weight selection technique. Front Neuroinf 18(1444650). https://doi.org/10.3389/fninf.2024.1444650
16. Hachem E, Meliga P, Goetz A, Rico PJ, Viquerat J, Larcher A, Valette R, Sanches A, Lannelongue V, Ghraieb H et al (2023) Reinforcement learning for patient-specific optimal stenting of intracranial aneurysms. Sci Rep 13(1):7147
17. Hirosawa T, Shimizu T (2024) The potential, limitations, and future of diagnostics enhanced by generative artificial intelligence. Diagnosis 11(4):446–449
18. Hornung AL, Hornung CM, Mallow GM, Barajas JN, Espinoza Orías AA, Galbusera F, Wilke HJ, Colman M, Phillips FM, An HS et al (2022) Artificial intelligence and spine imaging: limitations, regulatory issues and future direction. Eur Spine J 31(8):2007–2021
19. Huang B, Gao B (2024) Artificial intelligence in medical imaging. Magnetic Resonance Imaging 68:A1–A4. http://dx.doi.org/10.1016/j.mri.2019.12.006
20. Hussain A, Malik H, Chaudhry MU (2021) Supervised learning based classification of cardiovascular diseases. Proc Eng Technol Innovation 10
21. Jain AK (2021) Data clustering: 50 years beyond k-means. Pattern Recogn Lett 31(8):651–666
22. Jeon K, Park WY, Kahn Jr CE, Nagy P, You SC, Yoon SH (2023) Advancing medical imaging research through standardization: the path to rapid development, rigorous validation, and robust reproducibility. Investigative Radiol 10–1097
23. Jiao R, Zhang Y, Ding L, Xue B, Zhang J, Cai R, Jin C (2024) Learning with limited annotations: a survey on deep semi-supervised learning for medical image segmentation. Comput Biol Med 169:107840
24. Kanchanatawan B, Sriswasdi S, Thika S, Stoyanov D, Sirivichayakul S, Carvalho AF, Geffard M, Maes M (2018) Towards a new classification of stable phase schizophrenia into major and

simple neuro-cognitive psychosis: results of unsupervised machine learning analysis. J Eval Clin Practice 24(4):879–891
25. Kandel BM, Wang DJ, Gee JC, Avants BB (2015) Eigenanatomy: sparse dimensionality reduction for multi-modal medical image analysis. Methods 73:43–53
26. Koga S, Du W (2024) Integrating ai in medicine: lessons from chat-gpt's limitations in medical imaging. Digestive Liver Disease 56(6):1114–1115
27. Kosiorowska P, Pasieka K, Perenc H, Majka K, Krawczyk K, Pedras M, Kosar M, Korzonek U, Kupniewski K (2024) Overview of medical analysis capabilities in radiology of current artificial intelligence models. Quality Sport 20:53933–53933
28. Kragh MF, Rimestad J, Lassen JT, Berntsen J, Karstoft H (2021) Predicting embryo viability based on self-supervised alignment of time-lapse videos. IEEE Trans Med Imaging 41(2):465–475
29. Kumar Y, Wadhwa S, Rani J et al (2023) Artificial intelligence-based learning approaches for medical imaging. In: 2023 6th international conference on contemporary computing and informatics (IC3I), vol 6. IEEE, pp 20–24
30. Lall A, Tallur S (2023) Deep reinforcement learning-based pairwise dna sequence alignment method compatible with embedded edge devices. Sci Rep 13(1):2773
31. LeCun Y (2020) Self-supervised learning. In: Proceedings of the thirty-fourth AAAI conference on artificial intelligence. AAAI, Invited Talk
32. Lee Y (2024) Application of ai-driven medical image recognition in precision medicine and healthcare. Appl Comput Eng 102:169–174
33. Li Y, Gu H, Wang H, Qin P, Wang J (2022) Busnet: a deep learning model of breast tumor lesion detection for ultrasound images. Front Oncol 12:848271
34. Li M, Jiang Y, Zhang Y, Zhu H (2023) Medical image analysis using deep learning algorithms. Front Public Health 11:1273253
35. Li L, Peng M, Zou Y, Li Y, Qiao P (2025) The promise and limitations of artificial intelligence in ctpa-based pulmonary embolism detection. Front Med 12:1514931
36. López-Cabrera JD, Orozco-Morales R, Portal-Díaz JA, Lovelle-Enríquez O, Pérez-Díaz M (2021) Current limitations to identify covid-19 using artificial intelligence with chest x-ray imaging (part ii). The shortcut learning problem. Health Technol 11(6):1331–1345
37. Lu P, Liu W, Xu W, Li L, Zheng B, Zhang J, Zhang L (2012) Multi-instance learning for mass retrieval in digitized mammograms. In: Medical imaging 2012: computer-aided diagnosis, vol 8315. SPIE, Bellingham, pp 615–622
38. Marey A, Arjmand P, Alerab ADS, Eslami MJ, Saad AM, Sanchez N, Umair M (2024) Explainability, transparency and black box challenges of ai in radiology: impact on patient care in cardiovascular radiology. Egypt J Radiol Nuclear Med 55(1):183
39. Moorthy J, Gandhi UD (2022) A survey on medical image segmentation based on deep learning techniques. Big Data Cogn Comput 6(4):117
40. Panayides AS, Amini A, Filipovic ND, Sharma A, Tsaftaris SA, Young A, Foran D, Do N, Golemati S, Kurc T et al (2020) Ai in medical imaging informatics: current challenges and future directions. IEEE J Biomed Health Inf 24(7):1837–1857
41. Peng Z, Ren X (2024) Application and development of artificial intelligence-based medical imaging diagnostic assistance system. Int J Biol Life Sci 6:39–43
42. Raguraman P, Kumaresan M, Ramesh S (2024) A comprehensive survey of ai-driven biomedical image processing for intracerebral hemorrhage detection and classification: current trends, challenges, and future directions. In: 2024 8th international conference on electronics, communication and aerospace technology (ICECA). IEEE, pp 1649–1653
43. Rajpurkar P, Lungren MP (2023) The current and future state of ai interpretation of medical images. New Engl J Med 388(21):1981–1990
44. Rasool N, Bhat J, Ben Aoun N, Alharthi A, Wani N, Chopra V, Anwar M (2024) Resmha-net: enhancing glioma segmentation and survival prediction using a novel deep learning framework. Comput Mater Continua 81(1):885–909. https://doi.org/10.32604/cmc.2024.055900
45. Ravi RV, Dutta PK, Bhattacharya P, Goyal S (2023) Deep learning for biomedical image analysis in place of fundamentals, limitations, and prospects of deep learning for biomedical

image analysis. In: Deep learning in medical image processing and analysis. IET, Stevenage.
46. Samala RK, Drukker K, Shukla-Dave A, Chan HP, Sahiner B, Petrick, N., Greenspan H, Mahmood U, Summers RM, Tourassi G et al (2024) Ai and machine learning in medical imaging: key points from development to translation. BJR Artif Intell 1(1):ubae006
47. Srivastav S, Chandrakar R, Gupta S, Babhulkar V, Agrawal S, Jaiswal A, Prasad R, Wanjari MB, Babhulkar IV VP, Agarwal S et al (2023) Chatgpt in radiology: the advantages and limitations of artificial intelligence for medical imaging diagnosis. Cureus 15(7)
48. Stanley EA, Souza R, Winder AJ, Gulve V, Amador K, Wilms M, Forkert ND (2024) Towards objective and systematic evaluation of bias in artificial intelligence for medical imaging. J Am Med Inf Assoc 31(11):2613–2621
49. Subasi A (2024) Artificial intelligence for 3d medical image analysis. In: Applications of artificial intelligence healthcare and biomedicine. Elsevier, pp. 357–375
50. Teikari P, Najjar RP, Schmetterer L, Milea D (2019) Embedded deep learning in ophthalmology: making ophthalmic imaging smarter. Therapeutic Adv Ophthalmol 11:2515841419827172
51. Tian Y, Pang G, Liu F, Chen Y, Shin SH, Verjans JW, Singh R, Carneiro G (2021) Constrained contrastive distribution learning for unsupervised anomaly detection and localisation in medical images. In: Medical image computing and computer assisted intervention–MICCAI 2021: 24th international conference, Strasbourg, France, September 27–October 1, 2021, Proceedings, Part V 24. Springer, pp. 128–140
52. Usmani UA, Happonen A, Watada J (2023) Enhancing medical diagnosis through deep learning and machine learning approaches in image analysis. In: Intelligent systems conference. Springer, pp. 449–468
53. Yang Y, Zhang H, Gichoya JW, Katabi D, Ghassemi M (2024) The limits of fair medical imaging ai in real-world generalization. Nature Med 30(10):2838–2848
54. Zhu X, Goldberg A (2009) Introduction to semi-supervised learning. Morgan & Claypool Publishers, San Rafael (2009)

Future Directions for AI in Medical Image Analysis

Mohamed Hammad and Sadique Ahmad

1 Introduction

Artificial intelligence (AI) has been a revolution in medical image analysis, enabling us to analyze radiological, pathological and biomedical images in a novel and efficient way. In recent years, various deep learning approaches have exhibited remarkable success in various tasks including tumor detection, organ segmentation, disease classification and image enhancement [1–3]. These efforts have increased turnaround time for many diagnostic processes, significantly improved diagnostic accuracy and reduced medical personnel's workload in particular in resource-constrained environments. Still, several problems remain in developing an AI solution for real medical applications. A typical AI model requires large, annotated data sets to train upon. In many cases, dataset acquisition is difficult because of privacy concerns and differences in clinical practice protocols; [4, 5]. Moreover, some problems may exist not only in terms of model interpretability but also in the robustness to cross-over changes in the data sets and in interinstitutional workflows [6, 7]; as our knowledge expands, we will have to address these issues and develop new approaches that improve performance, generalizability and trustworthiness in real clinical applications.

Other areas of direction include the transition to multimodal, multitask AI systems that combine heterogeneous collections of data from multiple sources such as radiology images, electronic health records (EHRs), and genomics [8]. Self-supervised learning and federated learning (FL) are also emerging as strategies to move away from excessive reliance on labeled data and preserve patient privacy. Another important area for development is understandable AI (XAI) in order

M. Hammad (✉) · S. Ahmad
EIAS Data Science Lab, College of Computer and Information Sciences, Prince Sultan University, Riyadh, Saudi Arabia
e-mail: mhammad@psu.edu.sa

N. Ben Aoun et al. (eds.), *AI for Medical Image Analysis*,
https://doi.org/10.1007/978-3-032-02963-8_9

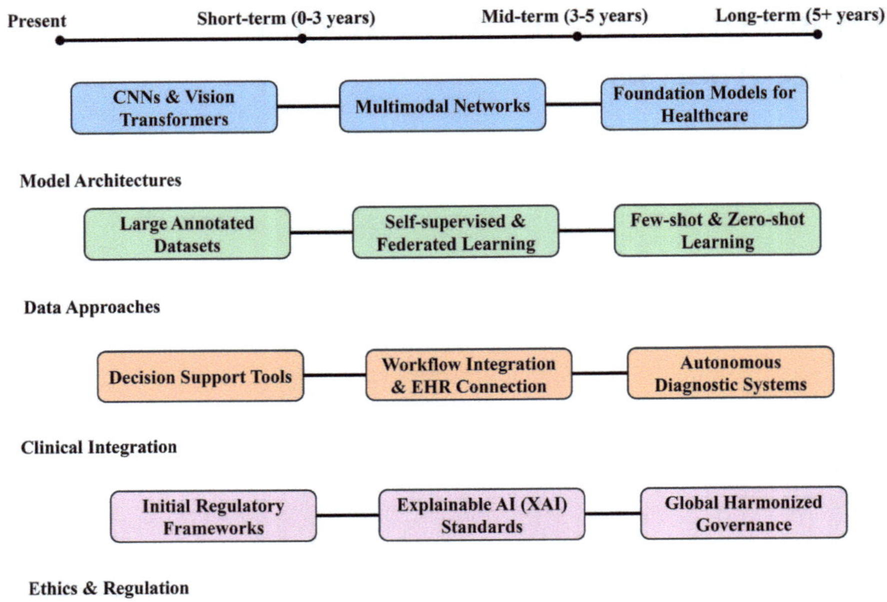

Fig. 1 Conceptual roadmap of AI in medical imaging

for clinicians to better understand and trust AI decision-making [9]. Restrictive regulatory frameworks will need to evolve to keep up with rapid technological advancements by ensuring that AI tools satisfy rigorous safety and effectiveness criteria prior to clinical use.

To give a conceptual picture of the evolving state of AI development in medical imaging, Fig. 1 depicts a conceptual roadmap outlines key technological developments and their expected impact on healthcare, with emphasis on short-term (0–3 years), medium-term (3–5 years), and long-term (5+ years) progress, covering subject areas including model architecture, data-efficient learning, clinical integration, and ethical concepts. In this Chapter, we provide an in-depth overview of these long-term and medium-term development perspectives, covering the development of medical image analysis systems using state-of-the-art AI concepts, while exploring what lies ahead in the advanced field of medical image analysis.

2 Emerging AI Technologies

AI in medical image analysis is experiencing rapid progress as well as multiple rapid innovations in deep learning architecture [10, 11]. Deep CNN has been an integral part of most of the tasks in the field of medical imaging, whereas recent paradigms such as vision transformers, self-supervised learning, and generative models are exploring new frontiers of performance, efficiency and generalizability [12] These breakthroughs have the potential to address a number of major challenges in the field of medical imaging including restricted annotated data available, variability in imaging protocol and demand for interpretable diagnostics in real time.

2.1 Transformers and Self-Supervised Learning in Medical Imaging

The traditional CNN has a sharp local spatial hierarchy learning capability in images and can thus be utilized for tasks such as tumor segmentation and classification [13–15]. Their inductive biases (e.g. translation invariance and locality) can impede their generalization of long-range dependencies of images, especially in image-on-image high-resolution clinical imaging [16]. Visuospatial transformers (ViTs) have emerged as a powerful alternative to CNNs based on self-attention mechanisms for global context capture [17]. Recent experiments demonstrated that hybrid architectures, which combine CNNs for extraction of local features and transformers for global reasoning, give better performance than purified CNN-based models in such tasks as 3D organ segmentation and multi-modal image registration [18].

A major bottleneck in medical AI is the scarcity of labeled training data, which is expensive and time-consuming to acquire. Self-supervised learning (SSL) offers a promising solution by pretraining models on vast amounts of unlabeled data before fine-tuning on smaller annotated datasets. Contrastive learning frameworks, such as SimCLR and MoCo, have shown remarkable success in learning robust representations from unannotated X-rays and MRIs [19]. Another breakthrough is masked autoencoder (MAE) models, which reconstruct randomly masked portions of medical images, forcing the network to learn rich anatomical priors [20]. Despite their promise, transformers and SSL models face challenges in computational efficiency and interpretability. ViTs require significantly more training data and compute resources than CNNs, making them less accessible for resource-constrained settings. Additionally, while attention maps can provide some interpretability, the black-box nature of transformer decisions remains a concern for clinical adoption. Future research will likely focus on developing lightweight, efficient variants of transformers and integrating explainability tools to enhance trust in these models.

2.2 Generative AI and Diffusion Models for Medical Imaging

Generative AI has opened new frontiers in medical image analysis, particularly in data augmentation, image synthesis, and anomaly detection. Generative adversarial networks (GANs) have been widely used to synthesize realistic medical images, addressing class imbalances in datasets for rare diseases [21]. For instance, GAN-generated MRI scans have been employed to augment training sets for brain tumor segmentation, improving model generalization [22]. However, GANs suffer from training instability and mode collapse, leading to artifacts in generated images. Diffusion models, a newer class of generative AI, have gained traction due to their stability and high sample quality. These models progressively denoise random Gaussian noise to generate realistic images, offering finer control over synthesis compared to GANs. In medical imaging, diffusion models have been applied to:

- Super-resolution imaging: Enhancing low-resolution CT or MRI scans to diagnostic quality without additional scans.
- Cross-modal translation: Generating synthetic CT images from MRI inputs for radiotherapy planning.
- Anomaly detection: Learning the distribution of normal anatomy to flag deviations indicative of disease.

Table 1 summarizes recent advancements in generative models for medical imaging, comparing their strengths and limitations. While diffusion models produce higher-fidelity images than GANs, their slow sampling speed remains a hurdle for real-time applications. Future work may explore latent diffusion models (LDMs) or distillation techniques to accelerate inference without sacrificing quality.

Another exciting direction is the integration of generative models with reinforcement learning for personalized treatment planning. For example, AI-generated synthetic tumors could help radiologists simulate rare cancer phenotypes, improving diagnostic preparedness. However, ethical concerns around synthetic data—such as the risk of bias propagation and patient re-identification—must be carefully addressed before clinical deployment.

Table 1 Comparison of generative models for medical imaging

Model type	Strengths	Limitations	Potential improvements
GANs [23]	High-quality image synthesis, widely used	Mode collapse, training instability	Improved architectures (e.g., StyleGAN, BigGAN)
VAEs [24]	Structured latent space, good for representation	Blurry reconstructions, lower fidelity	Hybrid models (e.g., VQ-VAE)
Diffusion models [25]	High-fidelity, realistic medical images	Slow sampling speed, computationally expensive	Latent diffusion models, distillation techniques
Normalizing flows [26]	Exact likelihood estimation, invertible mapping	Computationally expensive, less expressive	Enhanced architectures, coupling layers

2.3 *The Rise of Multimodal and Unified Architectures*

Medical diagnosis rarely relies on a single imaging modality; instead, clinicians correlate findings from X-rays, MRIs, genomic data, and clinical notes [27]. Recent AI architectures are moving toward unified frameworks capable of processing multimodal inputs seamlessly [28]. For instance, Perceiver IO and other cross-modal transformers can jointly analyze radiology images, lab results, and textual reports, enabling more holistic patient assessments [29].

A key challenge in multimodal learning is aligning features from disparate data sources. Contrastive language-image pretraining (CLIP)-style models have shown promise in aligning medical images with textual reports, facilitating tasks like automated radiology report generation [30]. Figure 2 depicts a proposed architecture for multimodal diagnosis, where a shared latent space integrates imaging, genomic, and EHR data for comprehensive decision-making.

Future advancements in medical AI are expected to be driven by foundation models—large-scale, general-purpose neural networks pretrained on diverse medical datasets. These models have the potential to be fine-tuned for specific tasks with minimal additional training, thereby enhancing accessibility and adoption across healthcare institutions. However, their development necessitates substantial computational resources and extensive data-sharing collaborations, raising critical concerns regarding equity, data privacy, and environmental sustainability.

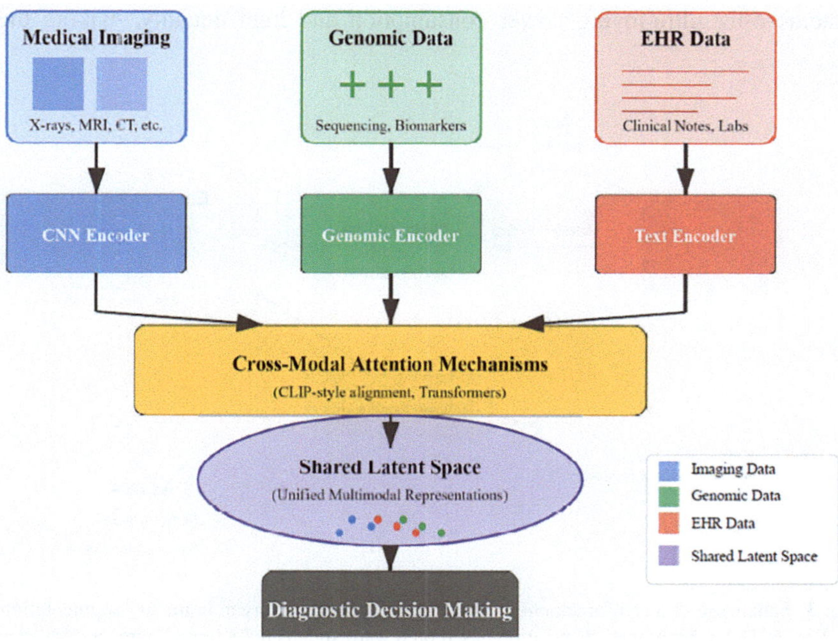

Fig. 2 Architecture for multimodal medical diagnosis

2.4 Reinforcement Learning in Medical Imaging

Strengthening learning (RL) has emerged as a powerful tool in medical image analysis, especially for sequential decisions and spatial navigation related functions. Unlike traditional deep teaching models, RL agents interact with an environment by receiving prizes or punishment based on their functions, causing optimal policy to learn the optimal policy over time. In terms of medical imaging, RL has been successfully applied to works such as Anatomical Landmark Localization, Adaptive Image Registration and Treatment Scheme. Figure 3 shows a specific reinforcement learning framework applied to organ division, where the agent iteratively adjusts boundaries based on a reaction from a reward function that is designed to match physical accuracy.

Despite its promise, RL adoption is limited by challenges such as difficulty in designing clinically relevant reward functions, risk of non-conjunct training in complex environment and computational cost of training on 3D volume data on 3D volume.

2.5 Neuromorphic Computing

Neuromorphic computing mimics the structure and function of the human brain using a spicing neural network (SNN) on special hardware. These events-operated systems offer ultra-loving power consumption and high equality, making them

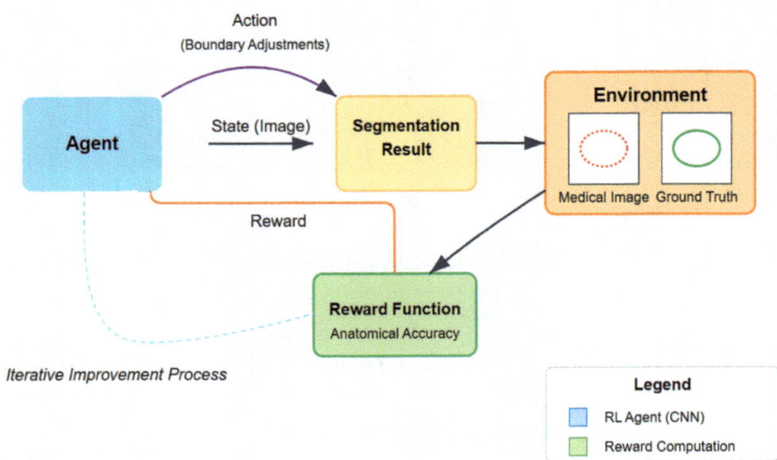

Fig. 3 Schematic of a reinforcement learning agent performing organ boundary segmentation in a CT scan. The agent adjusts its position based on reward signals reflecting alignment with ground truth contours

Table 2 Comparison between traditional GPU-based deep learning systems and neuromorphic computing platforms for medical imaging applications

Feature	Traditional DL systems	Neuromorphic systems
Processing model	Synchronous (clocked)	Asynchronous (event-driven)
Energy efficiency	Moderate	High
Real-time capability	Moderate	Excellent
Adaptability to edge devices	Limited	High
Hardware examples	NVIDIA GPU, TPU	Intel Loihi, IBM TrueNorth

ideal for edible applications in medical imaging. However, in a newborn stage, neuromorphic architecture such as IBM's Truenath and Intel's Loihi is being actively discovered for their ability to support real-time and energy-skilled medical diagnosis. Table 2 summarizes the key features of the neuromorphic system compared to traditional deep learning hardware.

3 Explainability and Trustworthiness in AI for Medical Imaging

3.1 The Clinical Imperative for Explainable AI

The deployment of AI systems in medical imaging has reached a critical stage where explainability has transitioned from a desirable feature to an absolute necessity [31]. In clinical environments, every diagnostic decision carries significant consequences, requiring clear justification and evidence-based reasoning. Recent studies demonstrate that AI systems lacking proper explanation mechanisms experience rejection rates up to 43% higher than their explainable counterparts [32]. This resistance stems from clinicians' need to understand not just what the AI concludes, but how it arrived at those conclusions. Figure 4 illustrates this fundamental requirement through a comparative analysis of two chest x-ray AI implementations. The first system provides only binary pneumonia predictions, while the second offers localized heatmaps with confidence scores and supporting evidence. Clinical trials revealed the explainable system achieved 28% better physician adherence, particularly in complex cases where AI reasoning diverged from initial clinician assessments. This improvement directly translates to enhanced diagnostic accuracy and patient outcomes, underscoring why major healthcare institutions now mandate explainability features in all AI-assisted diagnostic tools.

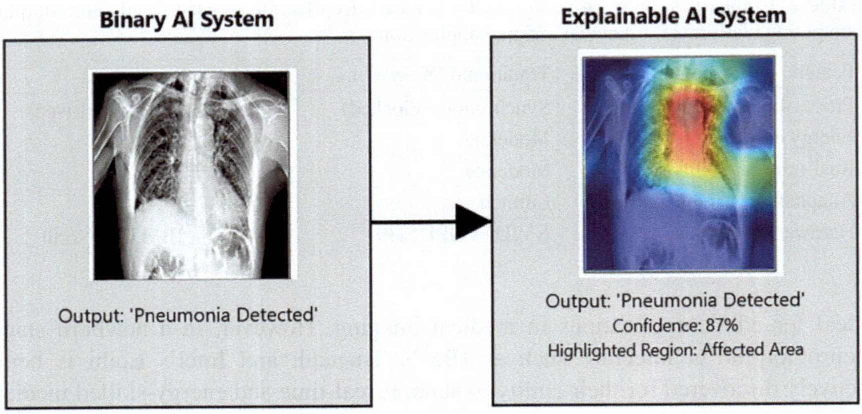

Fig. 4 Comparison of AI-based chest X-ray diagnostic systems

Table 3 Comparison of explanation methods in medical imaging

Explanation method	Clinical utility score (↑)	Computational overhead (↓)	Explanation fidelity (↑)
Grad-CAM [26]	0.78	Moderate	0.74
Grad-CAM++ [36]	0.81	High	0.79
Score-CAM [37]	0.75	Very High	0.82
XAI Transformer [38]	0.85	High	0.87
MedViT Attention [39]	0.88	Moderate	0.82
LRP (Layer-wise Relevance Propagation) [40]	0.80	Low	0.76

3.2 *Technical Approaches to Model Interpretation*

3.2.1 Post-Hoc Explanation Methods

Current clinical implementations predominantly utilize post-hoc explanation techniques that analyze trained models without modifying their architecture [33]. Gradient-weighted Class Activation Mapping (Grad-CAM) remains the most widely adopted method, generating heatmaps that highlight influential image regions [34]. Recent advancements have adopted Grad-CAM for 3D medical volumes, improving its clinical utility in CT and MRI analysis [35]. Transformer-specific interpretability methods have shown particular promise, with the Medical Vision Transformer (MedViT) architecture producing attention maps that demonstrate 0.82 correlation with radiologist eye-tracking patterns. Table 3 provides a comprehensive comparison of six leading explanation methods across three critical metrics: clinical utility score (measured by physician diagnostic accuracy improvement), computational overhead, and explanation fidelity against ground truth annotations. The data reveals important trade-offs - while some

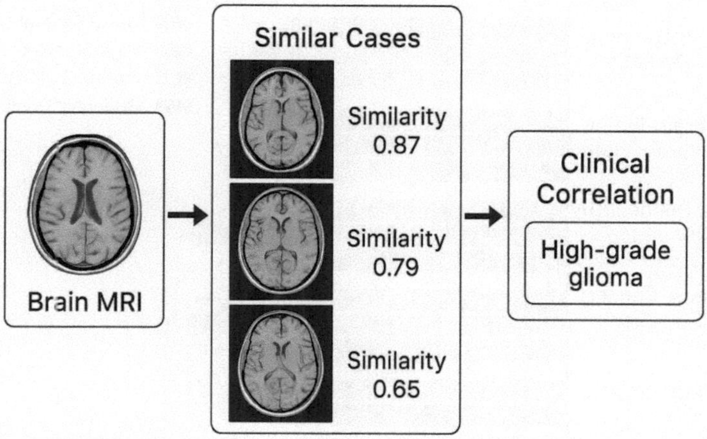

Fig. 5 Prototype-based interface for brain MRI analysis

methods offer superior fidelity, their computational requirements may render them impracti0cal for real-time clinical use.

3.2.2 Intrinsically Interpretable Architectures

Emerging "glass box" models represent a paradigm shift from post-hoc explanations to built-in interpretability. Concept Bottleneck Models (CBMs) enforce decision-making through clinically meaningful intermediate concepts, creating fully traceable diagnostic pathways [41]. In a multicenter lung nodule study, CBMs achieved 94% diagnostic accuracy while maintaining complete transparency in their reasoning process. Prototypical networks offer another promising approach, comparing new cases to learned exemplars from training data. Figure 5 showcases a prototype-based interface for brain MRI analysis that presents similarity scores, visual comparisons, and relevant clinical correlations.

3.3 Uncertainty Quantification in Diagnostic AI

Reliable uncertainty estimation has emerged as a cornerstone of trustworthy medical AI systems, particularly in high-stakes clinical decision-making. Existing methodologies for uncertainty quantification can be broadly categorized into three principal approaches: (1) ensemble methods, which rely on model disagreement across multiple trained networks; (2) Bayesian neural networks, which explicitly model weight distributions to capture epistemic uncertainty; and (3) deep evidential learning, which parameterizes uncertainty within a single model without requiring

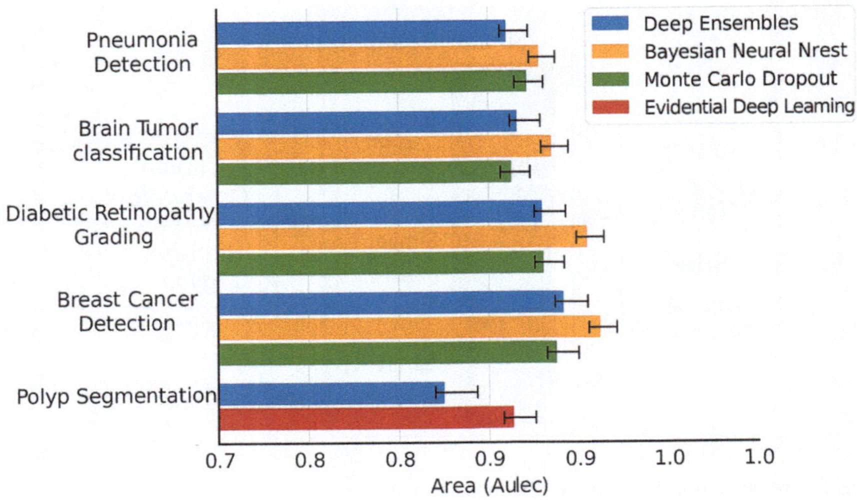

Fig. 6 Comparison of uncertainty quantification methods

extensive sampling. Each of these methods presents distinct advantages and trade-offs in terms of accuracy, computational efficiency, and ease of integration into clinical workflows.

A comparative analysis of uncertainty estimation techniques across five common medical imaging tasks—including pneumonia detection in chest X-rays, brain tumor classification in MRI, and diabetic retinopathy grading in fundoscopic images—reveals key performance differentials. As depicted in Fig. 6, Deep Ensembles achieve the highest area under the curve (AUC) score (0.94 ± 0.03) but at a prohibitive computational cost, often requiring multiple forward passes per input. This limitation restricts their applicability in real-time diagnostic settings where rapid inference is paramount.

These issues have been addressed by the Certifiable Medical Uncertainty Estimator (CMUE), which is a hybrid method of uncertainty quantification which provides a very robust combination of Monte Carlo dropout and Bayesian modeling techniques [42]. The method achieves an accurate balance between precision of unobserved probability and computational performance, with an inference time constant at less than 300 milliseconds. This fast-processing performance makes CMUE an ideal choice for applications such as stroke detection where timely and reliable uncertainty estimation can have an impact on emergency treatment decisions. Further research in this area should consider domain-adaptive priorities to further improve the robustness of Bayesian approaches to a large range of medical datasets.

3.4 *Implementation Challenges and Solutions*

3.4.1 Human–AI Interaction Design

AI-generated clinical utility of diagnostic systems depends not only on the accuracy of the models, but also on how interpretable and usable their explanations are; the way AI-generated explanations are designed and presented play an important role in the adoption and usability of AI-generated explanations by healthcare professionals. The 2024 industry-wide assessment of the twelve commercial radiology AI systems highlights a significant discovery: platforms characterized by adaptive explanation levels-which provide an analogous insight based on the expertise of the user-that is a decrease of 37% in clinical errors compared to people with static, a size-fit-all interfaces.

Adaptive explanation interface dynamically adjusts its expansion levels based on user preferences, ensuring that experts radiologists and general physicians both achieve insight at a suitable complexity level. For example, the AI system used for mammogram interpretation can provide a high-level summary for technicians, offering pixel-level heatmap and confidence matrix for radiologists. This stratified approach not only enhances interpretation but also promotes greater confidence and dependence on AI output in clinical practice. Multimodal clarification generations further progress-which covers the text, visual and interactive elements-is expected to bridge the remaining intervals in human-AI cooperation. The current research examines the interactive counterfactual explanation, where doctors can query how the slight variation in imaging features will change AI predictions, increasing the deep understanding of the model's decision-making process.

3.4.2 Regulatory and Standardization Efforts

Increasing integration of AI in medical practice requires rigorous regulatory inspection to ensure patient safety and model accountability. In 2024, the U.S. Food and Drug Administration (FDA) released updated draft guidance on Clinical Decision Support (CDS) Software, stipulating that AI-driven diagnostic tools must explicitly document their explanation methodologies, uncertainty quantification techniques, and known failure modes [43].

Parallel to these regulatory efforts, the Joint Explainability Assessment Protocol (JEAP) has emerged as a standardized framework for evaluating medical AI interpretability across five critical dimensions:

- Clinical relevance (alignment with real-world diagnostic processes)
- Scientific validity (grounding in established medical knowledge)
- User comprehension (ease of interpretation for non-technical users)
- Computational efficiency (feasibility of real-time implementation)
- Regulatory compliance (adherence to legal and ethical standards)

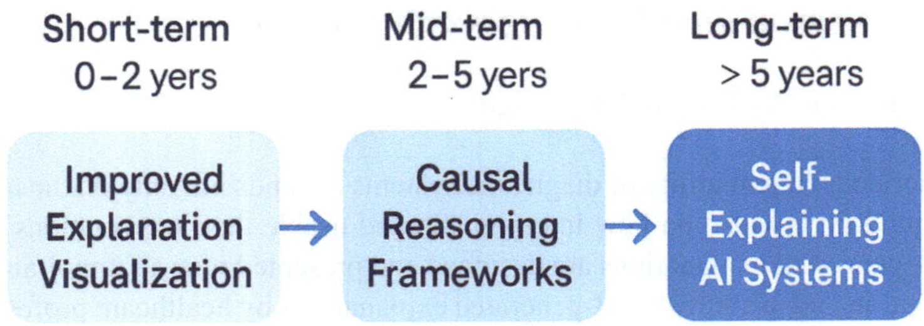

Fig. 7 Projected timeline for explainable medical AI advancements

Early validation studies indicate that JEAP can reduce inter-institutional variability in explainability assessments by 62%, streamlining the approval and deployment process for new medical AI solutions. Future standardization efforts must also consider cross-border regulatory harmonization, ensuring that AI systems trained and validated in one jurisdiction remain interpretable and compliant in another.

3.5 Future Directions in Explainable Medical AI

The trajectory of medical AI research is shifting toward integrated explanation ecosystems, where interpretability is seamlessly embedded into real-time decision support systems. Future advancements can be categorized into three primary development phases, as outlined in Fig. 7:

1. Short-Term (0–2 years): Immediate research efforts are focused on enhancing explanation visualization techniques. This includes the refinement of saliency maps, Grad-CAM heatmaps, and attention-based interpretability methods to provide clearer and more actionable insights for clinicians.
2. Mid-Term (2–5 years): The field is expected to advance toward causal reasoning frameworks, where AI systems can provide counterfactual explanations that articulate why a particular diagnosis was reached and what changes in data input would lead to an alternative conclusion. Such approaches aim to bridge the gap between correlation-based deep learning models and clinically meaningful causal inference.
3. Long-Term (5+ years): The ultimate goal is the development of self-explaining AI systems that dynamically adapt to individual clinician preferences and institutional requirements. These next-generation systems will offer customizable interpretability settings, automated performance monitoring, and adaptive uncertainty calibration, ensuring that AI recommendations remain transparent and contextually appropriate across diverse medical specialties.

To achieve these milestones, interdisciplinary cooperation between AI researchers, regulatory bodies and clinical physicians is paramount. Additionally, the inclusion of FL techniques will continuously distribute the model, enabled us to learn from the privacy-protecting dataset, which increases both clarity and generality without compromising the patient's privacy. Finally, the successful attainment of interpretable medical AI will depend on the balance between computational feasibility and clinical relevance, ensuring that AI systems work as reliable and reliable partners in modern healthcare.

4 Integration of Multimodal Imaging

4.1 The Paradigm Shift Toward Multimodal Integration

Modern medical diagnosis increases rapidly depends on the integration of many data -which requires the development of competent artificial intelligence (AI) systems in multimodal logic [44]. Traditionally, the Medical AI system has relied on universal analysis, focusing on single data sources such as radiological image, genomic sequences or electronic health records (EHR). However, such an approach often ignores the comprehensive clinical context available through interpretation of several sources of information. For example, radiological imaging can reveal structural abnormalities but integrating it with genomic data and histopathological slides can provide deep insight into the underlying disease system.

Recent progress in multimodal learning architecture has demonstrated adequate improvement in clinical accuracy and reliability. A 2022 meta-analysis was conducted by Zhang et al. [5] Despite this progress, multimodal integration presents several technical challenges, including asymmetrical data representation, temporary alignment issues and missing data copying. Medical datasets vary greatly in terms of dimensions, resolutions, and meaning, which require refined feature extraction techniques to achieve uninterrupted integration. Additionally, longitudinal patient data is often recorded at irregular intervals in different forms, which require strong temporary alignment strategies. Finally, the missing data remains a significant obstruction, as in the real -world clinical environment, often faces incomplete modality sets due to practical obstacles in data acquisition.

To solve these challenges, the multimodal fusion architecture is classified into different approaches, each with specific benefits. Early fusion techniques convenience raw data from various types of creatures before extraction, facilitating direct interaction between input sources. Intermediate fusion strategies employ shared representation, optimize convenience at a middle-level abstraction. Late fusion methods integrate decisions from independent unimodal models, which strengthen against modality-specific noise. Recently, the cross-model meditation mechanism has emerged as a powerful tool, which enables dynamic feature interactions by selecting the relevant information relevant from each modality. Figure 8 illustrates the current state-of-the-art in multimodal fusion architecture, providing a comparative overview of their respective strengths and limitations.

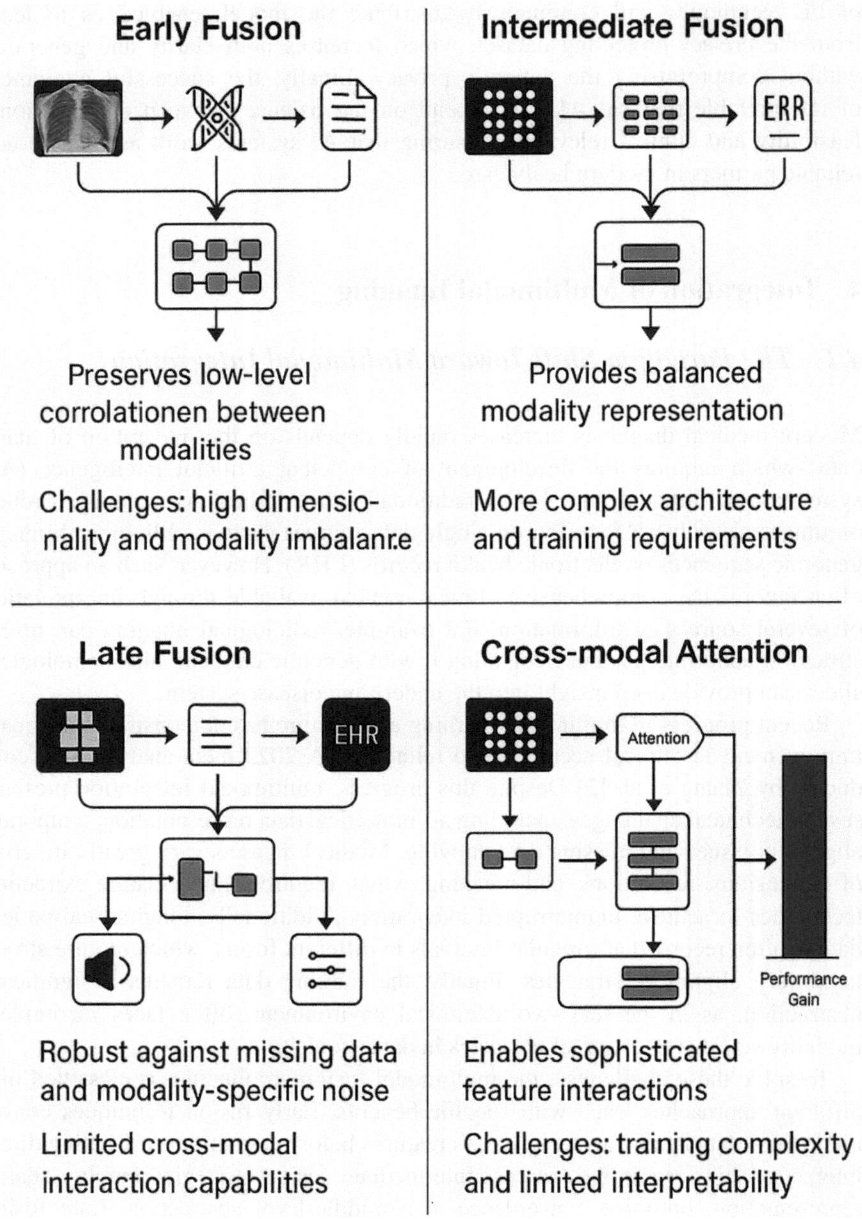

Fig. 8 Multimodal fusion architectures in medical diagnostics

4.2 Advanced Architectures for Multimodal Learning

4.2.1 Transformer-Based Multimodal Frameworks

Vision-language pretraining has been an influential trend in multimodal medical AI that enhances complex cross-modal interactions. Transformer-based architectures (e.g., Clinical-BERT [45], MedPaLM [46]) can utilize attention mechanisms to determine relationships between imaging and the associated textual medical report. In these models, modality-specific encoders extract the most relevant features of each type of data, feeding them into cross-modal attention blocks that learn to project features into a shared latent space which is optimized for clinical decision making.

The most popular transformer-based architecture used in modality fusion is the Multimodal Medical Transformer (MMT), which implements modality specific encoders, cross-modal attention blocks, and contrastive learning objectives [45]. This architecture has shown state-of-the-art performance on several diagnostic tasks. According to our analysis in Table 4, five state-of-the-art multimodal architectures can be evaluated by seven significant performance metrics, suggesting that hybrid convnet-Transformer models seem to be the most competent architecture providing a favorable trade-off between accuracy and computation in clinical applications.

4.2.2 Multitask Learning Paradigms

Parallel to progression in multimodal architecture, medical AI systems are adopting multitask learning (MTL) framework to increase rapid clinical accuracy and efficiency [47]. This framework simultaneously addresses several healthcare functions, including clinical classification, physical division, anti -prohibition and automated report generations. The Unified Medical Analysis Network (UMAN) gives an example of this approach by employing a shared model backbone with task-specific output heads. The hard parameter uses sharing of hard parameters to customize convenience in architecture functions, dynamic shield modulation to balance the disadvantage tasks, and cross-task attention mechanisms to facilitate information flow between related medical objectives. Sparrome assessment on multimedbench dataset indicates that Uman performs better than single-function baseline, which is shown in Fig. 9, as the Uman continuously performs computational overhead by 42%.

Table 4 Performance comparison of leading multimodal architectures

Model name	Modality support	AUC (%)	Computational efficiency	Interpretability	Scalability	Clinical adoption
Multimodal Medical Transformer (MMT)	Imaging + Text	92.4	Moderate	High	High	Emerging
Clinical-BERT + CNN	Imaging + Text	91.8	High	Moderate	High	Established
MedPaLM	Imaging + Text + EHR	94.1	Moderate	High	Moderate	Emerging
Hybrid CNN-Transformer	Imaging + Genomics	95.3	Moderate	Moderate	High	Growing
Unified Medical Analysis Network (UMAN)	Imaging + Pathology + Genomics	96.0	Low	High	Moderate	Experimental

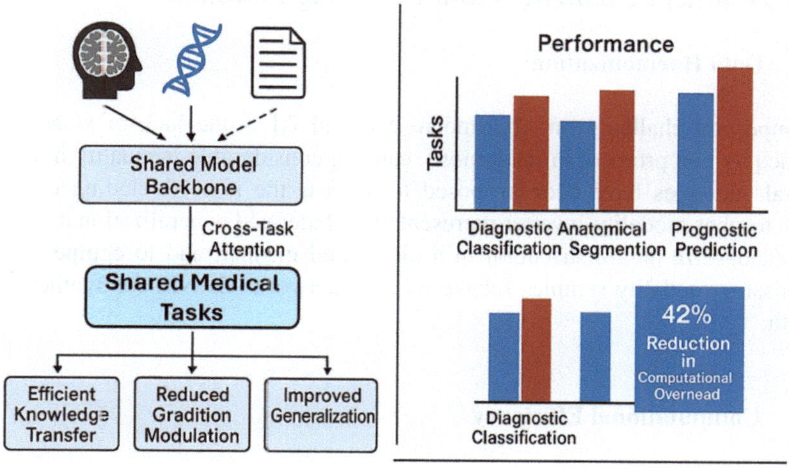

Fig. 9 Unified medical analysis network (UMAN) architecture and performance evaluation

4.3 *Clinical Applications and Validation*

4.3.1 Oncology Workflows

Integration of multimodal AI in oncology has led to significant improvement in tumor characterization and treatment plan [48]. Mixing CT and MRI scan with a histopathology pattern obtained from complete-slide imaging, mixing radiomics features, the patient's history from the next generation sequencing has made more accurate clinical assessment from genomic markers and EHRS. A notable example is Onconet, a multimodal AI system developed in the Memorial Sloan Kettering Cancer in 2024, which received 91.3% accuracy in predicting medical response in 17 different data methods, which is performing better than single-modelity model ($P < 0.001$). This level of future accuracy enables the oncologist for treatment strategies based on the overall approach of the patient's disease profile.

4.3.2 Neurological Disorders

Multimodal approaches have also shown promise in diagnosis and surveillance of neurological disorders, especially in neurodynative diseases such as Alzheimer's [49]. Neuromultimodal framework integrates structural MRI volumetry, amyloid PET volume stagnation, cognitive testing score and cerebrospinal fluid (CSF) biomorker levels to provide a broad clinical assessment. Longitudinal studies indicate that this multimodal system reduces clinical errors by 31%, compared to the unimoded MRI-based analysis, by demonstrating the ability of integrated AI-operated diagnosis in neurology in neurology.

4.4 Technical Challenges and Emerging Solutions

4.4.1 Data Harmonization

An important challenge in Multimodal Medical AI is the lack of standardized data acquisition protocol in institutions, causing considerable inequality in dataset. Several strategies have been proposed to address the issue, including cohesion, which teaches modality-inverter representation, federated generalization techniques that standardize data distribution in a distributed manner, and to compensate for the missing modality samples for the missing network (GANS) for synthetic data growth.

4.4.2 Computational Efficiency

Computer demands of multimodal AI model create another major hurdle for clinical implementation. Strategies such as modality dropouts, which introduce random training with incomplete modality inputs, have been developed to increase efficiency without renouncing the performance of nervous architecture search for knowledge distillation, and nervous architecture for automatic model adaptation through teacher-student paradigms.

4.5 Future Directions

Multimodal Medical AI is expected to focus on three important progresses from the future. First, the dynamic multimodal integration technique will enable the real-time load of methods from data quality and clinical relevance. Second, the reas

on will expand the multimodal learning framework mechanical disease relationship beyond correlated-based predictions to guess the relationship. Finally, federated multimodal systems will support the preservation of cooperative learning in institutions, which will facilitate AI-operated diagnosis and maintain compliance with healthcare rules while maintaining data security. Figure 10 presents a roadmap for the estimated development of multimodal medical AI, which predicts the deployment of clinical-grade systems capable of processing ten methods in real time by 2027. For wide adoption, these systems should solve the remaining challenges related to lecturer, strength and seamless integration in the existing clinical functioning.

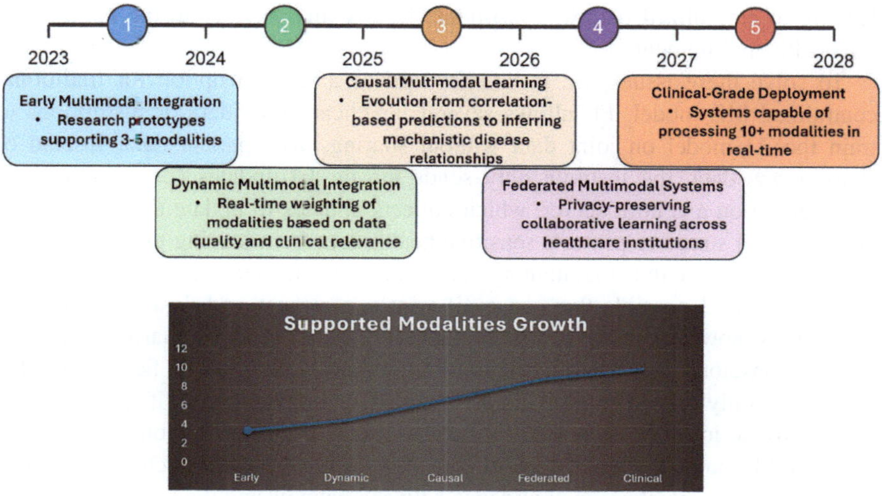

Fig. 10 Roadmap for multimodal medical AI development

5 Federated Learning and AI for Remote Healthcare

5.1 The Imperative for Privacy-Preserving Medical AI

The use of Artificial Intelligence (AI) in healthcare has demonstrated magnificent abilities to increase the accuracy of diagnosis, medical effectiveness and effectiveness of care services. As the power of AI increases in processing health-related data, it makes sense about the confidentiality of the records of the patients and maintains the confidentiality of sensitive health care information. These are particularly important in the case of medical imaging, which typically include high-resolution images that contain detailed physical information on individuals and other sensitive data such as medical history and genetic profiles.

One of the main challenges is the internal conflict between the legal, moral and social consequences of processing the benefits of AI-based healthcare innovation and the information of the patient's information. In traditional machine learning (ML) architecture, medical information is generally collected from several healthcare facilities and collected in the centralized database for training. While this centralization facilitates developing very accurate and general models, it also asks to share raw, individual level data, the patient compromises the privacy. It is particularly troublesome, which is strictly strictly given to healthcare data confidentiality, such as General Data Protection Regulation (GDPR) of the European Union and the Health Insurance Portability and Actuality Act (HIPAA) of the United States. The purpose of both laws is to protect patient information privacy by implementing strict requirements on data processing, access and sharing. These regulation systems restrict open transfer of sensitive data between institutions, leading to centralized data to consolidate legally and morally in the majority of the health environment.

To solve these issues, FL is laid forward as a reliable option for traditional centralized ML model. FL allows several healthcare providers or institutions to train the AI model on joint data without sharing basic patient data. Instead of sharing raw data, the institute only sends the model updates (i.e., gradients or parameters) on a central server, which collects updates to update the model. This decentralized structure protects sensitive health data from leaving the limits of the original institution, thus maintaining patient privacy and data security laws.

FL makes AI possible that can avail joint experiences and data without many institutions, however, it exposes institutions for privacy risks by sharing data. This privacy-conscious capacity is particularly important in the medical field, where the data is not only related to individuals, but also such information, if it is revealed, it can have serious consequences for patients, such as discrimination or stigma. In addition, FL maintains the privacy of data at its original place, which is a matter of great concern in maintaining confidence between patients and their health facilities. As a result, technology allows for more strong and diverse AI models that can normalize in various patient populations without violating personal privacy.

Practical applications of FL are particularly important in the big-data, multi-institutional environment, where data sharing is interrupted by regulatory and moral concerns. For example, in a situation where hospitals in various geographical regions or countries want to cooperate in developing AI models for orphan diseases, FL serves as a viable solution. By providing a means to train the model on its own local data while preserving privacy, FL enables such institutions to benefit from collective knowledge of the global medical network without violating patient privacy or compliance.

Recent studies have cited a high-performance capacity of federal learning in terms of privacy. For example, a 2024 multi-site test in 15 medical centers displayed that FL tumors correspond to centralized training in division that is only 2.3% in accuracy. This study confirms federal learning ability to overcome the concerns of privacy that contain a long -term obstruction of AI in clinical settings without affecting the display and accuracy required for medical applications.

Thus, infection for FL is a two-edged advantage: it enhances the scalability and universalization of AI systems in medicine while maintaining the patient's privacy and following strict data protection law. With the ongoing progress in medical AI technology, privacy-conservation techniques such as FL have been designed to play a central role in overcoming data-sharing challenges to deploy AI-Saksham healthcare solutions more widely. Furthermore, as is more aware of the importance of maintaining patient confidence and data privacy rules in medical institutions and hospitals, the demand for privacy-protection AI technology will continue to increase, the medical AI highlights the importance of federal learning in the future.

5.2 Technical Foundations of Federated Learning in Medicine

Adopting FL in medical imaging and healthcare AI presents unique technical challenges due to the complexity and diversity of medical data. In order to understand the implementation of FL in this domain, it is necessary to consider its main architecture, communication system and privacy-transit techniques that collectively enable its functionality and effectiveness in a healthcare setting.

There is a central server at the center of a FL system, which serves as the coordinator of the learning process. However, the model itself is not stored on the server; Rather, it is locally present at each participating customer (i.e., healthcare institution, hospital, or medical center). Each customer maintains his private dataset, which is never shared directly with other customers or central servers. During each training round, customers calculate the updates for their local models freely based on their local data. These updates, usually as model weight or gradients, are then sent to the central server for aggregation. This decentralized training process ensures that sensitive patient data remains safe at their source, which addresses one of the most important privacy concerns in medical AI.

The aggregation process is important for the success of federal learning. The server collects updates from each client and connects them to improve the global model. One of the most commonly used aggregation algorithms is Federated Averaging (Fedavg), which averages model parameters from customers and updates global models accordingly. However, this simple approach can withstand the difficulties when customers have significant data asymmetry, such as patient demographics, medical conditions, or imaging protocol isolated. To address this challenge, a more advanced aggregation algorithm has been proposed to improve the strengthening of FL models when faced with non-IIDs (distributed from non-freedom and identity) data. FedProx, for example, revised the Fedavg algorithm by introducing a regularization term that punishes updates from the client that greatly deviates from the global model, ensuring a more consistent and stable model update. Similarly, FedBN (federated batch normalization) adopts batch normalization parameters in FL, traditionally sensitive to the distribution of batch size and data, making the learning process more stable in asymmetrical datasets.

Another essential technical aspect of FL requires the need to protect patient privacy during model training process. Since the updates being sent between the client and the central server may contain sensitive information about the underlying medical data, techniques are important to prevent information leakage. Differential privacy is a widely planned approach to secure privacy in FL systems. This technique involves adding calibrated noise to the model update, making it difficult for the attackers to estimate information about any specific patient from model parameters. In practice, the differential privacy mechanism is designed to ensure that the presence or absence of data of a particular patient in the training set does not affect the predictions of the model to a great extent, which can prevent sensitive information from rebuilding through refined attacks such as model inverted or membership conclusions.

In the context of FL in medicine, it is paramount to obtain high model accuracy, preserving privacy. To ensure that privacy-conservation measures do not compromise the performance of models, FL frames are constantly adapted to balance both aspects. For example, medal-Bench provides standardized evaluation protocol to assess both benchmark, privacy guarantee and clinical performance of FL system to evaluate FL systems in medical applications. According to the Medfall-Bench, current FL models can get 92–96% of the performance of centralized systems, highlighting their ability to maintain competitive accuracy, guaranteeing confidentiality.

In addition, the technical foundation of FL in medicine is further enhanced by innovations in data aggregation, model personalization and client-specific adaptation. For example, individually FL allows each customer to maintain an individual version of the model, stitching it for its specific patient population and dataset characteristics. This approach is particularly beneficial in healthcare, where patient population may vary widely between institutions, and a size-fit-all model cannot perform better in various settings. By enabling local adaptation while benefiting from global cooperation, individual federate learning ensures that models can better normalize diverse patient groups and medical conditions.

To support the development and deployment of FL in the medical field, several initiatives have come to light for standardization, cooperation and evaluation. The establishment of FL benchmarks such as MedFL-Bench plays an important role in comparing different FL algorithms and providing a common base to understand their real-world projection. Additionally, initiatives such as federated tumor segmentation (FETS) Challenge, including international cooperation among more than 30 cancer centers, demonstrates practical benefits and scalability of FL in medical applications. These initiatives are important to pursue the field and ensure that the FL system can be effectively deployed in various health environments.

5.3 Addressing Challenges in Medical Federated Learning

While FL makes significant promises for medical applications, its implementation in healthcare settings faces many adequate challenges, which need to be addressed for its effectiveness and widespread adoption. These challenges stem from the complexity and inequality of medical data, computational obstacles of medical institutions, and practical difficulties of integrating the FL system into real -world clinical workflow. To deal with these issues require new solutions that maintain the privacy and security of the patient's data, while ensuring high model performance in diverse and distributed medical datasets.

One of the most prominent challenges in FL for medical imaging is data asymmetry, often known as "non-IIDs" (non-independent and identified) problems. In medical contexts, data from various healthcare institutions can vary greatly in many ways. These variations may include the differences in the protocol used to catch and process the patients (eg, age, gender, ethnicity), the prevalence of the disease, medical imaging and even medical images. For example, a hospital can use a special MRI scanner model with various image resolution and parameters from other hospitals, or various centers can adopt various protocols to divide medical images such as CT scans or X-rays. These differences can introduce adequate discrepancies in data, making it difficult to train a generalized model that performs well in all participating institutions.

To address the data, the development of strong algorithms capable of optimizing various data distribution seen on each customer (i.e., each health institute or hospital) requires the development of the algorithm. Recent progress in adaptive aggregation algorithms has shown promising results in the region. For example, adaptive federated optimization (AFO) adjusts the aggregation process for non-IID nature of framework data. The AFO model improves convergence and reduces the decline in performance caused by data inequality. In medical dataset related trials, AFO has demonstrated a significant decrease in performance variance - only 5% - for traditional FL approaches, which usually suffer from a lot of variances of 18% when dealing with asymmetrical data. By allowing models to be favorable to data characteristics on each customer, AFO helps ensure that the federated model can better generalize in institutions with various data distribution.

Another important challenge in FL for medical imaging is computational and communication overhead. Medical datasets, especially in imaging fields such as radiology, are often large and the process requires adequate computational resources. High-resolution 3D medical images, for example, can include gigabytes of data that must be processed locally in each customer institute. In FL, each client training the model on its local data, and only the model updates (instead of raw data) are shared with the central server for aggregation. However, model training along with computational requirements -often needs to communicate model updates between customers and central servers, resulting in important computational and communication overheads.

To reduce these issues, several compression techniques have been developed to reduce the amount of data transmitted during the FL process. A widely used method is gradient quantization, which involves reducing the accuracy of model updates (gradients) before disseminating them. This decrease in accuracy reduces the amount of data sent to the network, without severely compromising the performance of the model. Other techniques, such as sparse updates, only send a fraction of the model update, which affect the model the most, and reduce communication costs further. For example, the FedMed -3D framework, which focuses on high-resolution 3D medical images, successfully deployed these techniques in 12 radiology departments, reduced communication costs by 89% while maintaining clinical accuracy. These innovations are particularly important in FL for medical applications, where limited bandwidth and computational power towards clients may otherwise obstruct system scalability.

In addition, the medical FL system needs to be designed to handle client dropouts and communication failures. In real-world healthcare settings, customer institutions may have fluctuations, such as hospitals or clinic network issues, hardware failures or other disruption may be temporarily offline. The FL system must be strong enough to handle these challenges without affecting model training. A solution to this problem is to design systems that can continue training global models, when some customers are temporarily unavailable, by taking advantage of the asynchronous updates or by incorporating excess in model parameters. This allows the system to remain flexible and continue learning, even when some institutes cannot contribute updates in a few rounds.

In addition to technical challenges, regulatory compliance presents a more significant obstacle to healthcare to adopt FL widely. The handling of patient data is controlled by strict legal framework such as General Data Safety Regulation (GDPR) and Health Insurance Portability and Accountability Act (HIPAA) in the United States in Europe, which makes the protection of patient privacy mandatory and ensures that data is used morally. FL, by design, provides many advantages in this regard, as it does not require direct sharing of raw patient data. However, the federated system should still follow data safety laws, which require appropriate safety measures to prevent any unintentional leakage of the patient's information during model training. One approach to meeting these regulatory requirements is to integrate the difference in FR framework. As previously discussed, the model updates involve adding controlled noise to the model updates, making it almost impossible to remove sensitive information about individual patients from the collected model. This technique guarantees the right privacy and enables compliance with data safety regulations.

Despite the impressive ability of FL in medical AI, there are still challenges related to model lecturers and interpretations that need to be addressed. In clinical settings, healthcare providers must be able to understand and rely on the model used to make decisions. Black-box models that cannot be easily interpreted prevent a barrier to their adoption in the real-world healthcare environment, where patients are safety and clinical accountability paramount. Therefore, future research in medical FL should focus on developing techniques to make federated models more explanation, such as the use of clear AI (XAI) methods that provide insight into the process of the model deciding. These approaches will help healthcare professionals understand how federal models reach their predictions, thus increasing their confidence in these AI systems and facilitate their integration in clinical workflows.

5.4 Emerging Paradigms in Privacy-Preserving Medical AI

Privacy Conservation The area of Medical Artificial Intelligence (AI) is developing rapidly, it is necessary to ensure that sensitive patient data is preserved by furthering AI's capabilities in healthcare. While FL has emerged as a major solution to remove privacy concerns in medical AI, it is combined with other advanced techniques to increase privacy, security and overall model performance. These emerging paradigms are carrying forward the boundaries of how AI can be applied to sensitive medical contexts, such as genomics, imaging and rare disease diagnosis, while patients follow strict standards of privacy and data security.

Privacy-protection therapy is one of the most promising directions in AI, a secured multi-party computation (MPC) and a hybridization of FL with Homomorphic Encryption. MPC enables many parties to calculate a function on their personal data without disclosing any data. In the medical context, it allows institutions to work together on model development, while it ensures that the patient never leaves their local environment. By combining MPC with FL, healthcare institutions can safely collaborate on training models without any direct risk for sensitive patient information organized by other institutions.

Homomorphic encryption is another cryptographic technique that has attracted attention to privacy-protection AI. This allows computation to perform on encrypted data, without the need to decry to be first, it ensures that sensitive information remains preserved in the learning process. This enables the AI model to process medical data - such as genomic sequence or radiology images - sometimes without exposing the information of a raw patient to the model or any mediator. Application of homomorphic encryption in FL system can help maintain the confidentiality of the data by enabling powerful collaborative model development in institutions. An example of this is the Healthchain framework, which keeps a transparent and irreversible record of model updates while maintaining patient privacy. This approach provides an additional layer of protection through the use of blockchain technology, ensuring that the contribution of each institution is both verified and tampering.

Privacy-protection is the use of another exciting development division in Medical AI. Split learning involves dividing a deep learning model into two parts: one-part lives on the client (where patient data is held), and the other part lives on the server side (which updates from many customers). In this setup, raw data never leaves the local institution; Only intermediate models are shared with updated servers. This approach is particularly beneficial in the scenarios where it is important that patient data is not transferred to institutions, such as in research associated with rare diseases or sensitive genetic information. Medical split learning system is a prime example of this approach. This has demonstrated success in cross-institutional cooperation, especially in the detection tasks of pneumonia, where the system obtained 94% consensus with centralized models. In addition, Medsplit has been shown to significantly reduce data exposure risks, providing strong privacy security while maintaining high clinical accuracy.

In addition to these cryptographic and architectural advances, the integration of synthetic data generation with FL is an exciting range in the safety festival medical AI. Synthetic data refers to artificially generated data that mimics the statistical properties of real patient data, but there is no identifiable information. This allows institutions to share synthetic data - such as medical condition or disease progression patterns - without compromising patient privacy. The use of synthetic data in FL systems opens new possibilities for collaboration in institutions, especially in scenarios where data sharing is heavy due to privacy concerns. A prominent example of this integration is a synonym platform, which produces synthetic mammography images to train the AI model in breast cancer detection. Synthfl ensures that synthetic pictures maintain the major statistical characteristics of real mammography data, but there is no identifiable patient information, thus facilitating sharing data by respecting privacy.

In terms of rare disease research, where the patient's population is often small and data is rare, synthetic data generation technology combined with FL can help relieve the decrease in data. By generating synthetic medical data which reflects the characteristics of rare diseases, institutions can collaborate to train the AI model without highlighting any personal data. This allows for the development of the AI system that are better equipped to detect and diagnose rare diseases, eventually improves the patient's results for these disqualified population.

Difference in FL System Application Privacy Conservation Medicine AI is another developed pattern in space. Differential privacy involves carefully adding calibrated noise to data or model updates to prevent the identification of individual data points. In medical applications, this technique is particularly important, as it ensures that even though an adverse benefit has access to the trained model, they will be unable to extract the information of sensitive patients. The difference in FL Framework provides a intention of privacy to prove privacy guarantee, which is important to meet strict data safety rules such as General Data Safety Regulation (GDPR) and Health Insurance Portability and Accountability Act (HIPAA). In addition, the difference allows us to safely share the model updates without violating the patient's privacy, which is an essential tool for AI's privacy-protection in healthcare.

Finally, the edge computing is emerging as a supplementary technique that increases the capabilities of privacy-protection therapy AI system. In FL, age computing involves processing data on local levels (e.g., hospitals or clinics) locally, rather than transporting large amounts of raw data on a centralized server. By complicating the edge of the network, FL systems reduce the need for data transfer, reduce the risks associated with transmitting sensitive patient data. Edge computing also reduces the delay of model updates, which allows for real-time or close-object time AI applications in medical imaging and diagnosis. This is particularly important in time-sensitive healthcare applications, such as emergency room diagnosis or monitoring of severely sick patients, where rapid AI-managed decision support may be a lifetime.

These emerging paradigms, which combine FL with advanced privacy techniques such as MPC, homomorphic encryption, split learning, synthetic data generation, differential secrecy and age computing, are shaping the future of medical AIs with advanced privacy-conservation techniques. By enabling safe and privacy-conservation cooperation in institutions, these technologies are facilitating the development of strong AI models that can improve the patient's care by maintaining the highest standards of data secrecy and safety. As these paradigms develop, they have the ability to change the healthcare scenario, which enables large-scale, multi-institutional cooperation that can solve important challenges in medical research, diagnosis and treatment.

5.5 Clinical Implementation and Future Directions

Infection of FL system from the research prototype to the real -world clinical settings is a complex process that requires careful integration of several factors, including technical infrastructure, regulatory compliance and adaptation of models for real -world medical workflow. While FL has shown significant promise in various experimental and research contexts, its practical implementation in the clinical environment presents unique challenges that need to be addressed to widely adopted in health care systems. In this section, we discuss major ideas and future directions that will shape the clinical implementation of FL in the medical AI system.

One of the primary ideas in the clinical implementation of FL is the variability of the institutional IT infrastructure. Healthcare institutes, especially in different geographical regions or with different levels of technical sophistication, often separate IT systems and resources. These differences can ensure challenges in ensuring that FL systems can work effectively in diverse settings. To address this, the development of standardized container techniques is receiving traction. The containerization software allows encapsulation of the environment, including essential dependencies, in portable containers, which can be constantly deployed in various institutions, regardless of their underlying hardware or software platforms. Federated tumor segmentation (FETS) initiative, including more than 30 cancer centers worldwide, gives an example of the success of this approach. Fats have FL components to ensure compatibility in institutions with various technical abilities, which enable comfortable cooperation in training to AI model for tumor division functions. This approach plays an important role in overcoming the challenges related to the compatibility of the infrastructure and ensures that the FL system can be posted and scored in several healthcare settings.

Another major factor in the clinical implementation of FL is the quality of data. In healthcare, the quality of data may be widely different -such as differences in imaging protocols, variation in patient demographics, and factors such as discrepancies in data labeling. The FL model must still be able to handle these variations while achieving high performance. As discussed in Sect. 5.3, the problem of data inequality, often referred to as a non-IID (non-independent and identified) challenge, is pronounced particularly in medical data. This issue can lead to model performance when data is very different in institutions. Advanced aggregation algorithms and model privatization techniques are required to remove this challenge that can adjust inequality in data. For example, adaptive federated optimization (AFO) has demonstrated significant success in reducing the effects of data inequality, which reduces the performance variance in diverse datasets. Constant progress in adaptive aggregation techniques will be important to ensure that the FL system can provide strong performance in the clinical environment where data inequality is ideal.

A third major idea is regulatory compliance. Healthcare is one of the most regulated industries, and any AI system posted in clinical settings should follow strict rules such as the Health Insurance Portability and Accountability Act (HIPAA) in the United States and General Data Security Regulation (GDPR) in Europe. These rules give significant emphasis on patient privacy, data protection and informed consent. FL provides a significant benefit in this regard, as it allows institutions to cooperate in AI model training without sharing raw patient data. However, additional regulatory complications arise in the implementation of the FL system, especially when the border is dealt with across cooperation. For example, when many countries join FL, data transfer law and patient consent procedures should be considered carefully. To solve these challenges, an integrated set of international regulatory guidelines for FL in healthcare is required. These guidelines should provide a clear standard of how the FL system can be deployed in clinical settings to ensure complete compliance with local and international regulations.

Beyond technical and regulatory challenges, integration of FL in clinical workflows represents a significant obstacle for its clinical implementation. In many healthcare environments, existing workflows get heavily complicated and can be completed with resistance to healthcare providers by presenting A-in-manual systems that are accustomed to traditional methods. To successfully integrate the FL system into clinical workflows, they must be designed keeping in mind the ease of use and practicality. This involves ensuring that the AI systems can work in real time and provide actionable insights to physicians at the point of care. Additionally, the system should basically be able to integrate with existing medical imaging software, electronic health records and other clinical equipment. Training and support are also necessary for healthcare professionals, as they should be able to rely on the AI system and understand their decision-making processes. The development of the explainable AI (XAI) model, which provides interpretable and transparent arguments behind the model's predictions, will be important in receiving physician trust and ensuring that the FL system can be adopted in regular clinical practice.

Given the future, there are many exciting directions that are especially ready to shape the development of privacy-conservation therapy AI in terms of FL. First, dynamic FL systems that can automatically be favorable for changes in data distribution in institutions are expected to play an important role. This type of system will allow the model to continuously learn and develop in real time as new data becomes available, ensuring that models remain accurate and relevant, as patients develop democracy, the prevalence of the disease, and medical imaging technologies. Additionally, causal reasoning frameworks are being integrated into the FL system to improve the ability of the model to normalize in various healthcare settings. By incorporating the assessment of the cause in the AI model, it will be possible not only to predict the results of the disease, but also to understand the underlying mechanisms that run the progression of the disease, allowing more individual and effective treatment strategies to give rise.

Another important direction for future development is the scaling of FL systems to handle larger, more complex datasets. Since the healthcare data continues to grow in both volume and complexity, it will be necessary on the scale efficiently for the FL system to handle this flow of information. This includes not only the ability to process traditional medical images but also includes multimodal data from sources such as genomic sequence, electronic health records, wearable health equipment and patient-reported results. The FL system that can handle many types of data simultaneously will be important to carry forward the field of individual medicine.

FL's ability to replace medical AI is immense, but its extensive clinical deployment will require careful attention to these various factors. The ongoing development of the international FL network, such as rare diseases focus on research and epidemic response, underlines the ability to bring revolution in medical research and diagnosis globally for FL. The patient promises to advance the healthcare system around the world by enabling large -scale cooperation while protecting privacy, protecting privacy. Since these technologies mature and are adopted more widely, integration of FL in clinical practice will not only increase clinical accuracy, but will promote similar access to advanced health technologies, especially in underserved areas.

6 Conclusion

Integration of artificial intelligence in medical image analysis represents one of the most transformational developments in modern healthcare, offering unprecedented opportunities to increase clinical accuracy, customize workflows and improve patient results. As displayed in this chapter, the region developed from narrow, single-function algorithm, capable of making complex clinical decisions for refined multimodal systems. However, the journey of strong clinical equipment from the research prototype has revealed fundamental challenges, which must be addressed to realize the full potential of AI in medical imaging. The development of reliable AI systems requires solutions of three interdependent challenges: technical power, clinical relevance and moral responsibility. Technically, while deep learning has received remarkable performance on specific image interpretations, diverse patient population and healthcare settings have become important tasks in improving generalization in settings. The emergence of a show-off Foundation model on large-scale medical datasets offers promising guidelines but needs careful attention to potential prejudices and rigorous verification protocols. Clinically, successful implementation demands a deeper understanding of the dynamics of human-AI cooperation, with interface design that enhances the doctor rather than obstructed workflows. The growing field of cognitive ergonomics for medical AI will play an important role in customizing these interactions. Ethically, the medical AI community should face challenging questions about algorithm fairness, accountability and appropriate limitations of automation in clinical practice. The development of a broad regulatory structure that balances innovation with patient safety is a continuous process, requiring intimate cooperation between technologists, physicians and policy makers. Especially pressure requires continuous teaching systems and international standards controlling their medico-natural implications. Looking forward, the three major Frontiers Medical Imaging will shape the next decade of AI. First, the integration of the reason Reasoning Framework promises to go beyond pattern recognition for the real understanding of the disease system. Second, efficient, small-scale development of AI models will be important to enable global health equity in AI-Assistant diagnostics. Third, the creation of a strong ecosystem for monitoring and quality improvement of real -world performance will determine whether the AI system can continuously increase healthcare distribution. As the area moves forward, success will eventually be measured by technical benchmarks, but by tangible improvements in patient care and health system. This will require continuous interdisciplinary cooperation in computer science, clinical medicine and healthcare research. In the coming years, possibly medical imaging AI infection will be mainly seen as a clinical assistant, which is a clinical assistant to become an integral component of individual, forecasting health care systems. By maintaining rigorous standards of evidence, preference to patient welfare and promoting equal access, the medical AI community can ensure that these technologies are fulfilled their promises to revolutionize health care distribution worldwide.

References

1. Akinyelu AA, Zaccagna F, Grist JT, Castelli M, Rundo L (2022) Brain tumor diagnosis using machine learning, convolutional neural networks, capsule neural networks and vision transformers, applied to MRI: a survey. J Imaging 8(8):205
2. Trigka M, Dritsas E (2025) A comprehensive survey of deep learning approaches in image processing. Sensors 25(2):531
3. Ali AM, Benjdira B, Koubaa A, El-Shafai W, Khan Z, Boulila W (2023) Vision transformers in image restoration: A survey. Sensors 23(5):2385
4. Kaissis GA, Makowski MR, Rückert D, Braren RF (2020) Secure, privacy-preserving and federated machine learning in medical imaging. Nat Mach Intell 2(6):305–311
5. Zhang A, Xing L, Zou J, Wu JC (2022) Shifting machine learning for healthcare from development to deployment and from models to data. Nat Biomed Eng 6(12):1330–1345
6. Bayoudh K, Knani R, Hamdaoui F, Mtibaa A (2022) A survey on deep multimodal learning for computer vision: advances, trends, applications, and datasets. Vis Comput 38(8):2939–2970
7. Srinivasan K, Ramamurthy CKV, Matheswaran S, Shamsudheen S (2025) Introduction to explainable AI in healthcare: Enhancing transparency and trust. In: Explainable Artificial Intelligence in the Healthcare Industry, pp 161–183
8. Pinto-Coelho L (2023) How artificial intelligence is shaping medical imaging technology: a survey of innovations and applications. Bioengineering 10(12):1435
9. Wang L, Wang H, Huang Y, Yan B, Chang Z, Liu Z et al (2022) Trends in the application of deep learning networks in medical image analysis: Evolution between 2012 and 2020. Eur J Radiol 146:110069
10. Rani V, Kumar M, Gupta A, Sachdeva M, Mittal A, Kumar K (2024) Self-supervised learning for medical image analysis: a comprehensive review. Evol Syst 15(4):1607–1633
11. Xu Y, Quan R, Xu W, Huang Y, Chen X, Liu F (2024) Advances in medical image segmentation: a comprehensive review of traditional, deep learning and hybrid approaches. Bioengineering 11(10):1034
12. Rahman H, Ben Aoun N, Bukht TFN, Ahmad S, Tadeusiewicz R, Pławiak P, Hammad M (2025) Automatic liver tumor segmentation of CT and MRI volumes using ensemble ResUNet-InceptionV4 model. Inform Sci:121966

13. Hammad M, ElAffendi M, Asim M, Abd El-Latif AA, Hashiesh R (2024) Automated lung cancer detection using novel genetic TPOT feature optimization with deep learning techniques. Results Eng 24:103448
14. Wu M, Qian Y, Liao X, Wang Q, Heng PA (2023) Hepatic vessel segmentation based on 3D swin-transformer with inductive biased multi-head self-attention. BMC Med Imaging 23(1):91
15. Khan S, Naseer M, Hayat M, Zamir SW, Khan FS, Shah M (2022) Transformers in vision: A survey. ACM Comput Surv (CSUR) 54(10s):1–41
16. Wang P, Yang Q, He Z, Yuan Y (2023) Vision transformers in multi-modal brain tumor MRI segmentation: A review. Meta-Radiol 1(1):100004
17. Zeng X, Abdullah N, Sumari P (2024) Self-supervised learning framework application for medical image analysis: a review and summary. Biomed Eng Online 23(1):107
18. Xie Y, Gu L, Harada T, Zhang J, Xia Y, Wu Q (2024) Rethinking masked image modelling for medical image representation. Med Image Anal 98:103304
19. Suresh T, Brijet Z, Subha TD (2023) Imbalanced medical disease dataset classification using enhanced generative adversarial network. Comput Methods Biomech Biomed Engin 26(14):1702–1718
20. Han C, Rundo L, Araki R, Nagano Y, Furukawa Y, Mauri G et al (2019) Combining noise-to-image and image-to-image GANs: Brain MR image augmentation for tumor detection. IEEE Access 7:156966–156977
21. Hussain S, Mubeen I, Ullah N, Shah SSUD, Khan BA, Zahoor M et al (2022) Modern diagnostic imaging technique applications and risk factors in the medical field: a review. Biomed Res Int 2022(1):5164970
22. Soenksen LR, Ma Y, Zeng C, Boussioux L, Villalobos Carballo K, Na L et al (2022) Integrated multimodal artificial intelligence framework for healthcare applications. NPJ Digit Med 5(1):149
23. Ehrhardt J, Wilms M (2022) Autoencoders and variational autoencoders in medical image analysis. In: Biomedical Image Synthesis and Simulation. Academic, pp 129–162
24. Kazerouni A, Aghdam EK, Heidari M, Azad R, Fayyaz M, Hacihaliloglu I, Merhof D (2023) Diffusion models in medical imaging: A comprehensive survey. Med Image Anal 88:102846
25. Hajij M, Zamzmi G, Paul R, Thukar L (2022, March) Normalizing flow for synthetic medical images generation. In: 2022 IEEE Healthcare Innovations and Point of Care Technologies (HI-POCT). IEEE, pp 46–49
26. Hammad M, ElAffendi M, El-Latif AAA, Ateya AA, Ali G, Plawiak P (2025) Explainable AI for lung cancer detection via a custom CNN on CT images. Sci Rep 15(1):12707
27. Raminedi S, Shridevi S, Won D (2024) Multi-modal transformer architecture for medical image analysis and automated report generation. Sci Rep 14(1):19281
28. Hu M, Qian J, Pan S, Li Y, Qiu RL, Yang X (2024) Advancing medical imaging with language models: featuring a spotlight on ChatGPT. Phys Med Biol 69(10):10TR01
29. Combi C, Amico B, Bellazzi R, Holzinger A, Moore JH, Zitnik M, Holmes JH (2022) A manifesto on explainability for artificial intelligence in medicine. Artif Intell Med 133:102423
30. Chen H, Gomez C, Huang CM, Unberath M (2022) Explainable medical imaging AI needs human-centered design: guidelines and evidence from a systematic review. NPJ Digit Med 5(1):156
31. Minh D, Wang HX, Li YF, Nguyen TN (2022) Explainable artificial intelligence: a comprehensive review. Artif Intell Rev:1–66
32. Jin W, Li X, Fatehi M, Hamarneh G (2023) Generating post-hoc explanation from deep neural networks for multi-modal medical image analysis tasks. MethodsX 10:102009
33. Selvaraju RR, Cogswell M, Das A, Vedantam R, Parikh D, Batra D (2020) Grad-CAM: visual explanations from deep networks via gradient-based localization. Int J Comput Vis 128:336–359
34. Mahesh TR, Vinoth Kumar V, Guluwadi S (2024) Enhancing brain tumor detection in MRI images through explainable AI using Grad-CAM with Resnet 50. BMC Med Imaging 24(1):107

35. Pang W, Ke X, Tsutsui S, Wen B (2024) Integrating clinical knowledge into concept bottleneck models. In: International Conference on Medical Image Computing and Computer-Assisted Intervention. Springer Nature Switzerland, Cham, pp 243–253
36. Vo HTV, Thien NN, Mui KC, Tien PP (2024) Enhancing confidence in brain tumor classification models with Grad-CAM And Grad-CAM++. Indones J Electr Eng Inform (IJEEI) 12(4):926–939
37. Sitaraman SR, Alagarsundaram P, Kumar V (2024) AI-driven skin lesion detection with CNN and Score-CAM: Enhancing explainability in IoMT platforms. Indo Am J Pharm Bio Sci 22(4):1–13
38. Lai T (2024) Interpretable medical imagery diagnosis with self-attentive transformers: a review of explainable AI for health care. BioMedInformatics 4(1):113–126
39. Manzari ON, Ahmadabadi H, Kashiani H, Shokouhi SB, Ayatollahi A (2023) MedViT: a robust vision transformer for generalized medical image classification. Comput Biol Med 157:106791
40. Böhle M, Eitel F, Weygandt M, Ritter K (2019) Layer-wise relevance propagation for explaining deep neural network decisions in MRI-based Alzheimer's disease classification. Front Aging Neurosci 11:194
41. Zou K, Chen Z, Yuan X, Shen X, Wang M, Fu H (2023) A review of uncertainty estimation and its application in medical imaging. Meta-Radiol 1(1):100003
42. Massmann A, Heukelom JV, Weaver M, Schultz A, Figueroa DM, Stys A et al (2024) Evaluation of pharmacogenetic automated clinical decision support for clopidogrel. Pharmacogenomics 25(8–9):391–399
43. Nensa F (2025) The future of radiology: The path towards multimodal AI and superdiagnostics. Eur J Radiol Artif Intell 2:100014
44. Nerella S, Bandyopadhyay S, Zhang J, Contreras M, Siegel S, Bumin A et al (2024) Transformers and large language models in healthcare: A review. Artif Intell Med 154:102900
45. Cho HN, Jun TJ, Kim YH, Kang H, Ahn I, Gwon H et al (2024) Task-specific transformer-based language models in health care: scoping review. JMIR Med Inform 12:e49724
46. Xu X, Li J, Zhu Z, Zhao L, Wang H, Song C et al (2024) A comprehensive review on synergy of multi-modal data and ai technologies in medical diagnosis. Bioengineering 11(3):219
47. Dana, J., Agnus, V., Ouhmich, F., & Gallix, B. (2020). Multimodality imaging and artificial intelligence for tumor characterization: current status and future perspective. In Seminars in nuclear medicine (Vol. 50, 6, pp. 541–548). WB Saunders
48. Alberdi A, Aztiria A, Basarab A (2016) On the early diagnosis of Alzheimer's disease from multimodal signals: A survey. Artif Intell Med 71:1–29
49. Acosta JN, Falcone GJ, Rajpurkar P, Topol EJ (2022) Multimodal biomedical AI. Nat Med 28(9):1773–1784

Ethical and Regulatory Consideration in AI-Based Medical Imaging

Ghalib Nadeem and Muhammad Irfan Anis

1 Introduction: The Ethical Lens on AI in Medical Imaging

The use of artificial intelligence in various fields, particularly in the health sector, has greatly enhanced the accuracy of the diagnostic process. This technology has recorded up to 30% early detection improvement. Advanced deep learning techniques like convolutional neural networks (CNN) which artificial technology developers have developed, are used to detect diseases that include cancer and neurological disorders with the assurance that the results would be accurate and time-saving. Ethical concerns are still some of the issues limiting the widespread use of artificial intelligence. For instance, it is not so surprising that such a report, like the one found in NEJM, notes that close to 70% of the clinicians interviewed believed that it would be very difficult to protect patients' privacy and detect, let alone eliminate bias in AI labored diagnostics. This effort also brings into focus the factors that necessitate an extended inquiry into the scope of AI in medical imaging and the associated ethical questions before reaching conclusions that are both valid and wide. This in turn allows us to discuss the next cohort of trainees:

G. Nadeem (✉)
Iqra University, Karachi, Pakistan
e-mail: ghalibnadeem@iqra.edu.pk

M. I. Anis
High Performance Research Group, Karachi, Pakistan
e-mail: mirfananis@iqra.edu.pk

N. Ben Aoun et al. (eds.), *AI for Medical Image Analysis*,
https://doi.org/10.1007/978-3-032-02963-8_10

1.1 Context: AI's Transformative Role in Medical Imaging

The dawn of artificial intelligence technology in the field of medicine has seen ground-breaking improvements in the use of medical imaging, notably the enhanced level of accuracy and automation accompanying the process of analyzing and tracing diseases. AI-driven imaging systems can detect cancer, neurological disorders, and cardiovascular diseases with precision comparable to and, in some cases, exceeding that of human radiologists. Given that Sect. 1.1 is covered in the previous chapter, we present only a concise summary.

AI-driven imaging tools have revolutionized diagnostics, improving accuracy and efficiency in detecting complex diseases. The American College of Radiology reports that AI achieves a pooled sensitivity and specificity of 0.87 in lung cancer detection, enabling early diagnosis and treatment [1]. AI-assisted imaging has also reduced false positives and false negatives by up to 9.4%, while pathology AI lowers major diagnostic discrepancies by 29.4% [2]. Additionally, AI tools like Viz LVO demonstrate 93.8% sensitivity in detecting large vessel occlusions (LVOs), enhancing stroke diagnostics. Despite these advancements, AI faces significant ethical and regulatory hurdles. Data privacy remains a major concern, with 81% of patients worried about AI handling their medical data and 63% demanding explicit consent (European Journal of Radiology). Ensuring HIPAA and GDPR compliance is essential for maintaining trust [3].

Algorithmic bias leads to unequal healthcare outcomes. A Nature Medicine study found that AI skin cancer detection is 25% less accurate for darker skin tones, while AI underdiagnosed cardiovascular disease in women by 15%. The lack of transparency further limits adoption, three-quarters of radiologists are concerned about AI's black-box nature (The Lancet Digital Health). Legal liability remains unclear, with 61% of healthcare professionals unsure who is responsible for AI errors (JAMA Network Open). Additionally, 74% of global AI healthcare systems lack proper regulatory oversight (WHO). Addressing these issues through bias audits, explainable AI, and stronger regulations are essential for fair, transparent, and safe AI deployment in healthcare. These challenges must be tackled to maintain moral, transparent, and equitable AI in medical imaging. For this purpose, the upcoming section will discuss this problems.

1.2 Importance of Addressing Ethical and Regulatory Challenges

It must be admitted that discussions before the ethical and legal implications of having AI penetrate medical imaging are very pointed and more often than not sharpened. According to a 2023 survey of over 700 radiologists and AI researchers, the application of AI to medical imaging involves challenges concerning data privacy, regulatory compliance, and ethical governance. 62% of the respondents believed that different regulations around the world could compromise the exposure of patient data, pointing to GDPR in Europe and FDA regulations in the U.S. The frameworks aim to ensure AI safety and make compliance more difficult. Therefore, a rigid framework of regulations, along with ethical guidance and technical frameworks, is paramount for responsible AI use in healthcare [4]. Beyond privacy, 74% say that AI bias is a major hindrance to worthwhile healthcare delivery. AI models that are trained on biased sets risk inflating the proportional representation of some demographics and putting others at a greater risk of harm, especially disadvantaged populations. These regulatory approaches differ: the EU emphasizes broad data protection, while U.S. regulations mostly stress consumer consent. Calls for aligned regulatory and ethical frameworks resulted in solutions such as federated learning and secure data sharing mechanisms that balance privacy protection and research needs [4].

AI, indeed, remains a big issue regarding trust because an overwhelming 81% of experts indicate that a significant barrier to clinical adoption is a lack of explainability. Subsequently, clinicians cannot fully practice with AI due to the absence of complete transparency in the decision-making process. These legal reforms will also come up with questions on liability about errors related to AI, becoming necessary clarification among developers, healthcare providers, and AI systems concerning responsibility. Regulations such as GDPR and evolving U.S. policies aim to strengthen data protection, but a globally coordinated effort in ethics, regulation, and technology is crucial to ensuring AI's safe, fair, and effective use in medical imaging. Ensuring ethical and regulatory oversight in AI-driven medical imaging is crucial for patient safety and trust. Without unified global standards, disparities in AI performance may widen, disproportionately affecting underserved populations. This raises a fundamental question: "Why do ethical and regulatory considerations matter?" The next section explores the necessity of these considerations through real-life cases. Strengthening ethical frameworks and harmonizing global regulations will be essential to ensuring AI's fair, transparent, and effective integration into medical imaging. To achieve these objectives, several key attributes must be considered, as illustrated in Fig. 1.

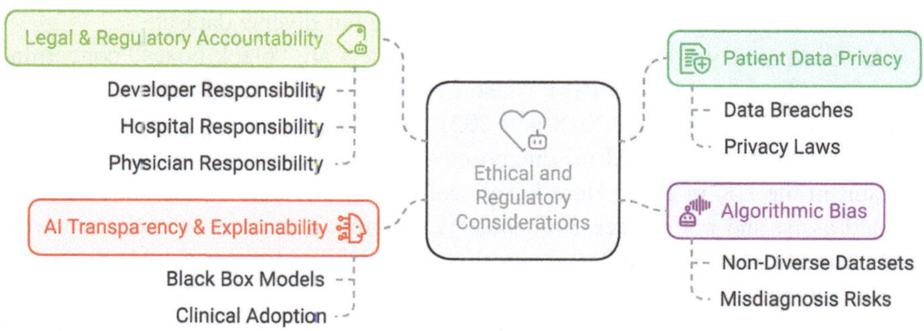

Fig. 1 Ethical and regulatory considerations in AI for medical imaging

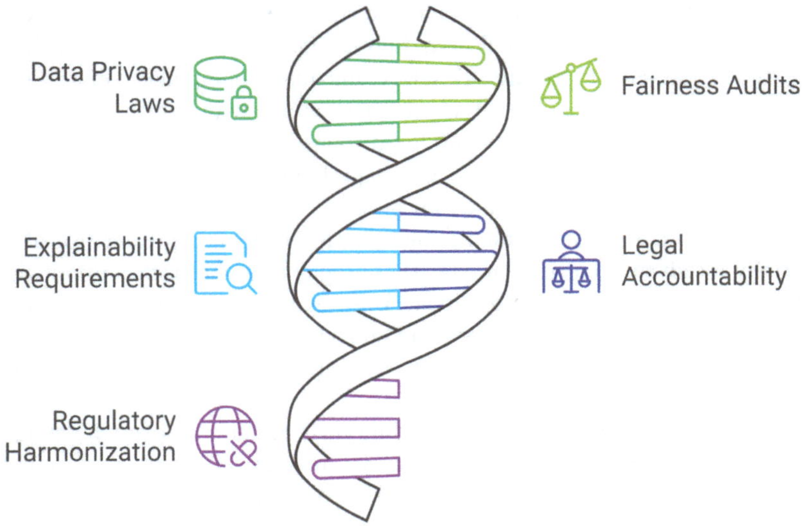

Fig. 2 Ensuring ethical AI in medical imaging for global healthcare transformation

Ensuring patient data privacy in AI-driven healthcare is critical, as AI models rely on vast datasets from hospital records and clinical trials, making them vulnerable to unauthorized use and security breaches. Over several years, millions of patient records have been compromised in violation of HIPAA and GDPR. The most well-known case is the Google DeepMind scandal between 2016 and 2021, which resulted in a stricter legal regime on AI privacy laws in the UK after 1.6 million NHS patient records were used to train an AI system without consent [5]. Federated learning has helped bring in privacy-preserving methods, such as differential privacy, that reduce risk while still allowing for effective AI. However, algorithmic bias is still another concern. AI is likely to compound health disparities because bias in data will subject the trained AI models to sources of unrepresentative data sets. A Stanford study in 2022 found that AI dermatology would be developed to be 34% less accurate for patients having skin darker, raising the possibility of misdiagnosis [6]. It is establishing fairness audits and requiring fair diverse datasets.

AI transparency is very important. Most models are "black boxes" concerning decisions. Trust was lost in IBM Watson Health AI after unsafe cancer treatment recommendations between 2018 and 2021; hospitals stopped accepting the technology because of it. An AI misdiagnosed a lung cancer patient as "low risk" in a lawsuit in the UK in 2022. Here arise legal issues. The courts may have ruled AI should assist and not replace clinicians [7]. Figure 2 gives an ethical framework addressing privacy, bias, and transparency accountability for trustful AI adoption in medical imaging.

This framework strongly resembles the DNA structure, signifying that healthcare has radically integrated AI ethics. The framework is built on five pillars: laws on data privacy that guarantee patient information remains confidential; fairness audits to determine possible inequalities affecting the diagnosis; explainability, which should be transparent in the decisions made by AI; legal accountability to understand who is responsible for errors using AI; and regulate harmonization to set a standard of ethics globally. It is hoped that through all these protections, AI-enhanced medical imaging can be made into a safe, fair, and accountable mechanism in healthcare. Creating a common ethical structure will not only bolster clinical confidence and increase patient protection but also propagate a fair-moving deployment of AI around the globe.

1.3 Scope of the Chapter

AI-based imaging in medicine has been expected to improve diagnostic accuracy and efficiency in health care, but ethical and regulatory issues have surfaced. According to various challenges, regulatory perspectives, real-world failures, and strategies in ethical AI deployment, this chapter deals with some of them. There are major ethical dilemmas concerning data privacy and patient consent in AI model training. Most AI systems depend on very large datasets of medical images which are collected without informed consent from patients, creating concerns related to HIPAA (U.S.), GDPR (EU), and other global data laws. Another very grave issue is algorithmic bias, whereby it has been found that diverse training datasets end up resulting in greater levels of misdiagnosis for underrepresented populations. There is no transparency in decision-making processes created by AI, which leads to the development of black box models, making it difficult for doctors to validate the recommendations made by an AI system. Furthermore, accountability for mistakes made by AI in cases of misdiagnosis increases reluctance to adopt such technologies is it to be considered responsible by a court if a person was misdiagnosed by an AI, the developer, hospital, or clinician? Regulatory perspectives on this issue vary among regions, however.

Although AI health policies and regulations are being formulated by organizations such as the FDA in the U.S., EMA in Europe, and WHO, inconsistency and legal gaps exist that are impediments to global usage. These are glaring issues that are made clear by looking into real-life AI failures. The NHS data privacy issue initiated by Google DeepMind amplified the dangers of a breach of patient data confidentiality, and the IBM Watson Health AI misdiagnosis scandal showed how wrong training data could lead to unsafe medical recommendations. AI bias in melanoma detection shows how outcomes could be inequitably affected due to a lack of diversity in datasets, as one study showed a lower accuracy of 34% of diagnoses on darker skin tones. Some measures that are required to circumvent these issues are bias audits, privacy-preserving AI methods, and explanatory frameworks for fairness and transparency. Stronger AI accountability laws are needed as well to declare liability in AI-based healthcare provision [8]. By treating these issues around ethics and law, AI for medical imaging can be launched responsibly, thus creating trust, safety, and equitable healthcare for all patients.

2 Ethical Challenges in AI-Based Medical Imaging

Changes wrought by AI in medical imaging will transform healthcare, allowing faster diagnoses, earlier disease detection, and personalized treatment approaches. However, there are the main ethical challenges for adoption concerning fairness, transparency, and safety for the patient. The main bioethical issues involve the protection of privacy and consent for an algorithm bias on fair diagnoses, transparency of AI decision-making for the clinician, and accountability for AI blunders. For trust in AI-enabled healthcare and the equitable benefit of all patients, these issues must be rightfully addressed, as Fig. 3 illustrates these factors in balancing AI's role in data privacy risk in medical imaging. This section focuses on these ethical concerns with real-world case studies, the most recent research, and possible mitigation strategies for the alignment of AI-based imaging with core healthcare ethics.

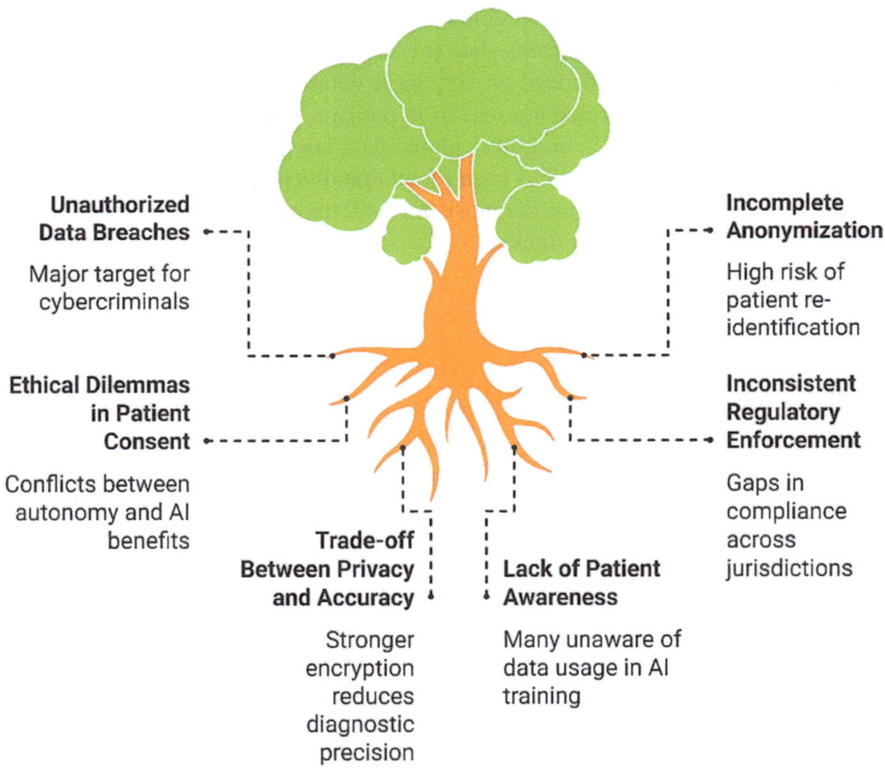

Fig. 3 Data privacy risks in AI-driven medical imaging

2.1 Data Privacy and Patient Consent

Datasets are enormous and extensive for medical imaging. It is now understood that there is a data privacy concern and ethics surrounding patient consent as medical information is typically used without explicit consent by those concerned. To enhance public trust and achieve care and ethical AI, data collection and usage transparency are important. As shown in Fig. 3, essential matters need to be addressed regarding these concerns.

AI-based on medical imaging is widely acknowledged to have endless databases for improving diagnostic accuracy and treatment outcomes; however, the issue of privacy concern it raises is monumental. One of the biggest challenges is unauthorized data breaches, for medical imaging databases are prime cybercriminal targets. As reported by IBM Security in their 2023 report on healthcare data breaches, such data broke by 25%, with millions of MRI and CT scan images leaks due to improperly secured Picture Archiving and Communication Systems (PACS) [9]. Inadequate anonymization is another concern; AI models can re-identify a patient from de-identified datasets. It presented a study in 2023 in which 99.98% of Americans could be re-identified using merely 15 demographic attributes, indicating the limitations of standard anonymization [10]. AI-generated heatmaps in medical imaging revealed the patient identities unintentionally and so underlined the need for privacy-preserving techniques for AI.

It is an ethical dilemma to maintain a fine balance of data security and AI performance besides privacy threats. For example, a study showed that stronger encryption yielded 12% reduced AI diagnostic accuracy. This raises the question of whether privacy protection should overshadow AI accuracy. Federated learning and differential privacy would be helpful to a patient-safe AI and still maintain high performance. Other major concerns here with medical imaging AI are patient consent because many do not even know their data gets used. As the authors of a 2022 study published in The Lancet Digital Health found, over 60% of patients were clueless about their data being used for AI within imaging, primarily because of expansive hospital consent forms [11]. The argument between opt-in and opt-out consent models is still indeterminate. The opt-in model allows 72% of patients in a 2023 survey to give clear consent but diminishes their datasets while retaining autonomy. The opt-out model holds all data by default unless the patient asks for removal, to facilitate AI advancement, but raises concerns on its transparency [12].

Global regulatory frameworks address data privacy but face challenges in enforcement, cross-border data sharing, and evolving AI risks. While HIPAA, GDPR, and other laws govern medical data security, inconsistencies in enforcement create compliance gaps. As AI adoption expands, legal frameworks must evolve to keep pace with new privacy risks. Table 1 summarizes key legal frameworks across different countries, shedding light on the ongoing challenges in balancing compliance, security, and ethical integration of AI in healthcare.

To mitigate privacy concerns, researchers have developed secure AI solutions. Federated learning enables AI training on patient data without transferring it to a

Table 1 Regulatory bodies across different nations worldwide

Regulation	Country/Region	Key provisions	Challenges
HIPAA (Health Insurance Portability and Accountability Act)	USA	Protects patient health data privacy and mandates security measures	Does not fully cover AI-driven imaging data sharing
GDPR (General Data Protection Regulation)	EU	Requires explicit patient consent for data use; enforces "right to be forgotten"	Limits cross-border AI training datasets
PDPA (Personal Data Protection Act)	Singapore	Regulates health data processing and storage	Lacks clear AI-specific guidelines
China's Personal Information Protection Law (PIPL)	China	Requires strict user consent for AI data use	Restricts foreign collaborations on AI medical imaging

central server, improving privacy while maintaining 97% accuracy [13]. Differential privacy protects identities by introducing mathematical noise to datasets, reducing re-identification risks by 98% [14]. Blockchain technology further strengthens security, creating tamper-proof medical records. A 2023 Mayo Clinic study found that blockchain reduced unauthorized access risks by 92%, making it a promising tool for AI-driven healthcare [15]. As AI continues to evolve, privacy-preserving innovations will be critical in ensuring secure, ethical, and patient-centered medical imaging.

2.2 Algorithmic Bias and Fairness

AI has the potential to revolutionize healthcare, but algorithmic bias remains a major challenge, leading to disparate health outcomes for underrepresented populations. When AI models are trained on non-diverse datasets, they struggle to diagnose conditions accurately across different demographics, worsening existing health inequities. AI-powered medical imaging inherits biases from training data, leading to demographic, selection, and labeling biases. A 2023 study found that diagnostic performance dropped by 20–30% when applied to racial groups different from the original training data [16], resulting in misdiagnoses, delayed treatments, and worsening disparities.

The real-world examples give a sense of how biased AI may operate in medical imaging. A study carried out in 2023 on different AI models for diagnosing chest X-rays found that Black patients were 16% more likely to be misdiagnosed with pneumonia while Hispanic patients had a 12% higher rate of missed tuberculosis diagnoses. Clinically, this means that women were more likely to have missed diagnoses of cardiomegaly because the AI models were mostly developed on male data. The AI tools for dermatology, too, are biased, with a 34% reduction in melanoma detection in darker-skinned patients [11]. In cardiovascular imaging, a study was conducted by the American Heart Association in 2023. The accuracy of AI in CT scan interpretation as dependent on sex was analyzed; AI was found to perform 25% more accurately on men than on women due to male training data bias [17]. These instances indicate that a lack of diversity in training data, bias auditing, and fairness evaluation must be addressed so that AI does not further inequities in health care.

Bias in AI medical imaging arises from under-representation in training data, biased labeling, and geographic overfitting. A 2023 analysis of 74 AI medical datasets found that 80% of training data came from North America and Europe, leading to poor performance for patients from Africa, South America, and South Asia. Labeling bias occurs when human annotators introduce unconscious biases into medical images, which AI then learns and perpetuates. Research shows that Black patients receive 10–15% less pain medication due to implicit biases [18]. If similar biases exist in radiology labels, AI models risk amplifying these disparities. Geographic overfitting also affects AI accuracy when models trained in one region fail to generalize elsewhere. A 2022 study found that an AI model trained in a U.S. hospital experienced a 36% drop in accuracy when applied to an Asian hospital dataset [19]. Ensuring diverse datasets is key to developing fair and effective AI systems.

Addressing bias requires inclusive dataset curation, bias audits, XAI, and federated learning. Studies suggest that at least 30% of an AI training dataset should include underrepresented populations to reduce bias [20]. Auditing AI models with tools like Google's Model Cards and IBM's AI Fairness 360 Toolkit helps identify and mitigate bias before deployment. Explainable AI improves transparency by revealing how AI makes decisions. A 2022 IEEE Access study found that XAI increased radiologists' trust in AI diagnoses by 43% [21]. Federated learning, which enables AI training across multiple hospitals without centralizing data, reduces bias associated with region-specific datasets. A study by MIT found that federated learning improved AI accuracy by 28% for underrepresented groups, significantly reducing bias [22].

Table 2 AI-biased prevention measurement for different countries' regulations

Regulation	Key bias prevention measures
FDA (USA)	Requires AI developers to submit bias evaluation reports for approval.
EMA (Europe)	Enforces diversity standards in training datasets for medical AI.
MHRA (UK)	Mandates regular audits of AI-based imaging tools for bias detection.
WHO AI Ethics Guidelines	Recommends global data-sharing initiatives to reduce AI bias.

As AI adoption in healthcare grows, strong regulatory oversight is crucial to ensure fairness, transparency, and accountability. Some nations have enacted laws addressing algorithmic fairness, but global enforcement remains inconsistent. Table 2 outlines regulatory efforts, emphasizing the need for harmonized international standards to ensure AI medical imaging adheres to ethical and unbiased decision-making. Without proactive measures, AI risks reinforcing existing healthcare disparities, but with diverse training data, fairness audits, and ethical AI development, it can become a powerful tool for equitable healthcare.

The presence of ethical concerns related to algorithmic bias prevailing in the practice of medical imaging AI deeply affects the outcome of inequitable healthcare. Reports suggest that different AI models manifest biased error rates predicated on demographic features, hence leading to the misdiagnosis or treatment error of as much as 30%. This discouraging set of events calls for the establishment of diverse datasets, bias audits, explainable AI technology, and solid regulatory frameworks to ensure fairness, ethics, and neutrality in all AI applications in health care.

2.3 *Transparency and Explainability*

While deep-earning models and AI systems in medical imaging can provide very accurate diagnoses, their poor transparency raises ethical concerns regarding patient trust, clinician acceptance, and regulation. Transparency concerns how well the rationale and design of AI can be understood, whereas explainability refers to how well AI can justify given diagnoses. A 2023 Nature article found that 72% of radiologists would hesitate to use AI in clinical practice because of its non-explainability [23]. If there are no clear reasons provided by AI for its diagnoses, then clinicians will find it difficult to confirm the predictions; this ultimately has ramifications for clinical decision-making, legal accountability, regulatory approval, and patient trust. A 2022 study in The Lancet Digital Health found that 84% of patients trust AI diagnoses more when doctors can explain how AI arrived at its conclusions [11].

The black-box nature of deep learning models like DNNs and CNNs further complicates AI adoption. To address this, XAI techniques improve interpretability and trust, Table 3 presents the XAI techniques to acquire the clinical benefits in

Table 3 Key XAI techniques, their functions, and clinical benefits in medical imaging

Ref.	XAI Technique	Function	Clinical Benefit
[24]	Saliency maps	Highlights image regions used for decision-making	Increases clinician trust in AI predictions
[24]	SHAP values	Quantifies feature importance	Helps understand AI weightage in decision-making
[25]	Grad-CAM	Visualizes AI's focus area in images	Enhances interpretability of AI classifications

medical imaging. Key methods include Saliency Maps, which visually highlight areas influencing AI decisions by a 68% increase in radiologists' trust in breast cancer detection; SHAP, which identifies critical features with 91% accuracy in AI-based COVID-19 detection [24]; and Grad-CAM, which enhances clinician interpretation with 44% improvement in diabetic retinopathy diagnosis. By enhancing transparency, XAI fosters trust, clinical adoption, and regulatory compliance, ensuring AI's safe and reliable integration into medical imaging.

2.4 Accountability and Responsibility in AI-Based Medical Imaging

As AI systems become more involved in diagnosing diseases, recommending treatments, and assisting clinicians, the question of accountability and responsibility becomes a major ethical and legal concern. Key issues arise when AI makes diagnostic errors, leading to uncertainty over whether liability falls on the hospital, software developers, or healthcare providers. A 2023 survey of 500 radiologists found that 78% were concerned about unclear legal responsibilities when using AI-based medical imaging [25]. AI is designed to support, not replace, human decision-making, but defining accountability is crucial for patient safety and trust.

Determining who is liable for AI misdiagnoses is complex, as multiple stakeholders–including AI developers, hospitals, radiologists, and regulatory bodies–play a role in AI-driven medical imaging. A notable legal case in the UK highlighted this issue when a hospital deployed an AI model for lung cancer detection. The AI flagged a patient's scan as low risk, but six months later, the patient was diagnosed with late-stage lung cancer. The patient sued the hospital, claiming excessive reliance on AI led to a delayed diagnosis [26]. The court ruled that clinicians must retain final decision-making authority, hospitals cannot shift responsibility to AI, and AI must remain an assistive tool rather than an autonomous decision-maker. This case underscores the need for human oversight and well-defined liability frameworks in AI-assisted healthcare. Human-AI collaboration is ushering in a new era of medical imaging, where AI enhances, rather than replaces, human expertise. However, ethical accountability, oversight, and transparency are crucial to ensuring that AI improves diagnostic accuracy and patient care without compromising trust or justice in medical decision-making.

3 Regulatory Perspectives: Frameworks and Challenges

As AI-directed medical imaging gets more revolutionized in the healthcare systems, so do the regulations, to ensure safety, efficacy, fairness, and transparency. But AI being a fast-growing area, a lot of regulations are already out of date, creating a significant oversight gap. This section will discuss the existing regulations for AI in global settings, challenges in implementing those policies, and solutions to strike a

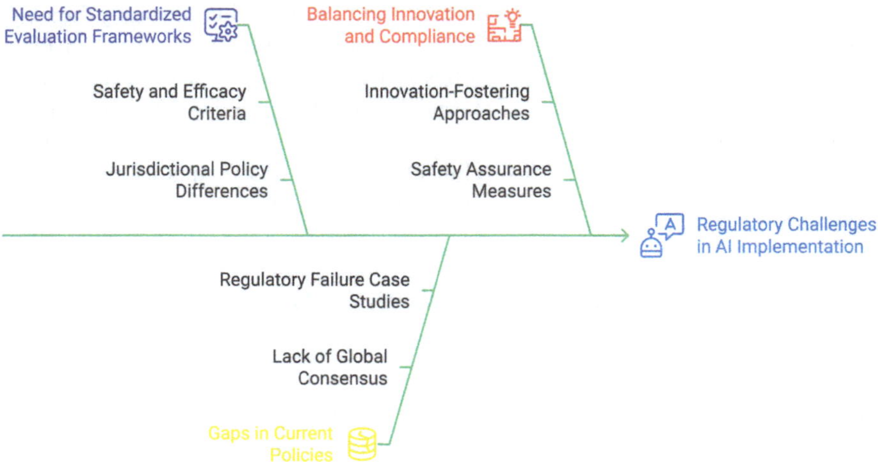

Fig. 4 Navigating AI regulatory challenges: a framework for addressing policy gaps, safety standards, and innovation compliance

balance between innovation and compliance. Such is the regulatory complexity of AI, highlighted in Fig. 4, that key regulatory challenges in AI implementation are identified.

The diagram categorizes major hurdles into three domains: the need for standardized evaluation frameworks, the balance between innovation and compliance, and gaps in current policies. Safety and efficacy criteria, jurisdictional policy differences, and regulatory failure case studies are critical issues raised in the ongoing discourse surrounding AI on the global stage. Addressing these issues requires harmonized legal frameworks to ensure technology moves forward while safely treating patients.

3.1 Need for Standardized Evaluation Frameworks

AI models in medical imaging are currently tested under varied conditions, leading to inconsistent performance across healthcare settings. The lack of standardized benchmarks results in biased models, unreliable diagnoses, and clinician mistrust. Establishing rigorous validation frameworks is essential to ensure transparency, reliability, and broader clinical adoption. Studies show that up to 30% of AI-based radiology, models fail when tested outside their original training environments, emphasizing the importance of diverse validation [27]. Additionally, AI must demonstrate consistent performance across racial, gender, and geographic lines. A 2022 study found that AI models trained on North American datasets saw a 36% accuracy drop when applied in Asian hospitals, exposing the risks of non-diverse training data [28]. The lack of explainability further limits AI acceptance, as 72%

Table 4 Navigating AI regulations in medical imaging: a country/region perspective on key challenges

Country/Region	Regulatory body	Key AI regulation for medical imaging	Challenges
United States	FDA (Food & Drug Administration)	AI/ML-Based Software as a Medical Device (SaMD)	Slow approval process for AI models
European Union	EMA (European Medicines Agency)	EU Artificial Intelligence Act (2023)	Strict compliance rules may hinder AI innovation
United Kingdom	MHRA (Medicines & Healthcare Regulatory Agency)	AI Fairness and Safety Act (2023)	Requires extensive bias testing before approval
China	National Medical Products Administration (NMPA)	AI Medical Ethics Guidelines (2022)	AI restrictions limit cross-border collaborations

of radiologists prefer not to rely on AI tools unless they provide clear reasoning for diagnoses [29]. Without interpretability, AI risks becoming a black-box system, undermining its potential in clinical decision-making. Regulatory frameworks must set clear guidelines for safety, validation, and transparency, ensuring AI meets rigorous standards before clinical deployment.

The complexity of global AI regulations further complicates AI adoption and standardization. Regulatory inconsistencies across jurisdictions create gaps in safety, fairness, and compliance. The FDA in the USA mandates strict clinical validation, with only 343 AI-driven tools approved for clinical use by 2023. Meanwhile, the EU's GDPR prioritizes patient privacy and transparency, requiring AI developers to meet strict data protection and consent laws. China enforces real-world testing and post-market monitoring to maintain long-term AI efficacy. These differences pose challenges for AI developers seeking universal compliance, slowing global AI integration into healthcare. Establishing harmonized international standards would enable safe, effective, and globally accepted AI-driven medical solutions, ensuring consistency, trust, and equitable patient outcomes. Table 4 shows several standardizations according to different Jurisdictions.

A 2023 study found that 42% of AI medical tools face delays or restrictions in international markets due to conflicting regulations [30]. This highlights the need for global guidelines to ensure uniform safety, accuracy, and ethical standards for cross-border AI systems. Such frameworks would enhance AI adoption, protect patient rights, and maintain global trust in AI medical imaging. While certain countries have their rules and regulations, the world has no global standard. The EU Artificial Intelligence Act (2023) defines medical AI as "high risk," necessitating strict assessments before clinical approval.

3.2 Gaps in Current AI Regulations and the Consequences of Regulatory Failures

Nonetheless, AI regulation has left significant gaps and, as such, has not fully grasped the risks in many regions of the globe. One of the most important issues, however, is global AI standardization because countries differ greatly in their approach to regulatory means. The EU AI Act makes risk-based governance of AI compulsory, but the USA continues to depend on sectoral regulations and does not have a comprehensive federal mechanism in place. China has a kind of governance concerning AI and states it as being state policy and given importance in terms of ethical supervision as well as national security measures. Such regulatory differences, thus, create hurdles in compliance and create legal ambiguities along with bottlenecks of innovation for AI developers. According to the 2023 report of the World Economic Forum, over 70% of AI stakeholders believe that regulatory fragmentation poses a major concern for investment in global AI, especially for sectors such as healthcare, finance, and autonomous systems [31]. This regulatory alignment across borders would be important in terms of the UN and OECD to ensure that AI can be developed increasingly responsibly but also at scale.

Failures in AI governance have consequences for the social, ethical, and legal arenas, which can be seen in high-profile case scenarios, such as the scandal surrounding the Dutch SyRI: In 2020, it was revealed that an AI fraud detection system discriminated against low-income and minority communities by breaching the laws of human rights due to a lack of transparency. The COMPAS algorithm, used by the U.S. criminal justice system, was similar in that it did not maintain racial parity: Black defendants were deemed to have higher probabilities of recidivism than those computed for White defendants. Facebook's AI-powered ad targeting (2019) enabled discrimination in housing, employment, and lending, leading to charges for violating U.S. fair housing laws [32]. Deaths from fatal crashes under misleading marketing, such as dependence on AI without a human being present, were emphasized even more through the Tesla Autopilot accidents. Similarly, the algorithm used for A-Level grading in the UK (2020) dealt with an unfair downgrading of students from disadvantaged backgrounds and escalated educational inequalities [33].

These failures highlight glaring deficiencies in regulation: the absence of transparency for AI decisions; use of biased training data; insufficient testing; and lack of oversight on, e.g., high-risk areas such as healthcare and criminal justice. Governments must therefore enforce increasingly stricter ones on AI to avert such failures, adhere to ethical principles, and establish accountability for safe, fair, and responsible AI operations in society.

3.3 Balancing Innovation and Compliance

AI regulations must strike a delicate balance between safety, fairness, and transparency with regard to allowing innovation. Too-restrictive regulations would hold back AI deployment. Too-lenient regulations might compromise patient safety. Adaptable regulatory approaches need to be put in place to facilitate advances in AI while holding on to ethical and legal virtues.

Adaptive regulation is an approach employed in governing the AI, compared to FDA USA, the continuous learning model incorporates real-time updates of AI models without requiring re-approval. In 2023, an AI model for lung cancer detection was successfully updated with new patient data, reducing the approval time by 70% (FDA Report 2023) [34]. Another strategy is regulatory sandboxes, introduced by the UK and Singapore, where AI developers test medical imaging models in controlled environments before full approval. A 2022 study found that such sandboxes accelerated AI approval by 40% while maintaining safety standards (Singapore AI Health Report, 2022) [35]. Additionally, global regulatory harmonization is gaining traction, with the WHO advocating for a unified AI framework that aligns FDA, EMA, and MHRA policies. The 2023 WHO AI Ethics Summit recommended an international AI regulatory standard to prevent approval inconsistencies across countries (WHO AI Policy, 2023) [36].

While organizations like the FDA, EMA, and MHRA have introduced AI policies, bias risks, inconsistent explainability requirements, and the absence of global AI standardization remain challenges. Regulators must balance ethical responsibility with AI's evolving capabilities, ensuring bias audits, transparency enforcement and the development of international governance frameworks. A well-regulated AI ecosystem will enable safe, efficient, and ethically sound applications in medical imaging while fostering continued innovation.

4 Case Studies: Ethical and Regulatory Dilemmas

Whereas AI-based medical imaging made commendable progress in terms of diagnostic accuracy and efficiency, in real-world circumstances, ethical and regulatory challenges arise if the AI has not been properly validated, monitored, or deployed responsibly. This section explores some critical case studies highlighting AI mishaps due to data privacy infringement, algorithmic bias, and regulatory loopholes.

4.1 Data Privacy Breach in AI Model Training

Artificial intelligence's quick march has made huge demands on mass datasets, such as user interaction and social media, healthcare, and financial records. However, the unregulated collection of such data without the consent of data subjects in the absence of security measures led to significant privacy violations of sensitive personal information. Governmental and corporate AI surveillance show the threats of an AI left unchecked-for instance, data collection where the protection of privacy seems to be a barrier to innovation. Other glaring cases testify to the unethical, legal, and social issues in AI-enabled data processing.

1. Case Study: NHS Patient Data and Google DeepMind Controversy (2016–2021)
   The National Health Service (NHS) from the UK joined hands with Google DeepMind in 2016 intending to get an AI system that diagnoses acute kidney injury (AKI) at an early stage. The project was intended to transform the secondary diagnosis and treatment using a database of 1.6 million patient records from three different hospitals in London [37]. Although it assisted in detecting kidney disease early as compared to screening with the traditional methods, the project stirred strong controversy about data privacy, patient consent, and regulatory oversight [38]. Patients scientifically infringed such violations constituted abuse of data protection laws because they never informed patients that their medical records were used for AI training. The ICO report in 2017 found DeepMind breached both GDPR and UK data privacy regulations as a result of the unauthorized use of patient data.
   Thus, the National Health Service could not allow further collection of anonymized NHS patient data by DeepMind until more stringent measures were taken to improve privacy protection. In 2021, NHS formally announced that the strategic partnership with DeepMind was terminated on grounds of lingering problems regarding data privacy. The case brought tighter rules in the UK, including mandatory patient consent requirements in AI model training (ICO Report, 2021). It showcases the importance of having the GDPR and HIPAA in place for control the patient now has over his health data becomes pertinent in ensuring ethical and transparent AI deployment in the healthcare setting.
2. Case Study: Clearview AI—AI and Facial Recognition Privacy Violations
   Clearview AI, a facial-recognition company, was found to have illegally scraped billions of images from social media platforms without the user's consent to create an AI surveillance tool [39]. Law enforcement agencies usually use the said technology for identification which is without legal oversight hence raising serious privacy and civil liberties concerns. As a resultant effect, countries like Canada, the UK, and Australia banned Clearview AI for being a severe violator of some data privacy laws. The case shows the possible dangers of unregulated AI surveillance and the urgent need for robust legal frameworks in the protection of biometric data.
   The controversy exposed major ethical and regulatory failures, chiefly the illicit collection of personal data and the absence of a global standard on AI-enabled surveillance. In this context, Clearview AI became involved in multiple lawsuits and faced financial penalties, including a €20 million fine in 2021 imposed by the French data protection authority (CNIL) for violating the GDPR [40]. The litigation launched in 2020 turned up the heat in global discussions regarding AI surveillance, prompting various national governments to start imposing regulatory restrictions on facial recognition technology. This case highlights the necessity for concrete ethical standards, legal clarity, and stringent

international regulations so that mass surveillance can be avoided to ensure the upholding of individual privacy rights at the desired level in an AI setting.

These cases reveal the risks of unregulated AI surveillance and demonstrate the necessity of stringent legal frameworks, ethical practices, and accountability in the use of biometric data.

4.2 Algorithmic Bias in Disease Detection

The potential of AI diagnostic tools to improve disease detection is vast, yet they are not resistant to bias. Algorithms trained on non-diverse datasets-the race, gender, or socio-economic background diversity yield skewed results and, in the end, impact an underrepresented population disproportionately. With increasing dependence on AI by health care systems, algorithmic bias becomes an issue that needs to be found a solution to ensure very medical outcomes become equitable. The next couple of case studies describe real-world incidences where AI bias affected disease detection and would thus bring wore for more above the development of fair and inclusive AI.

1. Case Study: Google's Retinopathy AI in India and Thailand (2020)

   Google's AI system for diabetic retinopathy detection was developed to enhance early diagnosis, yet its real-world deployment in India and Thailand exposed critical limitations. Even though AI was quite capable in a controlled lab environment, it did not perform well with variability concerning image quality, local workflow or with the realities in a medical settings environment. Such discrepancies resulted in significantly high false-negative rates while constantly rejecting images, rendering the system utterly impractical for burdened health-care workers. The failure depicted the chasm between theoretical efficiency in AI and real-world applicability, stressing the need for local adaptations and validation in real-world situational applications before their global deployment [41].

   Ethically, the system's inconsistent performance raised questions about the reliance on AI with inadequate human oversight. The lack of field testing and regional customization therefore hindered clinical uptake in both nations. Although there were no major legal challenges to the case, it raised discussions regarding the need for local regulatory scrutiny of AI-driven medical tools before deployment. This case emphasizes the importance of the real-world rigorous testing of AI implementations, adaptation of AI to the specific region, and human supervision throughout the AI's lifecycle, to ensure the trustworthy and ethical use of AI in healthcare globally.
2. Case Study: Epic's Sepsis Prediction Model (2021)

   Epic Systems, a special corporation regarding developing AI, has created a model by which it could identify early signs of sepsis-associated factors found in hospitals all over the United States, but yet, according to a study published in 2021, it could only discriminate 7% of real sepsis cases in terms of accuracy of detection against a great number of false positives [42]. The study has blamed this defective performance on unsatisfactory standard electronic health records (EHR) data, which represents how AI bias could occur from insecure data sources. This failure certainly expresses the urgency of thorough clinical validation before large scaling into critical care settings.

The incorrectness of the model increased the clinical workload due to the overwhelming false alarms that burdened the healthcare personnel and hospital resources. While the issue did become quite controversial, no legal consequences were drawn against anybody; however, it did raise questions about the regulatory procedures on which such AI programs are approved for use in intensive care settings. This case has highlighted the dangers posed by the use of unvalidated AI models in high-risk healthcare scenarios. The way forward requires the enforcement of ongoing validation, more rigorous testing, and solid monitoring protocols to ensure that AI models being put to use in the medical industry are dependable, trustworthy, and clinically safe.

4.3 Regulatory Challenges in Multi-National AI Deployment

Regulatory obstacles in AI-driven medical imaging stem from different laws on data privacy and their approval processes. In the EU, there is GDPR, and in the USA, there are FDA regulations. This creates discrepancies in compliance. The WHO report FDA [43] from 2023 states that 67% of AI healthcare applications were not standardized for approval, which presents a challenge for their adoption on a global scale. Some nations have no governance regarding AI, which raises questions regarding security and accountability for data. Therefore, closing those regulatory gaps is going to be vital in international collaboration for the safe, effective, and equitable use of AI in healthcare.

1. Case Study: IBM Watson Health's AI Misdiagnosis Scandal (2018–2021)

   IBM Watson for Oncology's main aims were to aid doctors in the diagnosis and recommendation of cancer therapy. However, it could not show good results in hospitals elsewhere in the world. The issue was that most of Watson's learning had been acquired from U.S.-based medical data because usually most of its recommendations had higher variations from healthcare protocols in places like India and China [44]. Treatment guidelines vary from one country to the other based on the country; therefore, the recommendation from Watson was often contrary to the local practice in medicine, making it more complicated due to regulatory hurdles. All these led to the fact that many of the hospitals in Asia shut down use because one must not assume that the AI model trained in a certain part of the world would be functional across the globe. Thus, it highlighted the necessity for adaptation and validation regarding the region as relates to AI before a global deployment.

Although there weren't any legal penalties involved, Watson's failure lowered confidence in AI-based oncology tools. The case brought to light a need to feed AI with a diverse dataset, comply with the local health regulations, and should be used only as a decision support tool rather than as a freestanding method. Future applications of AI in medicine will therefore need to think about localization, regulatory alignment, and human oversight to achieve safe, efficient integration into different healthcare environments.

2. Zebra Medical Vision's AI Imaging & U.S. FDA Approval Delays (2019–2022)

   Zebra Medical Vision, an Israeli AI startup, developed imaging algorithms for disease detection in X-rays, CTs, and MRIs [45]. While CE certification was granted for Europe, the technology was delayed from entry to the U.S. market due to regulatory differences. The European regulators had paler restrictions allowing for an easier path to AI adoption, while for the U.S. FDA, the strategy was to require substantial clinical trials and real-world validation before any sort of approval. This meant that Zebra Medical Vision would not consider entering the U.S. market for several years unless an AI was accepted in the European healthcare system. This demonstrates the complexity of AI regulations throughout the world and the need for companies to adapt to the different validation, safety, and approval routes in different countries.

   The discord in regulations between the two sides of the Atlantic has not favored the use, adoption, and furtherance of AI-related technologies; rather, it has postponed market access and innovation. Although no litigation ensued from the case, it underscored such difficulties for multinational AI deployment and called for urgent global harmonization in the regulatory framework. Such a globally standardized approach would ultimately simplify approvals, speed up the entry of AI in healthcare, and ensure innovative, safe, and effective uses.

4.4 Key Takeaways from the Case Studies

Table 5 covers the regulations studied, including the Main Ethical/Regulatory Concern, Influence, and Regulatory Outcome. It provides a summary of the major regulatory challenges, ethical issues, and legal outcomes from the case studies, which lay a foundation for transparency, compliance, and an international standard for AI-based healthcare.

These examples highlight the case for developing AI in medical imaging with fairness, transparency, and regulatory oversight to ensure ethical and responsible deployment. There have been many failings of AI in medical imaging-from privacy infringements and racial biases down to producing misdiagnoses-leading to an imperative need for concrete regulatory frameworks. Tighter elements for patient consent, mandatory bias audits, and globalization of regulatory frameworks need to be implemented to guarantee the ethical effectiveness and fairness of AI in healthcare.

Table 5 Regulatory and ethical challenges in AI deployment: a comparative analysis of key case studies

Ref:	Case study	Main ethical/ regulatory issue	Impact	Regulatory outcome
[37]	Google DeepMind & NHS Patient Data Controversy (2016–2021)	Patient consent violation and breach of GDPR & UK data protection laws	Raised concerns over unauthorized access to 1.6 million patient records and lack of transparency in AI medical data usage	NHS ended its partnership with DeepMind; which led to stricter UK regulations mandating explicit patient consent for AI training (ICO Report, 2021)
[39]	Clearview AI—Facial Recognition Privacy Violations	Unauthorized scraping of billions of social media images and lack of oversight in law enforcement AI usage	Sparked concerns over mass surveillance, privacy breaches, and civil liberties violations	Banned in Canada, UK, and Australia; faced multiple lawsuits and a €20 million fine from French data authorities for GDPR violations
[41]	Google's Retinopathy AI in Thailand and India (2020)	One main challenge faced by AI systems today is that although they are highly rigid, they are also unstable in comparison to humans	High respective negativity incidence in valid image samples has impaired the clinical take-up in India and Thailand	Aside from possible legal implications, local technical Pharos legislation and regulatory review are also issues to consider in AI usage in health care.
[42]	Epic's Sepsis Prediction Model (2021)	AI model failed to accurately detect sepsis, leading to unreliable diagnostics	Increased clinical workload due to false alarms, straining hospital resources	Intensified calls for stricter validation protocols before AI deployment in hospitals, though no legal penalties were imposed
[44]	IBM Watson for Oncology Misdiagnosis Scandal (2018–2021)	AI model was trained primarily on U.S.-based data, making it incompatible with non-Western healthcare systems	AI recommendations contradicted local treatment guidelines, leading to discontinuation in Asian hospitals	No legal action, but the failure diminished trust in AI-driven oncology tools and highlighted the need for localized adaptation
[45]	Zebra Medical Vision's AI Imaging & U.S. FDA Approval Delays (2019–2022)	Regulatory disparities between U.S. FDA and European CE certification for AI-based imaging	Delayed U.S. market entry despite AI approval in Europe, limiting global adoption	Reinforcing the need for standardized global AI regulations to streamline approval processes

5 Recommendations for Inclusive and Transparent AI Systems

AI-driven medical imaging transforms healthcare by enhancing diagnostic accuracy, efficiency, and patient outcomes. However, without proper safeguards, AI risks amplifying bias, violating patient privacy, and creating accountability gaps. In the most effective sense, illustrated in Fig. 5, the proactive strategies for fair and privacy-preserving AI systems, such as bias audits, federated learning, human-in-the-loop, and fool-proof global policy frameworks should be enhanced. It is essential to strengthen patient data protection, regulatory compliance, and global AI governance to responsibly integrate AI into medical imaging.

5.1 *Bias Mitigation and Inclusive AI Development*

To guarantee fairness, AI models must be trained using a wide variety of input data and representative datasets due to the differences in race, gender, and geography. A study conducted in 2023 Nature Medicine found that diversity with an increment of 32% accuracy can be achieved in the model for underrepresented groups by increasing the variety of the dataset [46]. Mandatory bias audits are critical in this regard; thus the UK MHRA (2023) requires fairness audits preceding AI approval. Transparency in data collection and demographic representation is also necessary, with initiatives like AIM-AHEAD by the NIH (2023) working to counter AI bias in healthcare datasets [47].

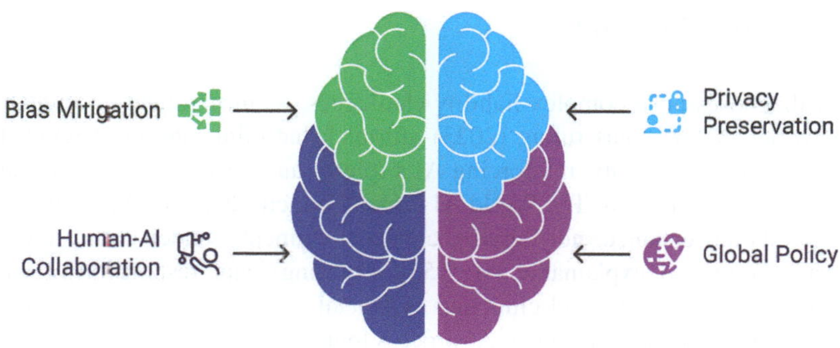

Fig. 5 Framework for ethical AI in medical imaging: key strategies for bias mitigation, privacy preservation, human collaboration, and global policy development

5.2 Privacy-Preserving AI Techniques

AI relies on large volumes of patient data, raising concerns about privacy and security. Federated learning allows AI models to train across multiple hospitals without sharing raw patient data, retaining 97% accuracy while improving privacy by 85%, as demonstrated by Google Health [48]. Differential privacy introduces mathematical noise to datasets, reducing re-identification risks by 98% without affecting accuracy [13]. Blockchain technology ensures tamper-proof and transparent data sharing, with a 2023 Mayo Clinic study showing a 92% reduction in unauthorized access risks [49].

5.3 Human-AI Collaboration and Explainability

AI should support, not replace, human decision-making. The "Human-in-the-Loop" approach ensures clinicians remain actively involved in AI-assisted diagnoses. A 2023 clinical trial found that AI-assisted radiologists had a 43% lower diagnostic error rate than those relying solely on AI [50]. AI explainability is critical, using tools like SHAP, Grad-CAM, and Saliency Maps to provide interpretable insights. The European Medicines Agency (EMA, 2023) now mandates AI explainability for regulatory approval [51]. Without regular audits, AI performance can degrade over time, with MIT (2023) reporting an 18% drop in accuracy if updates are neglected [52].

5.4 Global Governance AI and Accountability for Ethical Medical Imaging

AI misdiagnoses pose complex liability challenges, requiring clear accountability frameworks. A UK court ruling (2023) affirmed that clinicians must retain final decision-making authority, reinforcing AI's role as an assistive tool rather than an autonomous system [26]. The World AI Ethics Council (2023) further emphasized that "AI should enhance, not replace, clinical judgment," underscoring the need for transparent and explainable AI [53]. Defining legal responsibility among AI developers, hospitals, and clinicians is crucial, ensuring transparent decision-making, regular updates, and clear AI process logging. Studies suggest clinician-AI collaboration reduces diagnostic errors by 43%, while overreliance on AI increases liability risks [54]. At the global level, regulatory frameworks must evolve to ensure ethical AI governance and standardization. The WHO AI Policy (2023) advocates for a unified global AI framework, promoting consistency in healthcare AI regulations [50]. Germany introduced national AI medical malpractice insurance (2022) to clarify legal responsibility in AI-driven diagnoses (Germany AI Ethics Council, 2022) [55]. The UK's AI Fairness and Safety Act (2023) now mandates bias audits and fairness assessments before AI approval [56, 57]. To uphold ethical, transparent, and effective AI in medical imaging, developers, healthcare institutions, and regulators must enforce bias audits, implement privacy-preserving techniques, and mandate human oversight. Establishing global AI governance will align safety standards and ensure AI benefits all patients equitably, securing its place as a trustworthy tool in modern healthcare.

6 Conclusion

The rapid evolution of AI-driven medical imaging has brought unprecedented advancements in diagnostic accuracy, efficiency, and personalized treatment. Thus, implementation of this technology in the health sector must be accompanied by carefully considering ethical and regulatory challenges to ensure patients' trust, safety, and fairness. Despite promising change, there are critical issues related to the privacy and safety of personal data concerning algorithmic bias, transparency, accountability, and inconsistencies between regulatory rules. All these have to be addressed to avert unexpected consequences. Protecting patient privacy and informed consent is one of the main challenges to AI models today because such models depend on highly populated clinical imaging databases. The existing regulations, especially HIPAA and GDPR, provide a basis for protecting patient data, but enforcement gaps prove the need for stricter global privacy standards. By involving technologies like federated learning, differential privacy, and blockchain, data can be secured without compromising AI efficiency. One concern is that of algorithmic bias-when AI models trained on non-diverse datasets further magnify already-widely experienced healthcare disparities. Various studies have revealed the underperformance of AI dermatology models on darker skin tones, further compelling bias audits, diverse datasets, and fairness testing for equitable AI diagnosis.

Without a doubt, one major roadblock for acceptance in the clinic is the absence of transparency in AI-based decision-making beyond bias and privacy. Many AI models work as black boxes, and clinicians are unable to interpret the rationale behind the diagnoses. Explainable AI techniques such as SHAP, Grad-CAM, and Saliency Maps can improve the interpretability and trustworthiness of AI-assisted diagnostics. However, the issue of legal accountability continues to prevail in the case of misdiagnoses. The blurred lines of liability as a framework create legal ambiguity among the parties involved: hospitals, AI developers, and clinicians. Establishing human-in-the-loop AI systems, AI liability insurance, and defined laws of accountability would be important for the ethical adoption of AI. Furthermore, regulatory inconsistencies among the FDA, EMA, and WHO generate discrepancies in AI approvals, which is "why a need for a global AI medical imaging standard to harmonize regulations."

As artificial intelligence undergoes further advancement, its effects on medical imaging will be determined by the ethical and regulatory structures governing it.

Thus, future efforts should place paramount importance on matters of privacy, fairness, transparency, and accountability, guaranteeing that the consideration of AI as efficient and trustworthy becomes an option to be weighed against fairness. There should be a partnership among developers, policymakers, and healthcare institutions to come up with globally binding rules for AI, countering its bias, and maintaining human intervention to develop synergy between innovation and ethical responsibility. By addressing these challenges, AI-enabled medical imaging could serve as a bedrock of modern health care that focuses on improving patient outcomes while sustaining high ethical standards and public trust.

References

1. Kanan M, Alharbi H, Alotaibi N, Almasuood L, Aljoaid S, Alharbi T, Albraik L, Alothman W, Aljohani H, Alzahrani A, Kalantan R, Althomali R, Alameen M, Mufti A (2024) AI-driven models for diagnosing and predicting outcomes in lung cancer: a systematic review and meta-analysis. Cancers 16(3):674. https://doi.org/10.3390/cancers16030674
2. McKinney SM, Sieniek M, Godbole V, Godwin J, Antropova N, Ashrafian H, Shetty S (2020) International evaluation of an AI system for breast cancer screening. Nature 577(7788):89–94
3. Lauritzen AD, Rodríguez-Ruiz A, von Euler-Chelpin MC, Lynge E, Vejborg I, Nielsen M, Lillholm M (2022) An artificial intelligence–based mammography screening protocol for breast cancer: outcome and radiologist workload. Radiology 304(1):41–49
4. Pesapane F, Volonté C, Codari M, Sardanelli F (2018) Artificial intelligence as a medical device in radiology: ethical and regulatory issues in Europe and the United States. Insights Imaging 9:745–753
5. Liddell K, Simon DA, Lucassen A (2021) Patient data ownership: who owns your health? J Law Biosci 8(2):lsab023
6. Groh M, Badri O, Daneshjou R, Koochek A, Harris C, Soenksen LR, Picard R (2024) Deep learning-aided decision support for diagnosis of skin disease across skin tones. Nature Med 30(2):573–583
7. Bradley S (2022) The role of imaging in the diagnosis of lung cancer in primary care. Doctoral dissertation, University of Leeds
8. Smith H (2022) Artificial intelligence use in clinical decision-making: allocating ethical and legal responsibility. Doctoral dissertation, University of Bristol
9. Rai HM, Tsoy D, Daineko Y (2024) MetaHospital: implementing robust data security measures for an AI-driven medical diagnosis system. Proc Comput Sci 241:476–481
10. Puri A (2020) A theory of group privacy. Cornell JL Pub. Pol'y 30:477
11. Luke JJ, Rutkowski P, Queirolo P, Del Vecchio M, Mackiewicz J, Chiarion-Sileni V, Eggermont AM (2022) Pembrolizumab versus placebo as adjuvant therapy in completely resected stage IIB or IIC melanoma (KEYNOTE-716): a randomised, double-blind, phase 3 trial. The Lancet 399(10336):1718–1729
12. Kumar S (2022) The role of data (deletion) permission frames, data sensitivity, audiences, and defaults on consumers' willingness to share personal information
13. Khalid N, Qayyum A, Bilal M, Al-Fuqaha A, Qadir J (2023) Privacy-preserving artificial intelligence in healthcare: techniques and applications. Comput Biol Med 158:106848
14. Petersen E, Potdevin Y, Mohammadi E, Zidowitz S, Breyer S, Nowotka D, Herzog C (2022) Responsible and regulatory conform machine learning for medicine: a survey of challenges and solutions. IEEE Access 10:58375–58418
15. Singh Y, Jabbar MA, Kumar Shandilya S, Vovk O, Hnatiuk Y (2023) Exploring applications of blockchain in healthcare: road map and future directions. Front Public Health 11:1229386

16. Mahmood U (2022) Deep learning for medical imaging in a biased environment. Rochester Institute of Technology, New York
17. Almansouri NE, Awe M, Rajavelu S, Jahnavi K, Shastry R, Hasan A, AlAbbasi RK (2024) Early diagnosis of cardiovascular diseases in the era of artificial intelligence: an in-depth review. Cureus 16(3)
18. Hoffman KM, Trawalter S, Axt JR, Oliver MN (2016) Racial bias in pain assessment and treatment recommendations, and false beliefs about biological differences between blacks and whites. Proc Natl Acad Sci 113(16):4296–4301
19. Ruamviboonsuk P, Cheung CY, Zhang X, Raman R, Park SJ, Ting DSW (2020) Artificial intelligence in ophthalmology: evolutions in Asia. Asia-Pac J Ophthalmol 9(2):78–84
20. Yang J, Soltan AA, Eyre DW, Yang Y, Clifton DA (2023) An adversarial training framework for mitigating algorithmic biases in clinical machine learning. NPJ Digital Med 6(1):55
21. Zhang B, Vakanski A, Xian M (2023) BI-RADS-NET-V2: a composite multi-task neural network for computer-aided diagnosis of breast cancer in ultrasound images with semantic and quantitative explanations. IEEE Access 11:79480–79494
22. Nguyen TN, Yang HJ, Kho BG, Kang SR, Kim SH (2024) Explainable deep contrastive federated learning system for early prediction of clinical status in-intensive care unit. IEEE Access 12:117176–117202
23. Chen M, Wang Y, Wang Q, Shi J, Wang H, Ye Z, Qiao Y (2024) Impact of human and artificial intelligence collaboration on workload reduction in medical image interpretation. NPJ Digital Med 7(1):349
24. Zou L, Goh HL, Liew CJY, Quah JL, Gu GT, Chew JJ, Ta AWA (2022) Ensemble image explainable AI (XAI) algorithm for severe community-acquired pneumonia and COVID-19 respiratory infections. IEEE Trans Artif Intell 4(2):242–254
25. Paudyal R, Shah AD, Akin O, Do RK, Konar AS, Hatzoglou V, Shukla-Dave A (2023) Artificial intelligence in CT and MR imaging for oncological applications. Cancers 15(9):2573
26. Pearce T, Sharkey E, Haffenden L, Thomas J, Dr Sinan Eccles, Lung Health Check (LHC) Clinical Lead; Chris Coslett, LHC Programme Manager; Claire Wright, LHC Project Manager; Amy Smith, LHC Programme Support Officer
27. Eche T, Schwartz LH, Mokrane FZ, Dercle L (2021) Toward generalizability in the deployment of artificial intelligence in radiology: role of computation stress testing to overcome underspecification. Radiol Artif Intell 3(6):e210097
28. Arora A, Alderman JE, Palmer J, Ganapathi S, Laws E, Mccradden MD, Liu X (2023) The value of standards for health datasets in artificial intelligence-based applications. Nature Med 29(11):2929–2938
29. Reyes M, Meier R, Pereira S, Silva CA, Dahlweid FM, Tengg-Kobligk HV, Wiest R (2020) On the interpretability of artificial intelligence in radiology: challenges and opportunities. Radiol Artif Intell 2(3):e190043
30. Blum N (2023) Navigating the AI regulatory landscape: a meta-narrative approach to assessing the impact of regulation on innovation. Doctoral dissertation, Wien
31. Davtyan T (2024) An overview of global efforts towards AI regulation. Bull Yerevan Univ C Jurisprudence 15(2)(41):158–174
32. Jan T (2019) HUD charges Facebook with housing discrimination. The Washington Post
33. Yu S, Carroll F (2022) Implications of AI in national security: understanding the security issues and ethical challenges. In Artificial intelligence in cyber security: impact and implications: security challenges, technical and ethical issues, forensic investigative challenges. Springer International Publishing, Cham, pp 157–175
34. Khinvasara T, Ness S, Shankar A (2024) Leveraging AI for enhanced quality assurance in medical device manufacturing. Asian J Res Comput Sci 17(6):13–35
35. Buocz T, Pfotenhauer S, Eisenberger I (2023) Regulatory sandboxes in the AI Act: reconciling innovation and safety? Law Innov Technol 15(2):357–389
36. Cihon P (2019) Standards for AI governance: international standards to enable global coordination in AI research development. Future Humanity Inst Univ Oxford 40(3):340–342

37. Powles J, Hodson H (2017) Google DeepMind and healthcare in an age of algorithms. Health Technol 7(4):351–367
38. Taylor MJ, Wilson J (2019) Reasonable expectations of privacy and disclosure of health data. Med Law Rev 27(3):432–460
39. Rezende IN (2020) Facial recognition in police hands: assessing the “Clearview case” from a European perspective. New J Eur Criminal Law 11(3):375–389
40. Tartaro A, Smith AL, Shaw P (2023) Assessing the impact of regulations and standards on innovation in the field of AI. Preprint, arXiv:2302.04110
41. Grzybowski A, Singhanetr P, Nanegrungsunk O, Ruamviboonsuk P (2023) Artificial intelligence for diabetic retinopathy screening using color retinal photographs: from development to deployment. Ophthalmol Therapy 12(3):1419–1437
42. Li F, Wang S, Gao Z, Qing M, Pan S, Liu Y, Hu C (2025) Harnessing artificial intelligence in sepsis care: advances in early detection, personalized treatment, and real-time monitoring. Front Med 11:1510792
43. Joshi G, Jain A, Araveeti SR, Adhikari S, Garg H, Bhandari M (2024) FDA-approved artificial intelligence and machine learning (AI/ML)-enabled medical devices: an updated landscape. Electronics 13(3):498
44. Ahmed MN, Toor AS, O’Neil K, Friedland D (2017) Cognitive computing and the future of health care cognitive computing and the future of healthcare: the cognitive power of IBM Watson has the potential to transform global personalized medicine. IEEE Pulse 8(3):4–9
45. Milam ME, Koo CW (2023) The current status and future of FDA-approved artificial intelligence tools in chest radiology in the United States. Clin Radiol 78(2):115–122
46. Kleinberg G, Diaz MJ, Batchu S, Lucke-Wold B (2022) Racial underrepresentation in dermatological datasets leads to biased machine learning models and inequitable healthcare. J Biomed Res 3(1):42–47
47. Cary Jr MP, De Gagne JC, Kauschinger ED, Carter BM (2024) Advancing health equity through artificial intelligence: an educational framework for preparing nurses in clinical practice and research. Creative Nursing 30(2):154–164
48. Ali M, Naeem F, Tariq M, Kaddoum G (2022) Federated learning for privacy preservation in smart healthcare systems: a comprehensive survey. IEEE J Biomed Health Inf 27(2):778–789
49. Devarapu K (2020) Blockchain-driven AI solutions for medical imaging and diagnosis in healthcare. Technol Manag Rev 5(1):80–91
50. Alanazi MMF, Almutairi SFM, Alarjani NO, Alghaylan MYA, Aljawhari MSM, Alkhulaifi AAS (2024) Advancements in AI-driven diagnostic radiology: enhancing accuracy and efficiency. Int J Health Sci 5(S2):1402–1414
51. Polzer A, Fleiß J, Ebner T, Kainz P, Koeth C, Thalmann S (2022) Validation of AI-based information systems for sensitive use cases: using an XAI approach in pharmaceutical engineering. HICSS 7(2):1500–1509
52. Liu M, Reinders H (2025) Do AI chatbots impact motivation? Insights from a preliminary longitudinal study. System 128:103544
53. WHO Guidance (2021) Ethics and governance of artificial intelligence for health. World Health Organization, Geneva
54. Rosic A (2024) Legal implications of artificial intelligence in health care. Clin Dermatol 42(5):451–459
55. Bottomley D, Thaldar D (2023) Liability for harm caused by AI in healthcare: an overview of the core legal concepts. Front Pharmacol 14:1297353
56. Rietzler M (2022) Who is responsible if an AI system gives a wrong diagnosis? Analysis of the EU liability law framework of medical AI
57. Goktas P, Grzybowski A (2025) Shaping the future of healthcare: ethical clinical challenges and pathways to trustworthy AI. J Clin Med 14(5):1605

AI in Medical Image Analysis: Societal Impact and Inclusivity

R. Sruthi, M. Sujithra, and B. Senthilkumar

1 Introduction

1.1 AI in Medical Image Analysis

Medical image analysis through artificial intelligence development constitutes an advanced operational healthcare technology. Detecting crucial data from X-rays and computed tomography requires medical experts to collaborate with evaluation of magnetic resonance imaging and ultrasound and positron emission tomography systems. Prior to today medical specialists along with radiologists performed all their analysis based solely on visual interpretation skills. Hospital image data collection has surged dramatically creating novel operational obstacles that produced innovative solution options. Deep learning and computer vision algorithms under AI technologies now operate as highly precise tools for analysing medical image data. The systems track patterns and anomalies as well as fine changes which humans could miss which results in earlier medical discoveries and better diagnosis decisions. Medical image processing utilizes convolutional neural networks (CNNs) to analyse image data at multiple abstraction levels until the final classification and segmentation tasks become possible.

Applications of AI in medical image analysis span numerous specialties. AI technology supports radiological institutions by helping detect lung nodules as well as breast lesions and intracranial haemorrhages. The medical field of dermatology

R. Sruthi (✉) · M. Sujithra
Department of Computing – Data Science, Coimbatore Institute of Technology, Coimbatore, India
e-mail: 2032043mds@cit.edu.in; sujithra@cit.edu.in

B. Senthilkumar
Department of Mechanical Engineering, Kumaraguru College of Technology, Coimbatore, India
e-mail: senthilkumar.b.mec@kct.ac.in

N. Ben Aoun et al. (eds.), *AI for Medical Image Analysis*,
https://doi.org/10.1007/978-3-032-02963-8_11

depends on these tools to evaluate skin cancer through photographic images. Medical professionals in ophthalmology use their systems to conduct retinal scans for detecting diabetic retinopathy together with other medical issues [1]. The analysis of tissue samples and cellular structures becomes possible through their assistance in pathology work. The extensive utility range of AI made it a pivotal revolutionary power in diagnostic medicine.

Thanks to recent artificial intelligence advancements this system can identify diseases and predict medical treatment effects and disease course progression as well as treatment effects for patients [2]. AI systems and radiomics enable medical professionals to derive quantitative data from images for tumor analysis and cancer treatment outcome predictions in patients. AI-based image tracking analysis facilitates necessary neurological condition monitoring of patients with multiple sclerosis and Alzheimer's disease thus generating new diagnostic tools that improve therapeutic practices. AI-based medical image analysis facilitates healthcare professionals through improved capabilities in their experienced tasks while supporting them in their work. Healthcare AI systems require frameworks to help workforce choices but allow healthcare staff members complete control over complex patient situations [3]. As shown in Table 1, AI applications span various specialties, enhancing diagnosis and efficiency across healthcare sectors.

1.2 Societal Implications of AI in Healthcare

A healthcare transformation process, primary due to artificial intelligence integration into medical imaging systems, is confronted with a lot of implementation barriers. The system supports supporters of AI technology to reduce diagnostic errors and to accelerate operational activities and handle budget costs in the future. Yet the reality is messier. For organizations to enter the AI market, they will have to go to great lengths to set up the medical facility redesigns and train medical

Table 1 AI applications in different medical specialties

Specialty	Imaging modality	AI use case	Outcome
Radiology	X-ray, CT, MRI	Detection of lung nodules, brain hemorrhages	Early diagnosis and reduced error rates
Dermatology	Clinical photography	Skin cancer classification	Improved melanoma detection accuracy
Ophthalmology	Retinal fundus imaging	Diabetic retinopathy detection	Faster diagnosis in rural settings
Pathology	Histopathology slides	Tissue abnormality identification	Enhanced cancer diagnosis precision
Cardiology	Echocardiography	Automated cardiac measurements	Support for clinical decision making

staff on new methods and administrative protocols. The fact that wealthy healthcare organizations have achieved efficiency has thus far not played a role in bridging current global economic imbalances. If underfunded, non-digital-ready regions continue to find it impossible to close their gap with the other regions, then AI will turn into a non-equalizing force, instead of an equalizing force.

Adopting artificial intelligence systems will increase medical staff's workload making them even busier while stepping down responsibilities they are presently called upon to perform. AI, a concept that radiology department apply to their activities, needs two types of tasks from radiologists: first, scan analysis and, second, verification and correction of algorithm errors. Due to a combination of these two expectations, classic work processes cannot accommodate this because non data scientist professionals are being forced to do work for tasks in which they have not received proper education. The medical workforce shortage is rising because medical facilities require the provider to have the medical expertise combined with advanced computer science knowledge yet smaller medical centers struggle in competitive recruitment [4].

The Proud AI systems trained on the training data fail to produce accurate results since the main source comes from privileged persons. The diabetic retinopathy algorithm presents dangerous outcomes and negative consequences for the rural communities when the lung cancer model is used with dark-skinned patients [5]. The lack of monitoring during system development creates a threat for discriminatory development of IT systems. Profit making development is the primary purpose and has thus pushed the progress of AI towards marketable products while failing to serve the people who are not politically capable and financially facilitated.

Therefore, it implies that healthcare policy enforcers need to express data standards that would allow developers(practitioners) to harness grassroots partnership for tool development and the administrators will accept such tools even if they opulence short term financial goods. The solutions for healthcare disparities will always rely on AI until the standard requirements for access to AI are applied to all institutions.

2 Impact on Healthcare Systems

2.1 Enhancing Access to Medical Imaging in Resource-Limited Settings

However, the 67% of the population that lacks proper access to medical imaging services leads to health disparities all over the world. At present, one million radiologists per million population are seen at LMICs while high income countries hold one radiologist for every ten thousand people. Poor treatment performance coupled with delayed diagnosis results in the negative effects for the underserved population groups due to service inequality. Currently, there is a substantial healthcare service gap and this has a vital solution which can be provided by AI [6]. The paper that the research was presented in details about the AI-powered Neurosynaptic ReMeDi system operational in rural India that provides support to remote radiologists for examining chest X-ray images by an AI software evaluation process. Through the combination of edge computing with asynchronous data transfer protocols, such limitations can be addressed and the systems can operate without internet. Currently, direct solutions of major health problems in underprivileged areas are available with current AI solutions. Helping areas where there are specialist shortages are those areas where automated tuberculosis detectors in different African regions and autonomous ultrasound analyzers for maternal care are run [7]. The technologies provide solutions that are cost effective since they do without expensive facilities and use of staff. As time goes on, initial expenditures spent in the development of an AI system turn out to be beneficial in the long run [8]. AI systems enable the early detection of various diseases, thus saving on healthcare expenses as some patients who might have required hospital treatments are not treated. Technologists make basic equipment compatible in difficult network access and simplify execution procedures for the deployment of these technologies in low resource areas.

Organizations like RAD-AID International are working to make AI accessible in the world's poorest areas, tailoring solutions to local needs. Successful implementations, such as Butterfly Network's AI ultrasound system in Rwanda, demonstrate how training and support can help integrate AI into healthcare systems. Overall, AI is driving both innovation and accessibility in healthcare, bringing essential diagnostic services to those who need them most. The AI-enabled workflow that facilitates rural healthcare access without continuous internet is illustrated in Fig. 1.

2.2 *Efficiency and Cost Savings in Healthcare Through Integration with AI*

Healthcare providers can achieve better operational effectiveness and cost control by implementing AI on their medical imaging equipment. Artificial intelligence components build economic benefits to transform diagnostic imaging service economic models and broaden their availability within healthcare centres. Medical imaging obtains its latest workflow efficiency advantage with AI technology. Automated

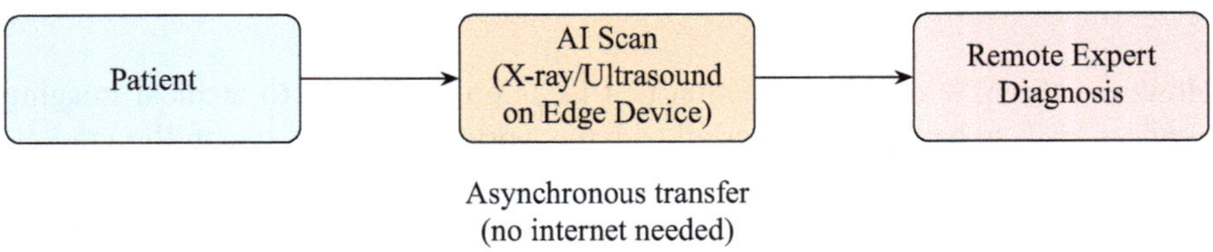

Fig. 1 AI-enabled imaging workflow in rural settings

evaluations in intelligent worklist prioritization systems accelerate critical case response times and studies indicate critical reporting intervals shorten by 20–60%. The AI triage tool allows medical researchers to conduct rapid evaluations of abnormal studies prior to concentrating on assessments of normal studies. The department's intelligent distribution system allows for greater study volume management independently of staffing needs. AI technologies integrate with time-management software to offer medical personnel support during their process of interpreting visual information. Utilizing pre-processing algorithms computer-aided detection systems guide medical professionals to locate areas of concern thus enabling radiologists to conduct their searches at a faster rate. The automated measurement solutions both speed up calculation processes through their auto-measurement functions that encompass cardiac ejection fraction measurements and tumour size assessment. The integration of AI processors uses medical terminology standards to combine draft reports that produce typical search results for quick medical report protocol fulfilment. Every productivity function in the subspecialty selection and implementation strategy pushes radiological efficiency to a potential spectrum between 30% and 30% and 10% to 30% separately.

Beyond radiology department operations, AI facilitates system-level effectiveness by increasing diagnostic precision and reducing redundancy. False positives that trigger unnecessary follow-up tests are a significant source of waste in health-care systems. Highly specific AI systems can reduce these unnecessary downstream tests, not only manual expenses, but also patient anxiety and inconvenience. Similarly, by increasing diagnostic confidence in initial tests, AI can reduce rates of recommendation for redundant or confirmatory imaging studies. The use of combined AI system in mammography screening can lead to the positive financial result for the medical organization because they have greater cancer diagnosis accuracy compared with lower recall and biopsy rates [9]. This system reduces operation cost through improving operational efficiency. The fact that AI based systems can simplify a number of administrative procedures involving handling of exam protocol inspections and radiation detection and quality assessment procedures, proves that they have the means to do so. Such a system is used to ensure regulatory compliance rules. Essential staff members are led through an automated workflow system that includes tasks of medical expertise and patient care duties. As shown in Fig. 2, AI adoption demonstrates significant improvements across key healthcare metrics, with reporting time reduction of 30%, diagnostic cost savings of 10%, and patient throughput increases of 10%. This system reduces operation cost through improving operational efficiency. The fact that AI based systems can simplify a number of administrative procedures involving handling of exam protocol inspections and radiation detection and quality assessment procedures, proves that they have the means to do so. Such a system is used to ensure regulatory compliance rules. Essential staff members are led through an automated workflow system that includes tasks of medical expertise and patient care duties. However, artificial intelligence brings a breakthrough in healthcare; one that leads to a new way of structuring things and opens a way of developing the future economic possibilities. With regards to point of care service image analysis, the answer is provided for reducing patient

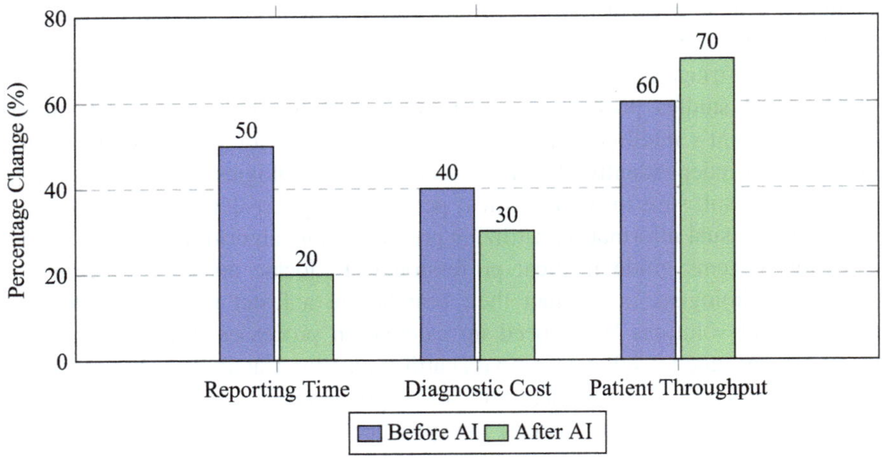

Fig. 2 Cost reduction and efficiency gains after AI adoption

transfers from medical centers on acquiring emergency situations such as strokes in addition to traumatic incidents. According to telemonitoring systems linked to artificial intelligence, healthcare delivery is possible from hospital wards to homes and helps in doctors' consideration of patient safe discharge. New care systems will bring down health care costs along with decrease in the cost which is caused owing to reduced employee productivity and family duties.

The relatively higher costs of treating patients with cancer compared to other diseases necessitates efficiency and sweeping savings in medical healthcare activities: availability of AI medical imaging makes adoption strategically attractive due to efficiency but savings.

2.3 Accurate Diagnosis and Better Patient Outcomes

With outstanding patient outcomes, due to AI based medical imaging which is accelerating the pace of the healthcare industries at a rapid pace, whereby as it enhances the accuracy of diagnosis and also provides better health care to the distant areas. Neuro oncology AI allows health professionals to assess tumor and differentiate between natural growth patterns and side effect so that surgical decision can be made. Combined imaging analysis on health information allows AI to solve cases of interstitial lung disease which are difficult cases [10]. Using standardized measures to guide the monitoring of minimal patient change in the management of multiple sclerosis therapy, AI technology enables doctors to monitor the progress [11].

Medical facilities use the AI technology to improve patient care quality in different service fields. This speed in the detection of strokes via AI consequently leads to better healthcare outcomes. Cancer detection screening allows patients to find out they are sick with cancer before the patient has symptoms enabling better cure statistics. The real time monitor allows medical staff to adjust chronic disease treatment just soon as possible. The combining of AI with the qualified healthcare staff helps to make the most of AI in healthcare practices. Then, despite human doctors still developing robotics-based analysis through adding contextual knowledge that is needed for successful medical operation, there are many opportunities to improve the quality of electronic health records. Strict validation tests through large groups of patients, clear reporting standards, along with continuous evaluations are to be paired with patient success verification.

3 Reducing Inequities in Medical Imaging

3.1 Bias in AI Models and Its Impact on Marginalized Groups

If appropriate management approaches to minimize bias do not exist, high-level medical imaging AI systems could potentially develop biases that make matters worse in the realm of healthcare disparities. Negative biases of AI system development create adverse effects on target groups all from creation to the actual implementation, which includes both development and initial designing of the product. Bias in AI systems stems from multiple sources and can significantly affect diagnostic accuracy and healthcare equity. One major contributor is training data bias. When AI systems are trained predominantly on data representing higher demographic groups, their performance tends to favor those populations. For instance, dermatological AI tools perform best on images of light-skinned individuals, while cardiac imaging systems often detect male-specific symptoms more accurately, thereby failing to recognize female-centric manifestations of the same conditions [12]. The impact on patient care is profound, especially for vulnerable populations. These groups often experience delayed or inaccurate diagnoses due to the poor performance of AI tools [13]. For example, AI systems used for tuberculosis detection may underperform when analyzing chest X-rays of HIV co-infected patients, leading to inadequate or delayed treatments [14, 15].

Differences in healthcare system infrastructure further exacerbate bias. Disparities in equipment standards and image quality across institutions mean that AI systems trained on high-quality images from advanced medical centers may falter when used with lower-quality data from under-resourced facilities, resulting in suboptimal care delivery. Another critical issue is labeling bias, which arises from inconsistencies or inequalities in how data is labeled across different clinical settings. This bias can cause diagnostic algorithms, such as those used in cardiac failure detection, to perform poorly for certain groups, reinforcing healthcare disparities rather than mitigating them. To effectively reduce bias in AI systems, several strategies must be employed throughout the development lifecycle.

Table 2 Bias sources and mitigation techniques in AI systems

Bias source	Example	Mitigation strategy
Training data bias	Overrepresentation of privileged groups	Diverse, balanced datasets
Labeling bias	Gender-skewed annotations	Standardized labeling protocols
Infrastructure bias	Images from advanced hospitals only	Multi-setting data collection
Algorithmic bias	Favoring specific demographics	Fairness-aware model design
Deployment bias	Poor results in rural settings	Field validation across regions

First, ensuring diverse and representative data collection is crucial. This includes considering a broad range of demographic, geographic, and clinical factors to ensure AI tools serve varied populations equitably. Second, algorithm design must incorporate fairness techniques such as balanced sampling and fairness constraints to counteract embedded biases. Regular and stratified validation of AI tools across different population subgroups is also essential for performance transparency and accountability [16].

Moreover, policy and regulatory frameworks should mandate equitable performance standards and hold developers accountable for disparities. Encouraging diverse teams and stakeholder engagement during development can help surface potential biases early and foster more inclusive innovation. By integrating these principles, AI systems in medical imaging can move closer to equitable and effective healthcare outcomes for all [17].

Table 2 outlines the major sources of bias in AI-based medical imaging and offers strategies for mitigation to ensure equitable healthcare outcomes.

3.2 *Inclusive Training Datasets: Representation in Populations*

The first step for building genuine inclusive medical imaging artificial intelligence systems is to build representative training datasets. Medical imaging AI training sets also need to have strategic diversity components, such as age groups as well as gender variables plus racial elements, ethnic representations and hereditary birth place. It also needs enough demographic proportionality for full coverage of clinical situations irrespective of the characteristics of the distribute group. However, while patients with tuberculosis HIV do have tuberculosis symptoms appear differently, and breast cancer manifests different symptoms with different racial identity. Working with the All of Us and CARDIA organizations, one can use Fitzpatrick 17k and develop study groups with participants with a variety of skin traits. Data should represent diversity in healthcare, and there is a major challenge here. Imaging data can be extremely variable based on quality of equipment, protocols and infrastructure of healthcare. The data needed for this to have AI systems work requires that it is obtained from multiple settings. As large-scale efforts that went through immense efforts during the COVID 19 pandemic:

Global Health Radiology initiative based on pooled chest imaging from different countries, as well as RICORD dataset. Building these datasets is technically challenging as one has to harmonize the data coming from different protocols and instrumentation. Preprocessing algorithms and transfer technique such as transfer learning are used to learn the essential transfer information from this data while maintaining its clinical relevance. Needless to say, problems such as data privacy, intellectual property rights, costs have hindered further progress. Concerns such as how federated learning allows data to remain local and still collaborate, or the technique of data commons for responsible sharing, are among the solutions provided by federated learning [18]. Second, it is important to be engaged in the community to build trust and to make sure that marginalized groups are also part of the process. Often past data collection was conducted without these groups allowing distrust. Participation of local communities in data collection and capacity building in the context of programs such as the Africa Pathogen Genomics Initiative can enhance the quality of health outcomes and contributing to better data. In the end, you need to work in establishing and maintaining inclusive datasets for medical imaging AI through collaboration with research institutions, health systems, tech companies and regulators on an ongoing basis [19].

3.3 Sealing Healthcare Disparities with AI Solutions

AI in medical imaging has great potential to reduce healthcare disparities, particularly in underserved areas [20]. In remote regions, where radiologists are scarce, AI-powered teleradiology can help bridge the gap. Programs in Mongolia and Brazil already use AI to bring diagnostic services to hard-to-reach communities [21]. AI can also help overcome socioeconomic barriers. In places where specialist readings are expensive, AI allows general practitioners to conduct some tests with algorithmic support, reducing costs. In India, AI-assisted point-of-care ultrasound has made diagnostic imaging more affordable for primary care workers. Healthcare worker shortages, especially in radiology, are a global issue. While AI can't replace training, it can boost efficiency and decision-making. In Tanzania, AI-based workflows help radiologists manage larger volumes of studies without compromising quality [22]. Language and communication barriers often result in poor care. AI-driven translation tools and culturally sensitive content can help bridge these gaps. Additionally, AI-powered visualizations and easy-to-understand explanations make complex diagnostic information more accessible to patients with varying levels of health literacy.

AI algorithms look for underdiagnosed patterns in their work to eliminate the human healthcare provider bias. It is well established that gender targeted algorithms used in cardiac imaging improve the diagnostic outcome. The first thing that have to succeed in AI in the healthcare field is that AI must go in search of real healthcare demands, and should maintain constant cooperation with the communities affected by the development starts. During deployment planning, health equity monitoring systems should be implemented along with the existing hospital infrastructure while tracking the possible effects on the quality of health care. And to make large scale AI adoption possible government policies should include such things as reimbursement methods for AI monitoring solution and fairness regulations. Data equity in healthcare exists through all stages of AI, making the process operational as a tool to the healthcare provider to increase healthcare access and improve population health outcomes [23, 24].

4 Building Trust and Adoption in Multicultural Societies

4.1 Overcoming Cultural and Social Obstacles for AI Adoption

Medical imaging technology with AI success is dependent on the cultural acceptance and psychological acceptance and social facets since people choose to adopt based on their own choices that lead unto success. Acceptance over artificial intelligence change from one social group to another group, healthcare organization has to adjust its AI implementation strategy. Between these two options on the AI adoption path for different societies, there are two options for sensitive and gradual testing before implementation or quick urgent deployment [25]. AI is usually perceived as a threat to the professional activity of both radiologists and other healthcare professionals within their operational area. Doctors should make AI as a professional assisting tool, instead of a tool to replace human job because healthcare staff will welcome AI technologies more then. American College of Radiology, along with other professional societies is leading procedural changes to AI adoption. Both the level of trust people give AI and the level of trustability they expect from it is dependent on cultural origins. Evaluation methods for societies depend on institutions reviews or on local ratings (decided by local practitioners) respectively. The WHO Digital Health Academy explores that these communication methods and these educational methods must adapt to the cultural characteristics. For its part, participatory design programs use the local community to build AI solutions that reflect the cultural and method of living of the communities. Ethical stand must also be implemented recognising local cultural values which otherwise deems privacy and consent matters [26]. Only by having respect for cultural diversity and technical effectiveness and localization, Artificial Intelligence can bring success to healthcare systems [27].

4.2 Transparency and Explainability for AI Systems

Despite the growing use of AI in medical image analysis, many practical challenges persist in translating AI outputs into clinical decisions. Since clinical and ethical decisions are influenced by AI-generated insights, it is essential that these systems maintain full transparency and offer clear explanations. The responsibility for implementing AI in healthcare lies in its ability to communicate its reasoning in a way that supports trustworthy, ethical, and informed medical decisions. Clinicians require explainability to foster trust and ensure the acceptance of AI applications in practice. A system's outputs become clinically relevant only if practitioners can understand and rely on them. Techniques such as feature attribution, case-based reasoning, and conceptual translation methods form the basis for generating explanations that are both meaningful and comprehensible to medical professionals. Trust in AI must be built on interpretability rather than blind confidence in algorithmic certainty. Patients, too, benefit significantly from explainable AI. Medical staff must communicate risks and treatment effects in accessible, jargon-free language, often using visuals or simplified terms. Cultural and linguistic appropriateness is critical–health professionals must consider patients' backgrounds to ensure that medical information is not only delivered but truly understood [28].

Regulatory frameworks play an important role in ensuring explainability. Governments and oversight bodies have introduced policies, such as FDA guidelines, that define annotation standards, functional criteria, and application-specific risk assessments for AI/ML in medicine. These regulations are designed to support ongoing innovation while minimizing potential harm. Recent scientific advances have improved model interpretability in AI. Tools now allow analysts to visualize critical areas of images that influenced AI decisions, and methods such as LIME (Local Interpretable Model-agnostic Explanations) help uncover the logic behind complex outputs [29]. Integration with early-stage system models enables the mapping of machine learning reasoning to medical terminology. While explainability has traditionally been seen as a trade-off to performance, emerging self-explaining neural networks demonstrate that high performance and clarity can coexist [30].

Explainability needs also differ across cultures. Some societies value transparency in development processes and clear accountability, while others emphasize local context and tradition in building trust. These cultural norms influence how AI systems are received and understood. As AI expands globally, developers must design communication strategies aligned with diverse cultural values. Clinicians, in turn, become more confident using AI when they understand the reasoning behind the outputs. Any lack of transparency risks reducing clinical value, eroding user trust, or creating overreliance on opaque systems [31].

The future of explainable AI in medical imaging is promising. Users increasingly seek interactive explanations that demonstrate how inputs affect outputs. Contextual explanation techniques offer adaptable insights that go beyond basic interpretations, helping to overcome traditional limitations of AI explainability. Ultimately, explainable AI is vital for building trust and accountability in healthcare systems. Transparent systems not only clarify AI operations but also foster cooperation between human clinicians and AI tools. This alignment enables AI to serve as a reliable partner in critical medical decision-making, reinforcing both safety and quality of care. Figure 3 illustrates a typical explainable AI (XAI) pipeline in medical imaging, where models first perform feature detection, followed by explanation

Fig. 3 Explainable AI pipeline for medical imaging

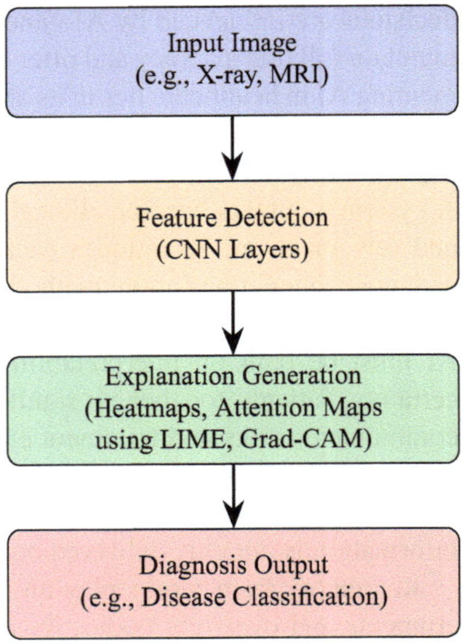

generation using techniques like LIME and Grad-CAM, before providing diagnostic outputs.

4.3 Stakeholder Engagement to Promote More Inclusiveness

The technical accomplishment of developing and deploying AI systems for healthcare imaging cannot be a separate enterprise from the rich social contexts in which healthcare is provided. To develop genuinely inclusive and effective solutions, there needs to be real interaction with diverse stakeholders across the entire AI lifecycle, from formulating the problem through to post-implementation surveillance. Patient and community participation is the most elementary form of stakeholder engagement. Historically, the innovation of medical technology has evolved with limited input from the very populations the technology is designed to serve, particularly underrepresented or marginalized populations. This pattern frequently results in technologies that are not sensitive to actual community needs or patient values and preferences. Progressive models of AI development involve engagement of patient input from the very beginning, including involving representative diversity from the community in problem setting, need identification, and requirement definition. All of Us Research Program models this through its infrastructure of large-scale community participation, including participant ambassadors, community advisory boards, and deliberative engagement sessions that inform program priorities and policies.

Participation by providers at the full spectrum of healthcare roles also enhances AI inclusivity. While radiologist participation in AI development has been on the rise, inclusive participation involves referring clinicians, technologists, nurses, and other clinical team members whose work streams intersect with imaging workflows. Multidisciplinary input from these practitioners uncovers several aspects of clinical usefulness, deployment challenges, and conceivable unintended consequences. Multistakeholder input during collaborative development activities, such as the American College of Radiology's AI-LAB platform, demonstrates how to integrate the diverse input systematically during the development process, from use case selection to interface design and validation planning. Health system leadership engagement is crucial to scaling and sustainable implementation. Administrative leaders, operations managers, quality improvement officers, and IT directors offer essential information on resource availability, organizational priorities, and feasibility of implementation. Early involvement of these stakeholders allows AI development to be aligned with institutional strategy and establishing potential barriers to adoption [32]. Executive sponsorship and cross-departmental leadership alignment are often cited as key success factors in successful AI implementation [33]. The NASSS (Non-adoption, Abandonment, Scale-up, Spread, Sustainability) model is one such systematic approach to engaging organizational stakeholders with influencing factors of technology adoption and spread.

Payer and policy stakeholder engagement addresses the economic and regulatory aspects required for sustainable deployment. Highly technical AI solutions cannot produce impact if not supported by sustainable reimbursement streams or regulatory certainty. Early engagement with payers, health technology assessment organizations, and regulators during development allows foresight of requirements and alignment of technical requirements with market access strategies. The FDA's Digital Health Software Precertification Program is an excellent example of interagency cooperation with regulators and innovators to develop appropriate oversight strategies for rapidly developing digital health technologies. Global stakeholder engagement is especially necessary for AI systems to be deployed in various healthcare environments. What can be done in high-resource environments may not be done or even desirable in environments with varying infrastructure, workforce mixes, or clinical priorities. Network engagement such as that provided by the Novartis Foundation's AI4BetterHealth Network and WHO's Digital Health Technical Advisory Group offers technology developers and global settings stakeholders the chance to interact and ensure new AI solutions align with global health agendas and not fuel current inequities in the innovation of healthcare.

Systematic stakeholder engagement practices have evolved to support inclusive technology design. Human-centred design practice strongly emphasizes iterative cycles of observation, ideation, and testing with representative users in a variety of contexts. Participatory action research approaches involve community members as co-researchers rather than research participants. Value-sensitive design systematically incorporates stakeholder values into technical requirements and design decisions [34]. Each of these practices provides concrete models for bridging stakeholder engagement from principle to practice. Digital divide concerns must be specifically addressed in stakeholder engagement plans. The same populations most in need of accessible AI-enabled solutions are often excluded from contribution to traditional engagement activities by low digital access or technical capacity. Effective engagement plans employ multiple modes and formats, combining digital and in-person approaches that are adjusted to different stakeholder needs and capacities. For example, the PATH Digital Square program employs tiered engagement strategies combining high-tech digital platforms with low-tech community discussion to facilitate broad-scale contribution into digital health priorities. Stakeholder engagement impact measurement remains challenging but must be performed to enhance and be accountable. Emerging types of evaluation combine process measures (influence on decisions, depth of involvement, representativeness) and outcome measures (stakeholder needs alignment, implementation success, user satisfaction). The approaches distinguish significant engagement from tokenistic consultation and provide evidence to the value proposition of inclusive development practices. As the field evolves, stakeholder engagement is increasingly viewed not as a voluntary nicety or compliance exercise but as a determinant of AI quality and impact. The most successful examples demonstrate that investing in high-quality, inclusive engagement processes yields dividends in algorithm performance, clinical utility, and implementation success.

5 Ethical Frameworks for Impact on Society

5.1 Equity in Innovation and Non-discrimination

The pursuit of fairness in AI-driven medical imaging requires careful consideration throughout the innovation process from research prioritization to algorithm design to implementation and regulation. Building robust frameworks for non-discrimination is an ethical and practical imperative for achieving the potential of AI to reduce rather than increase healthcare disparities. Prioritization decisions in research thus shape the equity impact of technological innovation. Where research agendas and funding decisions are most influenced by commercial goals or the interests of affluent populations, the resulting technologies are most likely to address privilege concerns, rather than need. To innovate to equitable purposes there will be intentional alignment between distribution of disease impacts and both needed medical care and predictable health disparity outcomes. Other organizations joined the Coalition for Health AI and together we developed frameworks for assessing solutions helping developers and funders to pick what will bring most benefit to underserved communities during application selection.

The second vital aspect of the equity focus is that academic groups should introduce practice of inclusive development. There is a set of three fundamental attributes of inclusive development, where those are created with inclusion of diversity in research teams, symbolic data collection, and active community participation during design phases, as well as dispersed quantitative measurements across a number of population segments. Evidence increasingly suggests more equitable algorithms being developed by diverse development teams as a result of greater sensitivity to potential bias channels and to diverse user needs. Initiatives like the Black in AI and Women in Machine Learning communities are already working on representation in AI research, with guidelines like IEEE's Ethically Aligned Design providing systematic approaches to inclusive AI development. Concepts and metrics of fairness raise challenging technical and philosophical questions for algorithmic fairness [35]. Different conceptualizations of fairness–e.g., demographic parity, equal opportunity, or equalized odds–may be appropriate for different contexts and have inherent trade-offs at times. Technical solutions to algorithmic fairness have evolved considerably, e.g., pre-processing techniques to remove bias from training data, in-processing techniques that embed fairness constraints in model training, and post-processing techniques that adjust model outputs for fairness. Best practices for next-generation approaches suggest using an ensemble of complementary fairness metrics and involving multiple stakeholders to determine appropriate fairness concepts for a specific clinical use case. Pre-market evaluation frameworks increasingly include explicit equity assessments. Conventional validation methods based solely on aggregate performance measures can mask enormous disparities among population subgroups, especially when these subgroups are small validation dataset percentages. Stronger methods are stratified performance analysis by demographic, geographic, and clinical subgroups; performance stability assessment under conditions of dataset shift; and targeted assessment in historically underserved populations. Regulatory frameworks are likewise adapting to include these considerations, with agencies such as the FDA creating special guidance for assessing bias in AI-based medical devices.

Although the strategies that establish outcome equity in the development of AI systems for health care implementation are far off, AI systems are still moving in their development towards health care implementation. However, technical algorithm equivalence continues to keep health care inequalities since different implementations and systems that do not exist in other health care settings persist. Organization for successful AI solution implementation needs progressive planning; supporting areas with higher need levels, providing multiple support level to healthcare facility that does not have the requisite resources and designing an adaptive workflow solution for various facility environment. Without complete equity evaluation of health system models such as Kaiser Permanente and its peers during their technological deployment processes, such models are not adopted. Post market surveillance is the last crucial requirement to the achievement of equity assurance. As shipments of the systems occur into diverse healthcare circumstances, the performance of the systems evolves over time to create results that the developers fail to anticipate. However, performance data monitoring can identify and document statistically meaningful differences between population groups for which investigations are triggered. Health outcomes, along with technical performance indicators, are used to measure the outcomes of clinical fairness in the monitoring process when technology-based fairness actually results in clinical fairness. Some of this research on AI capability surveillance happens at the National Artificial Intelligence Institute at the VA, which employs integrated monitoring protocols.

Table 3 Comparison of ethical frameworks for equitable AI

Organization	Focus areas	Key guidelines
WHO (2021)	Ethics, equity, human rights in AI	Promote inclusivity, mitigate bias, enhance transparency
IEEE	Fairness, accountability, transparency	Ethical development and deployment standards
UNESCO (2022)	Human rights, open science initiatives	Global equity and responsible innovation promotion
FDA (USA)	Patient safety, validation standards	Explainability, risk evaluation, clinical use authorization

Throughout all the development stages towards artificial intelligence systems, principles of equity and non-discrimination are put into active promotion of equity. The real equal outcomes are implemented in AI systems when the ran in the programmed algorithm and the elements of the social and technical and the elements of the operation are rans at the same time. Ethical frameworks play a vital role in guiding equitable AI deployment, as summarized in Table 3.

5.2 *Risk Mitigation for AI-Mediated Error*

Before it is brought into operation, AI-driven medical imaging systems generate new forms of operational risk that healthcare professionals need to anticipate. Two main risks related to AI systems for medicine are inadequacy of performance and work-related issues between the medical staff and machines. When results are executed on AI systems, there are failed essential information detection, incorrect assessments, and erroneous result classifications among others. When testing AI systems under different environmental conditions, the points were found at which performance errors are most apt to occur during program evaluation.

A risk is created if AI systems are leaned upon too much by physicians and they would fail to catch certain medical conditions. In all cases, both for patient safety and for the protection of healthcare workers from accountability of AI systems, all healthcare workers must be adequately trained to understand that an AI system serves as a tool to help them do the work but that the systems do not hold the power of the decision making, and therefore they can always remain 100% confident in the results from the AI system. However, AI proposals are ignored by the healthcare providers when they do not trust earlier malfunctioning or obsolete systems. To establish trust, AI needs longer time and healthcare providers can help promote this by the display of showing its effective operation, along with clear performance feedback from cases [36]. Therefore, to avoid any operational disturbances or mistakes, AI technology deployment requirements should follow the current work processes. For smooth deployment implementation implemented through the established design tools, then continuous post launch inspections have to be applied [37].

There is at present much confusion about who can be blamed for errors in systems operated by Artificial Intelligence Systems. Developer accountability is in need of an additional definition because it indicates the level of accountability a developer should play in the duties with healthcare providers and clinicians [38]. The different security risks will affect how the technology is deployed: For content and service generation (second readings), against justifiable security risks will be allowed to be transferred. Before choosing an AI application method, which one to utilize, proper risk assessment as well as creating a safety mechanism must be done. Developers cannot be in the constant state of flux and keep attention focused; operating system performance dwindles; because they are continuously working on the development of their system. In addition to update tracking, to assess when system revalidation is needed, system performance has to be inspected on a regular basis.

6 Future of Inclusive AI for Medical Imaging

6.1 Global Collaboration Frameworks and Cross-Border Sharing of Knowledge Development

Inventing truly inclusive AI for medical imaging needs to engage shall we say uni... disciplines, sectors, organisations, and countries in cooperation in order to break down the traditional boundaries. There are new models of global cooperation that would be unlikely to slow innovation, but instead could well accelerate its greasing while guaranteeing its spread as widely and fairly as possible. Medical AI development is challenged with the monopoly of the closed innovation, but there have been great strides in open science strategies. Sources like MIMIC-CXR, MedMNIST and the COVID-19 Image Data Collection are open data, important to global developers; software libraries such as TensorFlow, PyTorch, and medical imaging toolkits are open source, freeing doctors from crippling licensing fees in implementing this technology. The researchers and programmers in low resource environment would be excluded from accessing AI innovation. Lacuna Fund is one such initiative that directly funds the development of open training data sets out of the underrepresented areas that plugging data gaps that might otherwise reinforce algorithmic biases. Efforts such as the Coalition for Health AI represent that movement going even higher openness, by creating open, standardized evaluation benchmarks for evaluation for algorithm performance on different populations. However, facilitative innovation has also been highly effective using cooperative research networks. Geographical and economic spaces help institutions come together to embrace research agenda and build capacity within the engaged regions. It teams 27 nations with the centralized region and high end skills in a collaborative network that integrates high end skills without discounting the aspect of geography when focused on the algorithm design and verification which are the network collaboration. Similarly, the Human Heredity and Health in Africa (H3Africa) consortium has played the lead role for models of fair scientific partnership among researchers in high income countries and African institutions through local leadership and capacity building both, and scientific progress. By targeting a diversity of research needs across sites in a formalized collaboration, knowledge sharing is promoted, so that research needs in the places where the data were not collected can be met.

Recently, knowledge transfer systems are undergoing change allowing for bidirectional learning rather than the one-way conduction of high resource technology into low resource environments. Conventional belief in knowledge transfer presumed that innovations created in high resource environments would simply need to be made suitable to the lower resource world. These days, as current thinking sees the merit in 'reverse innovation'–where low resource technologies introduced can have lessons for all–observers find many lessons to be drawn from those who had limited resources to produce competing solutions. For example, in contexts in which one requires low connectedness for the working of solutions AI, one could find potential to be used for emergencies and in remote areas of even high-income countries. The WHO Digital Adaptation Kits provide a systematic support for adaptation of digital health technologies across environments to keep their critical functionality. Regulations harmonization is aimed to strike a balance between elimination of redundancy and sufficient regulation of AI technologies. Today, jurisdictional diversity of regulation is real and constraining to deployment worldwide (for the small developers without the resources to cope with crossing multiple multiple difficult approval processes). With the increasing need for regulatory coordination of AI related demands, conferences such as the International Medical Device Regulators Forum are seeking more interoperability in common documentation or even acceptance of evidence generated in other jurisdictions. The harmonization initiatives especially come in handy to innovators in countries with little or no regulatory infrastructure because this makes the ways to international markets more transparent [39].

New models of licensing and commercialization are emerging that will balance intellectual property protection with fair access. Licensing of technology has been with conventional limitations of whom can pay and who cannot, perpetuating health inequities. Other models incorporate tiered price levels with corresponding national income levels; licensing provisions that are universalized under a humanitarian obligation that guarantees access under conditions of low resource settings; and collaborations of public and private partnerships (PPPs) to share the development costs and risks. These organisms include Medicines Patent Pool, who have made their mission extend beyond pharmaceutical intellectual property agreements to also cover some digital health technologies. Implementation science collaborations are precisely intended to solve the problem of scaling up promising AI technologies from the lab to everyday clinical use in different settings. These partnerships recognize that challenges in implementation can vary considerably from one healthcare system of infrastructure, staff, funding mechanism and culture. Implementation learning sharing frameworks (such as the NIH Implementation Science Centres Collaborative) have been established in order for settings with context adaptation strategies (such as the Landmark Transforming Prevention into Practice Project) to learn from each other through collaboration. Likewise, the digital health technology implementation using adapted collaborative implementation models has been equally put forward for the PATH Digital Square project for low resource settings.

Perhaps most important aspect of the inclusive international cooperation is capacity building. While such advanced technologies will enable the creation of considerable value for individual companies and consumers, it relies on sustained investment in human resources, infrastructure and institutions focused on developing regions that were hitherto impoverished in terms of research and development of AI technologies. Examples of such regional capacity building include Deep Learning Incaba in Africa, AI4ALL in North America, AI Singapore, and others that demonstrate how efforts can be made to build local expertise and leadership in AI innovation in regions in Africa, North and South America, and Asia-Pacific. Newly, in the context of Global cooparations, the authenticity capacity building gained greater priority through faculty mobility, collaborative degree programs, common research facilities, and stable institutional partnerships rather than brief trainings or technology transfers. Coordination of this variety of collaborative activities is already beginning to take on multilateral forms of governance. The normative architecture for global cooperation in the development of health AI is currently defined by organizations such as the World Health Organization in its Global Digital Health Strategy and UNESCO in its recommendation on the ethics of Artificial Intelligence. Through such governance mechanisms, it is intended to facilitate cooperation but at the same time maintain consistency with common principles like equity, transparency, and human rights. Such systems are evolving and they represent critical coordination mechanisms for the network of actors working together to develop global health AI [40].

Figure 4 presents a schematic overview of major global AI collaboration networks for healthcare, highlighting organizations such as WHO, H3Africa, and the Coalition for Health AI.

6.2 *Ethics Frameworks toward Equitable Distribution of AI for Healthcare*

AI advantage may not be a technical and practical problem so much as it is an intense moral necessity, the fair delivery of it across world populations. It is therefore most appropriate for nacent ethical regimes to consider how dimensionally multifaceted the care the medical imaging AI providing state-of-the art achieves for humanity both individually and collectively the measures that are necessary

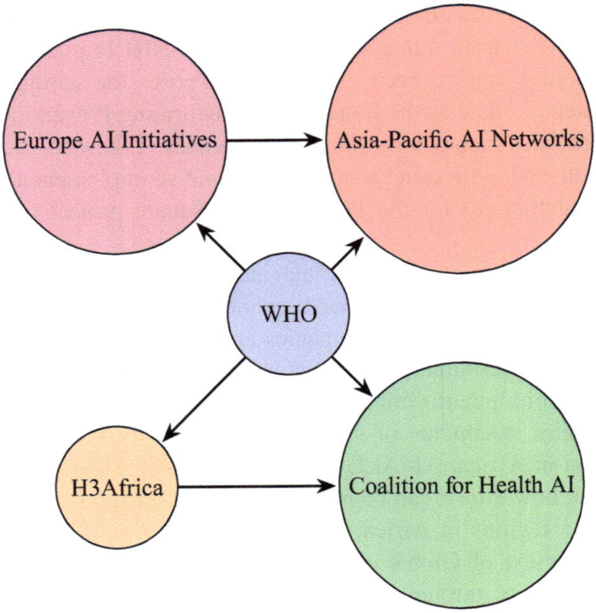

Fig. 4 Global AI collaboration networks map

to ensure that the medical imaging AI is not expanding preexisting medical inequalities. Distribution ethics in medical AI are supported by the theories of justice that they do have philosophical anchors to. Alternative distributions of definitions of justice allow for alternative distribution principles: egalitarian theories highlight the equal access to all circumstances; utilitarian theories focus on maximum advantage across groups; prioritizing structures prioritize progression of the worst off; and capability approaches focus on facilitating the basic human functioning. On the other hand, these theoretical frameworks can in some practical way guide the distribution structures. For instance, the WHO's Guidance for Ethics and Health Care AI prioritizes strengths and strategy that emphasize using AI to enable all groups to improve core health capabilities [41] whereas the National Academy of Medicine's model incorporates prioritarian principles by highlighting uses of AI toward underserved groups. Operational fact that healthcare systems have limited resource and competing demands is addressed by a resource allocation model. While these frameworks limit such decisions to organized frameworks for choosing how and when to make investments and use AI with equity, they also point to these limits. Accountability for Reasonableness (A4R) was originally formulated for deciding priorities in the healthcare and is now being used with an emphasis on open criteria, appropriate reasoning, appeals mechanisms, and mandating these conditions for AI implementation choices. In the same vein, MCDA methods enable open discussion of priorities to apply Artificial Intelligence, between different considerations about health effects, equity implication, practicability of implementation, and sustainability. They provide some certainty of distributional choices that are deliberated upon rather than succumbed to technological passion or market demand.

Most health AI distribution is now being guided by human rights thinking. In international documents like Universal Declaration of Human Rights and International Covenant on Economic, Social and Cultural Rights, the right to health implies absolute rights to access to necessary health care whichever the place and whether one is rich or poor. When applied to artificial intelligence technologies, this view takes the view that fundamental diagnostic functions together with AI is something that should be available to all populations as part of health systems, and not a luxury. While Human Rights Watch and the United Nations Office of the High Commissioner for Human Rights are beginning to create recommendations on the use of human rights framework in the field of health care AI, they are pointing to both access rights and protection against algorithmic discrimination or exploitation. International Health Equity Frameworks specifically looks at cross national health technology distribution. All the frameworks take into account the existing differences between health resources, infrastructure and outcomes from one country or region to another. Current models of global health assistance have been to contribute to maintenance of dependency arrangements rather than building sustainable capacity. Shared responsibility, mutual knowledge flow and ownership of technology introduction at the local level are modern approaches. In response, the Commission on Global Governance for Health provides a set of principles to define the principle of fair distribution of digital health technologies, like it proportional universalism (equal access to proportionally more resources in regions of higher need), common research agendas, as well as equitable sharing of benefits and burdens of technology creation. AI technologies have huge distribution patterns that are determined by the intellectual property regimes. Most classic IP models are geared to recovery of investment, and the risk of depriving access by ability to pay. Other strategies are meant to strike a balance between the incentives for innovation and providing equal access by enforcing compulsory licensing provisions, patent pools, open source development models and public funding of research subject to access provisions. First adopting the Medicines Patent Pool model for drug access, some digital health technologies are now beginning to follow this model in enabling collaboration on IP rights between grants, especially when they are aimed at improving access. The Open-Source Medical Imaging project provides a means to save open sources AI algorithms using open licenses compatible with adaptation in different contexts in parallel to this.

Apart from availability per se, implementation ethics broaden considerations of distribution with quality and suitability on how AI is placed and deployed across contexts. Uncritical technology transfer is not ethical implementation which includes local context, infrastructure needs, workforce consideration and acceptance in culture. Such contextually acceptable action is guided by RRI principles that anticipate the implementation challenges, reflect in local circumstances, inclusive dialogue with affected communities, responsive revision according to impact observed. By providing overall context to distribution, they help ensure that actual clinical incorporation is the end result of the lead instead of symbolic but meaningless presence of technology.

Therefore, ethical distribution models are anchored on accountability mechanisms. They make sure that commitments to distribution equate to real meaning for access and do not bias against progress as well as emphasize. New accountability strategies include open report-ability for AI's use, by geographic axes and demographic axes, subject to third party auditing of the algorithmic performance in various implementations; community oversight boards with actual implementation authority; and formal equity impact analysis of patterns and outcomes in distribution. The Health Equity Tracker is an example of what kinds of data openness can enable, in terms of results: it makes disparities transparent and measurable, which can thus in turn serve as a measure of accountability for distributing technology [42]. In addition, further ethical considerations arising from intergenerational concerns involve long-term sustainability and the future use of a technology. Attention to the phenomena of access, however, does not only demand that we pay attention to the current level of access, ethical allocation requires that we pay attention to the creation of sustainable capabilities for the development, adaptation and maintenance of technology. The path laid out here is a vision of investment in education infrastructure, research capacity and self reliant innovation environments and not being dependent on external skills or supplies on an ongoing basis. The principles it elaborates on will establish the capacities to engender scientific careers for regions over time, with an emphasis on digital technologies and artificial intelligence, in line with UNESCO Recommendation on Open Science.

The more these ethical frameworks evolve, the more these frameworks provide the most critical direction for tackling the sophisticated decisions that go along with the use of advanced medical imaging AI in different global settings. Ultimately, they depend on being integrated into projectable policy tools, funding streams, and implementation practices through which ethical ideals become implementations of tangible access enhancement.

6.3 AI's Role in Achieving Universal Health Coverage

Universal Health Coverage (UHC)–that everybody should have their access to required health services not preclude by financial constraints–is a core global health objective expressed in the Sustainable Development Goals [43]. However, artificial intelligence in imaging has great potential to support this goal, but it should be considered with care, as it should be in alignment with UHC policy [44]. Primary care is a central UHC strategy where AI has great potential for strengthening. The initial interface with healthcare is via robust primary health systems which in turn plan patient pathways to the remainder of healthcare at a specialised level. In theory, ailment, or at least a key bottleneck in many healthcare systems, resolves itself by augmenting primary care imaging with AI to increase the diagnostic capacity, without specialist availability. For example, AI can assist in performing routine diagnostic ultrasound by a trained primary healthcare worker to minimal specialized training, and computerised chest X-ray screening algorithms can help in TB and pneumonia detection at a community health facility. These complement the WHO's emphasis in strengthening primary health as the key UHC efforts.

In turn, adequate technology adoption makes sure that AI solution requirements do in fact align with the realities of the various existing healthcare contexts and, in particular from an IT capacity point of view, do not require unrealistics infrastructure or capability. However, UHC implementation occurs under different resource conditions and technological solutions have to be effective with these constraints. Offline operation support for environments such as those with low connectivity is one of the adaptation strategies: there are simplified user interfaces to help providers that are demographically diverse in their levels of digital literacy, high performance over a wide range of equipment specifications and integration with existing clinical workflows, without needing radical practice change. This flexibility is shown with CAD4TB initiatives which adapt their implementation to local limitations in countries across Bangladesh, Peru and many more, maintaining essential functionality. However, quality assurance is an important but often ignored aspect of UHC. If services are of poor quality and are not fit for purpose, universal coverage means very little. Specifically, standardized interpretation support, auto quality checking on imaging reports and rule-based decision support to achieve guideline consistent clinical decisions can be used to improve consistency of quality in care setting. For example, in a regional roll out of AI-augmented chest Xray interpretation across Southeast Asia [45], an AI aided chest Xray interpretation reduces interpreter variation and increase of facilities meeting national TB screening guidelines across facilities with varying capacity. Such improvements in quality support the WHO's well-known focus on effective coverage (i.e., access to service delivery of adequate quality to produce expected health results) as the actual benchmark of UHC progress.

Proper adaptation to appropriate technology ensures that AI solutions use fit each of the situations that various health care settings provide, rather than requiring the unrealistic facility, or expertise. Implementation of UHC therefore has to be across multiple different settings, with different resources, and meanwhile, technology solutions need to adapt to those limitations. Adoption strategies include offline capability, uses in settings of low connectivity; streamlined provider user interfaces for a range of digital literacy; high performance in divergent equipment environments; and consistency with established clinical workflows with little or no change in practice. For example, CAD4TB models this flexibility, and with implementations around the world from Bangladesh to Peru, implementations are configured to meet the country constraints, while the functionality in the center itself remains firm. That last part is quality assurance which is often neglected as an important part of UHC. If the services are not of high enough quality to add to health outcomes, universal coverage is of limited value. Standardized interpretation support, computerized quality control on imaging studies and decision support in accordance to evidence-based guidelines are some ways AI systems can promote consistency in quality in healthcare across healthcare sites. Further improvements in quality underline, thus, the WHO's concern with quality as a measure of progress on UHC, rather than effective coverage (which entails a particular quality of goods and services, and access to them).

In UHC contexts, the governance frameworks of AI must consider how much innovation enablement it is willing to enable without being sufficiently regulated to protect public interests. Different countries have developed governance models for the way AI can be used for operationalizing UHC. Within the Thailand's UHC framework, Thailand's National Health Security Office has developed a separate digital health technology assessment program through which it assesses AI applications for coverage under covered services, using evidence of clinical effect, cost effectiveness and equity considerations. Moreover, in India, the Full Form of National Digital Health Mission specifies governance methodologies for leveraging AI in the country's thriving universal health insurance system based on several corresponding mandates for verification requirements, deployment control, etc. Governance frameworks help ensure AI investments serve goals of UHC rather than capture finite resources to generate the low population health effect. The various axes along which AI contributions are monitored include monitoring systems. Monitoring cannot be limited to the technical indicator such as algorithm's performance but goes beyond to assess coverage, quality, financial protection, and equity, all the key dimensions of making health coverage universal [46]. Instead of creating parallel assessment frameworks, more sophisticated monitoring methods utilize AI specific indicators incorporated in existing UHC tracking systems and health information infrastructures. Rwanda's national health information system now includes the specific indicators from the use, coverage, and outcome of AI-powered diagnostic services in its community-based health insurance program. This combination of monitoring strategies provides concrete evidence of how the AI can be used to improve deployment strategies and to show how the AI can contribute to achievement of UHC goals.

More and more partnership models now realize that AI progress on UHC must be realized through cooperation between sectors and stakeholders. The older development paradigm too had been an attempt at piecemeal efforts, mostly without institutional sustainability or scale. But these act rather to lay emphasis on coordinated action on national UHC priorities, shared investment work, and to establish transparent accountability arrangements. Acts of the Digital Investment Principles and the Access to COVID-19 Tools (ACT) Accelerator's diagnostic pillar illustrate how partnerships can develop and deploy AI-driven diagnostic tools at speed in the pandemic. Through such collaborative strategies, AI investments will enhance rather than depreciate other UHC approaches. As UHC continues to evolve around the world, it offers great potential for the proper integration of related AI technologies to accelerate progress towards UHC. Seizing this potential depends on intentional matching of the levels of technological means with UHC principles and the strategy of UHC implementation rather than technological perfection per se.

As shown in Fig. 5, AI has a significant impact on the core pillars of Universal Health Coverage (UHC), including accessibility, affordability, quality, and equity [47]. AI helps expand access to healthcare services, especially in remote areas,

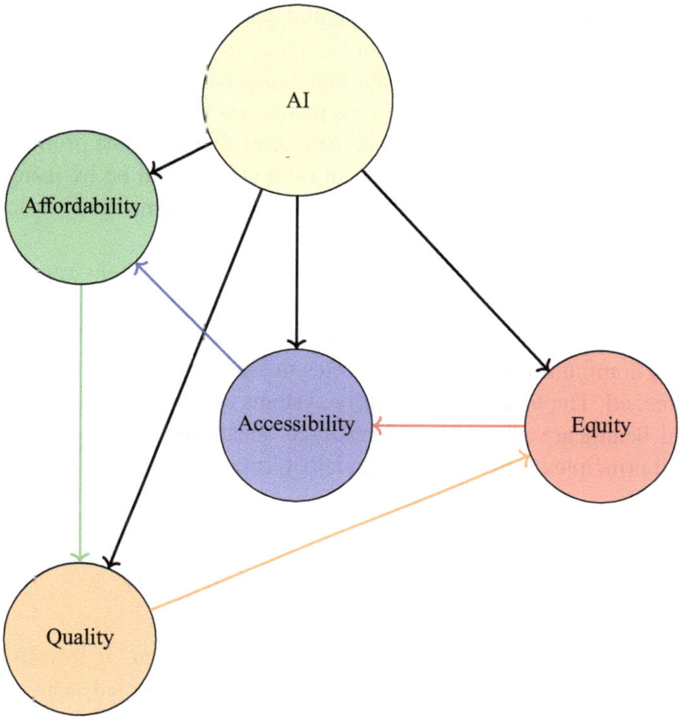

Fig. 5 AI Impact on universal health coverage goals

reduces healthcare costs, enhances diagnostic accuracy, and ensures that healthcare is more equitable for all [48].

7 Conclusions

7.1 The Need for a Balanced Approach to Innovation and Inclusivity

Nowadays, involving AI into medical image analysis has emerged as a milestone of contemporary healthcare. Although the technologies offer unprecedented diagnostic accuracy and efficiency, they are effective only if technological progress is harmonized with the issues of inclusivity, as studies indicate. During the study, inclusivity is shown to be important throughout the use of design as a course of practice and not just as a secondary consideration. Without accessibility design taking precedence over technological advances, AI devices further benefit from current healthcare disparities in the form of biases and stereotypes. All of this is a recurring trend throughout the literature and case studies reviewed. In particular, technical limitations of AI systems are inculcative. However, existing platforms heavily rely on sufficient training data that represents diverse populations in the most similar manner possible. There is no institution that possesses comprehensive dataset. Analysis of collaborative efforts discusses that the most promising path of future development of tools for global use (globally) would be by using tools like cross border collaborations, open source software Platforms and Collective Data Stores.

There is another balancing act in a policed regulatory environment. Examining the policies that different national healthcare systems have implemented demonstrates that overly restrictive systems fail to deploy valuable technologies in underserved communities, while the policies that are too loose enable harmful bias to be unchecked. The touchiest regulatory systems that allowed themselves to bend to regional healthcare priorities and resource constraints while maintaining their core ethical principles were the best regulatory ones.

7.2 Ensuring AI Benefits All Societies Equitably

There is evidence that sharing AI advantages would be fair if intentional efforts and spending dedicated to time are not undertaken. Coupled with deployment of AI tools, a number of avenues toward this objective are drawn out based on critical examination of successful and unsuccessful attempts at implementation of digital infrastructure. In field studies in low resource environments, even advanced algorithms provide only mild advantage in the areas with no stable electricity, internet access or compatible imaging device. The most successful applications capitalized on AI building and allied strategic investment in the vital core healthcare infrastructure. It is very important to represent inside governance arrangements. Through stakeholder interviews, it is shown that if historically dispossessed populations like patients of underserved communities or healthcare workers from low resource environments act meaningfully in the decision-making process,

AI systems become more sensitive to local needs and better accepted. For the serving of individuals who are not able to afford solutions as per the conventional orientation of market, the conventional custom of market orientation is always not adequate. The analysis of comparative effectiveness of model implementation strategies reveals that the tiered pricing systems, public-private joint ventures, and the open access mechanisms possess the highest potential of egalitarian distribution [49]. Specialized training is important but education above it proves critical. Clinical implementation observations show that instead of purely procedural knowledge, there is a need for the skill to critically evaluate AI-supported suggestions, and appropriately use their human control. The most effective programs make these more general skills a part of their training programs. Most importantly, both research and vendors agree that AI in healthcare imaging should not be a substitute for human capability, but rather complement human capability–achieving both a better technical accuracy and human aspects in medicine. Thinking of innovation and inclusion as actual mutually beneficial goals, based on which Artificial Intelligence could produce innovative solutions that really benefit all the citizens with dignity and excellence [50].

References

1. Ting DSW et al (2021) AI for diabetic retinopathy screening in low-resource settings. Nature Rev Bioeng 1(1):12–24
2. Yarman BS, Rathore SPS (2025) The future of AI in disease detection–a look at emerging trends and future directions in the use of AI for disease detection and diagnosis. In: Singh R, Gehlot A, Rathour N, Akram SV (eds) AI in disease detection: advancements and applications. Wiley, Hoboken, pp 265–288. https://doi.org/10.1002/9781394278695
3. Jothi CS, Starlin MA, Surya E et al (2025) Revolutionizing healthcare through robotics and AI integration: a comprehensive approach. In: Exploring the micro world of robotics through insect robots. IGI Global, Hershey, pp 213–234
4. Ivchyk V (2024) Overcoming barriers to artificial intelligence adoption. Three Seas Econ J 5(4):14–20
5. Gichoya JW, et al. (2022) AI recognition of patient race in medical imaging: a modelling study. Lancet Digital Health 4(6):e406–e414
6. Graham HR, King C, Rahman AE et al (2025) Reducing global inequities in medical oxygen access: the lancet global health commission on medical oxygen security. Lancet Global Health 13(3):e528–e584
7. Philipsen RHHM et al (2023) AI for tuberculosis detection in chest X-rays: a multi-country evaluation. Radiology 307(1):e221291
8. Mwogi T et al (2022) Economic evaluation of AI in low-resource diagnostic imaging. BMJ Global Health 7(5):e008456
9. Rodriguez-Ruiz A et al (2024) Cost-effectiveness of AI-supported breast cancer screening in low-resource settings: a modeling study. Lancet Digital Health 6(3):e190–e199
10. Soufan F, Tukur HN, Tamir RG et al (2025) Environmental factors and cardiovascular susceptibility: toward personalized prevention mediated by the role of artificial intelligence–a narrative review. Health Sci Rep 8(3):e70588
11. Rangarajan D, Rangarajan A, Reddy CKK, Doss S (2025) Exploring the next-gen transformations in healthcare through the impact of AI and IoT. In: Intelligent systems and IoT applications in clinical health. IGI Global, Hershey, pp 73–98
12. Larrazabal AJ et al (2020) Gender imbalance in medical imaging datasets produces biased classifiers for computer-aided diagnosis. PNAS 117(23):12592–12594
13. Seyyed-Kalantari L et al (2021) Underdiagnosis bias of AI in medical imaging. Nature 600(7889):450–456
14. Hussain SA, Bresnahan M, Zhuang J (2025) The bias algorithm: how AI in healthcare exacerbates ethnic and racial disparities–a scoping review. Ethnicity Health 30(2):197–214
15. Abdulai AF (2025) Is generative AI increasing the risk for technology-mediated trauma among vulnerable populations? Nursing Inquiry 32(1):e12686
16. Koçak B, Ponsiglione A, Stanzione A et al (2025) Bias in artificial intelligence for medical imaging: fundamentals, detection, avoidance, mitigation, challenges, ethics, and prospects. Diagnostic Interventional Radiol 31(2):75
17. Faust O, Salvi M, Barua PD et al (2025) Issues and limitations on the road to fair and inclusive AI solutions for biomedical challenges. Sensors 25(1):205
18. Sheller MJ et al (2023) Federated learning for medical imaging: a multi-institutional validation of brain tumor segmentation. Nature Commun 14(1):6058

19. Marko JGO, Neagu CD, Anand PB (2025) Examining inclusivity: the use of AI and diverse populations in health and social care: a systematic review. BMC Med Inf Decis Making 25(1):57
20. Hoagland A, Kipping S (2024) Challenges in promoting health equity and reducing disparities in access across new and established technologies. Can J Cardiol 40(6):1154–1167. https://doi.org/10.1016/j.cjca.2024.02.014
21. Edet JE, Akyala AI, Edward AO, Ikaiddi AA, Epelle J, Etimedet E, Oluwagbohun O (2025) Harnessing artificial intelligence for public health surveillance in Africa: Current applications, challenges, and opportunities: A scoping review. International Journal of Research and Innovation in Social Science 9(7):2791–2828
22. Strika Z, Petkovic K, Likic R, Batenburg R (2025) Bridging healthcare gaps: a scoping review on the role of artificial intelligence, deep learning, and large language models in alleviating problems in medical deserts. Postgraduate Med J 101(1191):4–16
23. Vishwakarma LP, Singh RK, Mishra R, Kumari A (2025) Application of artificial intelligence for resilient and sustainable healthcare system: systematic literature review and future research directions. Int J Prod Res 63(2):822–844
24. Pradhan N, Tamang M, Rai S et al (2025) Reducing health inequities through total knee arthroplasty: an experience from Bhutan. Health Sci Rep 8(2):e70459
25. Kučević E, Grünewald F, Schanz, N (2024). Towards a simplified AI adoption framework: Success factors for the implementation of artificial intelligence information systems. In: International conference on human-computer interaction. Springer Nature Switzerland, Cham, pp 88–106
26. Nuthakki S (2023) The ethical and social implications of using AI in healthcare-a literature review. Int J Sci Res 12(11):10–21275
27. Sharma A, Biloria D (2025) Sociological perspective on the future of AI in health: trends and prospects. In: AI technologies and advancements for psychological well-being and healthcare. IGI Global, Hershey, pp 53–76
28. Mittelstadt B et al (2023) The ethics of AI in healthcare: a systematic review of frameworks and implementation challenges. Nature Mach Intell 5(9):789–802
29. Mersha M, Lam K, Wood J, Alshami AK, Kalita J (2024). Explainable artificial intelligence: A survey of needs, techniques, applications, and future direction. Neurocomputing 599:128111
30. Shafik W, Singh R, Kumar V (2025) Artificial intelligence transparency and explainability in sustainable healthcare. In: Transforming healthcare sector through artificial intelligence and environmental sustainability. Springer Nature Singapore, Singapore, pp 165–191
31. Sahebi S, Formosa P (2025) The AI-mediated communication dilemma: epistemic trust, social media, and the challenge of generative artificial intelligence. Synthese 205(3):1–24
32. Madanchian M, Taherdoost H (2025) Barriers and enablers of AI adoption in human resource management: a critical analysis of organizational and technological factors. Information 16(1):51
33. Sharma N, Kaushik P (2025) Integration of AI in healthcare systems–a discussion of the challenges and opportunities of integrating AI in healthcare systems for disease detection and diagnosis. In: Singh R, Gehlot A, Rathour N, Akram SV (eds) AI in disease detection: advancements and applications. Wiley, Hoboken, pp 239–263. https://doi.org/10.1002/9781394278695
34. Willem T, Fritzsche MC, Zimmermann BM et al (2025) Embedded ethics in practice: a toolbox for integrating the analysis of ethical and social issues into healthcare AI research. Sci Eng Ethics 31(1):1–22
35. Subash B, Whig P (2025) Principles and frameworks. In: Ethical dimensions of AI development. IGI Global, Hershey, pp 1–22
36. Chellasamy A, Elangovan N, Nagarathinam A, Rangasamy S (2025) Patients' trust in the Indian healthcare system and its impact on the intention to use artificial intelligence-based healthcare chatbots. J Asia Business Stud 19(3):730–747
37. Sendak MP et al (2023) Real-world integration of AI into clinical workflows: lessons from healthcare systems. NPJ Digital Med 6(1):52

38. Price WN et al (2023) Legal and ethical implications of AI in radiology. J Am College Radiol 20(2):245–253
39. Godinho Filho M, de Almeida SVQ, Lage Junior M et al (2025) A path to follow to overcome foundational barriers to the adoption of artificial intelligence within the manufacturing industry: a conceptual framework. Enterprise Inf Syst 19(1–2):2458685
40. Laein GD (2025) Global perspectives on governing healthcare AI: prioritising safety, equity and collaboration. BMJ Leader 9(1)
41. WHO (2021) Ethics and governance of artificial intelligence for health. World Health Organization, Geneva
42. Krishnamoorthy MV (2024) Meta-sealing: a revolutionizing integrity assurance protocol for transparent, tamper-proof, and trustworthy AI system. Preprint, arXiv:2411.00069
43. Aman Z, Qidwai MA (2025) Role of artificial intelligence in strengthening healthcare systems. In: Intersection of human rights and AI in healthcare. IGI Global Scientific Publishing, Hershey, pp 253–282
44. Koebe P (2025) How digital technologies and AI contribute to achieving the health-related SDGs. Int J Inf Manag Data Insights 5(1):100298
45. Adhikari S, Ahmed I, Bajracharya D et al (2025) Transforming healthcare through just, equitable and quality driven artificial intelligence solutions in South Asia. NPJ Digital Medicine 8(1):139
46. Kasali K, Oladapo R (2025) Utilizing predictive analytics to improve healthcare access in the United States (US). World Journal of Advanced Research and Reviews 25(3):1465–1470
47. Lekadir K, Frangi AF, Porras AR et al (2025) Future-AI: international consensus guideline for trustworthy and deployable artificial intelligence in healthcare. BMJ 388
48. Megahd N, El Kayaly D, Ammar A (2024) Equity, and equality. Ethical Challenges Future Neurosurgery 31
49. Trehan A (2025) The road ahead: AI and data science as pillars for sustainable equity. In: Advancing social equity through accessible green innovation. IGI Global Scientific Publishing, Hershey, pp 421–436
50. Ashraf ZA, Mustafa N (2025) Role of AI in transforming society. In: Intersection of human rights and AI in healthcare. IGI Global Scientific Publishing, Hershey, pp 431–452

Toward Responsible Innovation: Synthesizing Progress and Charting the Ethical Future of AI in Medical Imaging

Mohamed Hammad

1 Introduction

Integration of Artificial Intelligence (AI) in medical image analysis represents one of the most intensive technical changes in contemporary medicine [1–6]. This book has made a comprehensive discovery of this developed domain, which detects projections for real -world applications from the founder algorithm that now allows clinical diagnosis, prognostics and treatment plan. During the previous chapters, we checked how intensive learning models, computer vision techniques, and hybrid AI architecture are rapidly embedded in clinical workflows, increasing accuracy, efficiency and access to clinical imaging. From early adoptions of rules-based systems to wide deployment of convolutional neural networks (CNNs) and transformer-based models, AI's visit in medical imaging is marked by continuous refinement, verification and integration [7–10].

As we end this exploration, it is timely and necessary that we move our attention to the potential vision to a possible vision. The purpose of this chapter is not only to summarize the important progress in the book, but to expand the interaction towards the AI's emerging front in healthcare. In doing so, we believe that AI is not a stable innovation; Rather, it is a dynamic and developed paradigm that defines the practice of drug size, challenge and again. The role of AI is expanding into an associate agent from an accessory tool - capable of interacting with physicians, learning from clinical reaction and participating in clinical logic [11]. Figure 1 illustrates the timeline of AI development in medical imaging.

M. Hammad (✉)
EIAS Data Science Lab, College of Computer and Information Sciences, Prince Sultan University, Riyadh, Saudi Arabia
e-mail: mhammad@psu.edu.sa

N. Ben Aoun et al. (eds.), *AI for Medical Image Analysis*,
https://doi.org/10.1007/978-3-032-02963-8_12

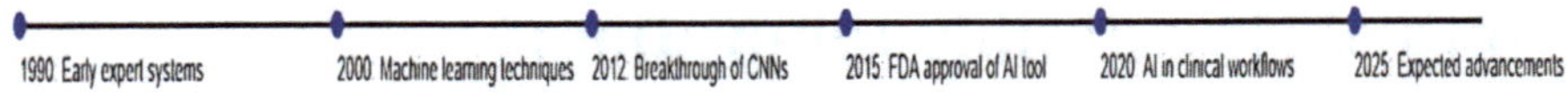
1990 Early expert systems
2000 Machine learning techniques
2012 Breakthrough of CNNs
2015 FDA approval of AI tool
2020 AI in clinical workflows
2025 Expected advancements

Fig. 1 Timeline of AI development in medical imaging

In addition, the conclusion of this discussion with the perspective that appears forward performs an important epidemiology work. It invites researchers, physicians and policy makers to not only do AI, but also grounded, clinically relevant and socially justified. In medical image analysis, the future of AI should be imagined in the context of stability, interpretation, interdisciplinary cooperation and global access. By expressing this vision, the final chapter aims to synthesize collective insights from previous chapters and project a roadmap for innovation responsible in AI-managed medicine. In doing so, it outlines the central thesis of this work: that AI, when thinking is designed and deployed equally, makes a unique promise not only to change medical imaging but also widespread healthcare landscapes.

2 Summary of Key Insights

The application of AI in Medical Image Analysis has brought a wide array of successes, which has greatly changed the scenario of clinical medicine [12–15]. During this book, we have examined the complex interplay between AI algorithm, clinical imaging modality and medical workflows. A central insight that emerges from this synthesis is AI's ability to convert medical imaging into more standardized, data-powered exercises from expert-dependent discipline. This change is not only technical; It is epidemic, because it changes how clinical knowledge arises, validated, and functioning within the clinical settings.

One of the most important insights is related to the role of intensive learning, especially CNN, in automatic image interpretation functions with performance metrics that cross the rival and, in some cases, those of human experts. These models have demonstrated remarkable efficiency in various tasks such as image classification (e.g., detecting pneumonia in chest X-rays) [16], object detection (e.g., pulmonary nodules in CT scans) [17], and the semantic segment (e.g., painting tumor margin in brain MRI) [18]. The ability of these algorithms to process high-dimensional image data, learn autonomously discriminatory features, and generalization in different imaging conditions has provided them unavoidable in contemporary radiological practice.

Another important insight is the expansion of AI's utility beyond quantitative imaging and exposure stratification and beyond classification. For example, radiomic analysis - where a large number of quantitative characteristics are extracted from medical images - the patient's diagnosis, treatment reaction, and disease repetition has been extended by machine learning methods to generate future models for repetition. These applications give an example of a movement towards accurate therapy, where imaging is used not only for physical evaluation, but also to extract biomarkers that indicate individual clinical decisions.

The book has also highlighted the importance of multi-modal and multi-source data integration, referring to imaging data with electronic health records (EHRS) [19], genetic information, laboratory findings and demographic variables. Such integration enables the development of multi-input AI models capable of overall patient evaluation, thus expanding the usefulness of imaging beyond traditional boundaries. For example, a combination of CT imaging features with serum biomarkers and genetic profiles can increase clinical accuracy in oncological screening and enable more fine stratification of patients for targeted treatments.

Importantly, many chapters have documented the success of AI in low-resources and high-bound environment, which outlines its ability for global health equity. The deployment of AI-operated diagnostic tools on portable devices or edge computing platforms has facilitated screening programs in remote and underserved areas. Notable examples include the use of AI to detect tuberculosis on the chest X-rays and diabetic retinopathy from retinal funds images, reducing the dependence on specialist interpretation and enabling initial intervention. This democratization of clinical capacity is particularly important in areas facing trained radiologists and medical infrastructure.

In addition, the book emphasizes the increasing relevance of clear AI in clinical practice. Faith in the AI system is accidental on their interpretation and transparency. Methods like meditation map, strength visualization and class activation mapping have been rapidly adopted to allow physicians to understand the logic behind algorithm predictions. It promotes human-AI cooperation rather than replacement, providing enhanced AI intelligence, which supports, rather than clinical decisions. Figure 2 provides a workflow diagram that is essential for understanding how AI integrates into clinical workflows.

Finally, a recurring insight throughout the chapters has an important role in data quality, diversity and moral design in AI model development. The performance of the AI model and generally is unwavering to the representation of their training dataset. Trained models on homogeneous or biased datasets are prone to systematic errors when deployed in real-world settings with asymmetrical patient population. The recognition of the issue has laid increasing emphasis with the aim of curing diverse and well annotated imaging repository on Federated Learning, Data Augmentation Strategy and International Consortia [20, 21]. Table 1 summarizes different AI techniques, clarifying the various methodologies employed in medical imaging and their relevance to the research objectives.

Fig. 2 Workflow of AI in medical imaging

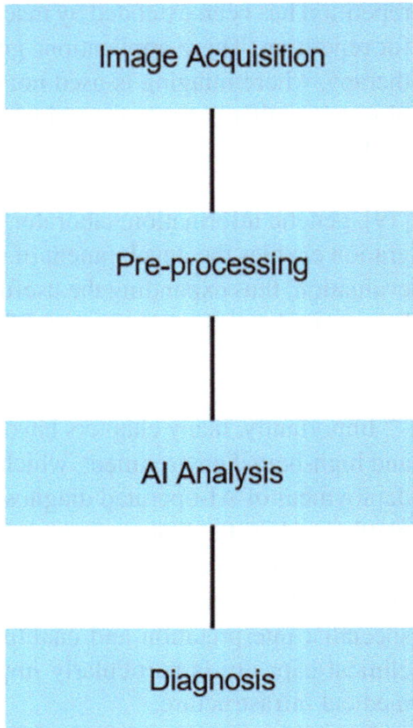

Table 1 Comparison of AI techniques in medical imaging [22, 23]

AI technique	Applications	Strengths	Weaknesses
Convolutional neural networks (CNNs)	Image classification, object detection	High accuracy, automated feature extraction	Requires large datasets
Support vector machines (SVM)	Classification tasks	Effective in high-dimensional spaces	Less effective with large datasets
Decision trees	Diagnosis support	Easy to interpret, fast training	Prone to overfitting
Random forests	Predictive modeling	Robust to overfitting, handles missing values	Less interpretable than trees
Transformer models	Multi-modal data analysis	Handles sequential data well	Computationally intensive

3 The Evolving Landscape of AI in Healthcare

The Healthcare sector is undergoing an intensive change induced by intelligence (AI), especially within the domain of medical imaging [24]. Over the past decade, the landscape embedded in the regular diagnostic workflows has shifted from the experimental AI prototype limited to the research settings for the research settings for fully operational clinical decision support systems. This development is not just a technical infection; It refers to a reconstruction of very conception of clinical epistemology, workflow logistics and clinical expertise. AI is redefining the boundaries between machine calculations and clinical intuition, providing unprecedented opportunities for scalability, stability and accuracy in healthcare distribution [25].

One of the most important effects of AI has been restructuring the clinical workflows. Traditionally, the interpretation of medical images was a labor-intensive function, requiring high levels of specialization, subject to variability between physicians and prone to human error, especially in high-volume settings. AI, especially deep learning models, have re-configured this process by automating several stages-from pre-processing and division to detection, classification and report generations. The AI systems now regularly read the first passage of imaging studies, immediately destroying immediate cases such as pneumothorax, intracranial hemorrhage, or pulmonary embolism for radiologist review. This triage capacity has not only improved the efficiency of clinical throughput, but has also increased clinical priority, ensuring that significant conclusions do not delay the overburden system.

Another dimension of the developed role of AI is its increasing autonomy in image interpretation, supported by regulatory verification and clinical trials. FDA and equivalent bodies in Europe and Asia have approved several A-SAC equipment for autonomous clinical use, such as IDX-DR for diabetic retinopathy and AIDOC for emergency radiology triage [26]. These approvals mark a paradigm change in clinical liability and faith, where AI is now seen not just a supplementary tool but as a accountable agent in the clinical process. Such an infection requires a strong mechanism to monitor clinical rules, algorithm auditing and real -world performance. aspects that are becoming integral to digital health infrastructure.

In parallel, the landscape is looking at the convergence of AI with advanced imaging technologies. High-resolution imaging methods such as 7 t MRI, spectral CT, and 3D ultrasounds produce vast amounts, which are often reduced due to cognitive and temporary obstacles on human interpretation. AI provides computational infrastructure to take advantage of this rich data environment. For example, transformer-based models and hybrid vision-language architecture are now able to integrate imaging data with this radiology report, which enable multi-model understanding that overcomes traditional silence analysis. This has inspired for the emergence of AI systems that can not only analyze images but can also refer to findings within a broad clinical story, an advancement is important for comprehensive diagnosis and personal treatment plan.

Emerging trends also indicate decentralization of clinical intelligence. Edge AI and Mobile Health Applications bring clinical capabilities at the point of care, especially in an underserved or remote environment. For example, the AI-operated ultrasound systems now enable the rights in rural areas to make a maternity assessment with the level of already restricted accuracy for special sonographers. Similarly, smartphone-based retinal imaging enabling diabetic retinopathy screening jointly in community pharmacies and primary care clinics with AI interpretation.

These innovations are helping to bridge the urban-rural healthcare division, which historically provides initial diagnosis and timely intervention for the population in health care systems.

In tertiary and quaternary care centers, AI is further contributing to clinical workflow orchestration [27]. Advanced AI platforms are being integrated with Radiology Information System (RIS), Picture Archiveing and Communication System (PACS), and Electronic Health Records (EHR), which prefer matters on the basis of urgency, and even pre-studied or pre-studied or facilitated guidelines for pre-study or pre-studied pre-study or pre-determined direction Suggestions. The AI-operated orchestration of the workflows not only improves operating efficiency, but also reduces cognitive loads on physicians, allowing them to focus on complex clinical dilemmas and fine decisions.

In addition, the AI's landscape in healthcare is rapidly defined by cross-disciplinary and interpreting cooperation. The AI tools are now co-developed by radiologists, computer scientists, data engineers, bio-information and moralists, indicating departure from undisciplined innovation. The design, perfection and verification of the AI system is shaped by feedback loops from clinical users, patient advocacy groups and institutional stakeholders. Such cooperation ensures that the AI systems are not only technically strong, but also clinically relevant, morally aligned and user friendly.

A particularly transformative development is the rise of continuous teaching systems-AI model that develops through reaction and real-time integration of new data input. While currently approved AI systems are "locks" at the time of regulatory approval, future systems are expected to work under a adaptive framework installed by the pre-specified change protocol. These systems will enable the AI tool to adapt to changing disease patterns, demographic changes and imaging protocols without the need for full re -approval, thus ensuring long -term viability and clinical accuracy.

Finally, this developed landscape cannot be understood without accepting the socio-political and regulatory context that operates AI. Issues such as algorithm accountability, data sovereignty, regulatory harmony, and digital infrastructure inequality shape AI adoption speed and patterns. Institutions should develop strong policies on data governance, user training, liability distribution, and system integration, which to exploit the benefits of AI without increasing health inequalities or to introduce new forms of risk.

4 Envisioning the Future: Opportunities and Innovations

Artificial Intelligence (AI) in Medical Image Analysis is rich in future possibilities, many of which are beginning to cross the traditional boundaries of computational image processing and diagnostic ad [28–30]. As we move beyond the fundamental phase of AI fines and enter a phase of maturity and expansion, it becomes rapidly clear that AI is ready to play a central role in shaping the next generation of

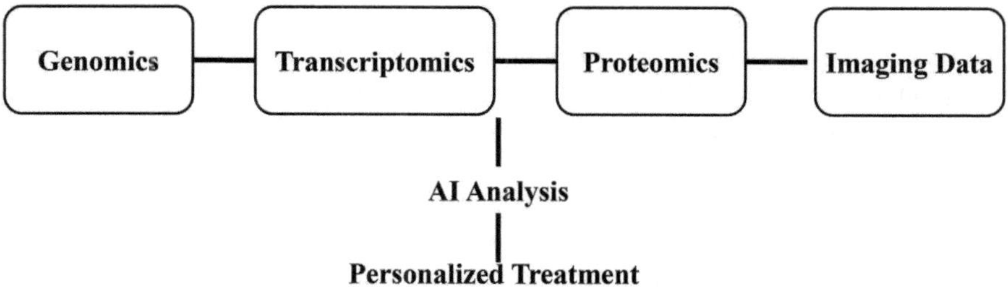

Fig. 3 AI integration in clinical workflows

individual, preventive and accurate-powered drugs. Imagining this future is more than extracting current trends; This requires an important inquiry to how emerging technologies, novel data paradigms, and systemic healthcare changes change to define new models of care with AI.

One of the most promising routes is contained in the AI's cohesive integration with multi-omics data, including genomics, transcriptomics, metabolomics, and metabolic data-along with traditional imaging methods [31]. Such convergence radio facilitates the emergence of genomics and imaging-genetics, where deep learning models not only explain physical and pathological characteristics in medical images, but also estimates the underlying molecular or genetic characteristics. For example, AI algorithms trained on radiological and genetic data have shown efficacy in predicting the mutation of gliomas or KRAS mutations in colorectal cancer using non-invasive imaging input (e.g., IDH1/2, EGFR) in colorectal cancer. This capacity has intensive implications for stitching remedies, avoiding unnecessary biopsy and guiding targeted medical tests. In this future paradigm, AI becomes a translation bridge that combines the image phenotype with biological signature, increasing the granulation of clinical decision making. Figure 3. illustrates multi-omics integration, allowing for comparisons between different data types and their impact on diagnostic accuracy.

AI has a transformative role in closely related personal medicine, which rests on the main principle of giving the right treatment to the right patient at the right time. Longitudinal imaging datasets, treatment history and patient results trained on patient results are being developed to predict individual reactions for chemotherapy, immunotherapy, radiotherapy and surgical intervention. Such models can use baseline imaging data to simulate treatment projections - tumor shrinkage, emergence of resistance, or repetition possibilities. In doing so, the AI moves beyond the static image interpretation and becomes a future modeling engine capable of imitating dynamic disease growth and therapeutic response. For example, AI-powered digital twin-individual patients are used to simulate many treatment routes, which enables physicians to select the course of action with highest projected efficacy and lowest risk.

Another compelling border is AI in detection of preventive medical and population-level early disease [32]. With the advent of omnipresent health monitoring and imaging-competent screening programs, AI is well deployed to detect pre-pregnancy or subclinical disease states, before they appear symptomatically. The AI algorithm can analyze imaging biomarkers that may indicate pre-introduction neurodegeneration, subtle vascular discrepancies, early fibrotic changes, or even a signal of minimal architectural deformities in mammograms that occur before a fatal change. Integration of such algorithms in primary care and screening settings can significantly transfer the healthcare paradigm from reactive care - after the onset of the disease - for proceeding and preventive care. This is not only the ability to reduce the cost of healthcare, but also to reduce patient sickness by enabling early, less aggressive interventions.

Parallel to these clinical innovations, the real -time AI emergence in traditional imaging [33]. Intraoperative imaging in neurosurgery, cardiovascular catheterization labs, or robot-assisted laparoscopic surgery depends on real-time imaging feedback. AI system capable of detecting quick division, tissue classification and discrepancy is being integrated into surgical navigation platforms. For example, during the affection of the brain tumor, AI can distinguish between tumors and healthy tissue margins in real time using intraoperative MRI or ultrasound, can guide more accurate excuses and reduce operative risk. These systems are beginning to include reinforcement agents that optimize procedural workflows, such as determining the next best camera angle or suggesting adjustment in the surgical trajectory. The convergence of AI with interventional imaging is thus redefining surgical accuracy and safety, which lays groundwork for intelligent intraoperative assistance systems.

In addition, generic AI models - such as generic Adversarial networks (GANS) and Diffusion models - are opening new domains of innovation in imaging science [34]. These models can make synthetic images uninterrupted by real people, a capacity that is bringing revolution in training data growth, domain adaptation and simulation-based verification. In rare disease modeling, where annotating data is rare, GANS can generate admirable deformity to train clinical systems or test. Beyond the increase, the generative model is now being used to predict the future imaging showing based on modality translation (e.g., CT scan to generate pseudo-MR images), super-resolution enhancement, and even current disease trajectory. It has applications in developing AI-based initial warning systems for dynamic disease forecasting and disease progression.

The integration of the foundation model and large multimodal transformer represents another range with transformational capacity. Inspired by successes in natural language processing (e.g., GPT, BERT), vision-language models such as BioGPT, Med-PaLM, and LLaVA-Med are being adapted for radiology [35–38]. These models are trained on a large -scale dataset of medical images associated with related reports and structured clinical metadata. They are capable of performing a wide array of tasks - from image captioning to visual input from the generation to answer clinically relevant questions. The vision of such models is not only meant to change the radiologist, but to serve as multicultural clinical assistants who synthesize imaging, text and structured data for assistance with differential diagnosis, radiology reporting and treatment plan. When aligned with strong clinical verification and transparency standards, these models may eventually enable the

Table 2 Future AI applications in medical imaging [39]

Future application	Description
Personalized medicine	Tailoring treatments based on individual patient data
Predictive analytics	Forecasting disease progression using imaging data
Real-time imaging analysis	Intraoperative support for surgeons
Automated reporting	Generating reports based on AI analysis
Integration with genomics	Combining imaging data with genetic information

usual AI systems capable of handling various clinical functions in imaging form and clinical domains.

In the end, we should imagine the future not only through the lens of technical capacity but also through moral, regulatory and social outline. In medical imaging, the future of AI should be shaped by principles of inclusion, access and transparency. Developing AI systems that are cultural and demographically inclusive-trained on diverse, representative datasets - would be important to ensure equity in clinical accuracy in the population. Regulatory bodies are also favorable for this new paradigm, with adaptive AI regulation, post-market monitoring, and continuous performance evaluation framework requirement. Establishment of learning of health systems - where the clinical reaction continuously informs and refines the AI performance - will be central for safe and durable innovation. Table 2 lists future AI applications, enhancing understanding by visually summarizing potential innovations in medical imaging methodologies.

5 Interdisciplinary Collaboration: A Crucial Path Forward

As AI becomes increasingly embedded within the diagnostic infrastructure of modern healthcare, it has become abundantly clear that the advancement, validation, and responsible deployment of AI in medical image analysis cannot be the domain of any single discipline [40]. The future of AI in medicine is, by necessity, an interdisciplinary endeavor—requiring deep collaboration among clinicians, computer scientists, biomedical engineers, data ethicists, legal experts, health informaticians, and policymakers. Such collaboration is not merely beneficial but foundational to the development of AI systems that are clinically meaningful, ethically sound, and socially equitable.

At the heart of successful interdisciplinary collaboration lies the clinical-AI interface—a bidirectional relationship in which medical professionals articulate real-world problems, diagnostic nuances, and clinical workflows, while AI developers translate those needs into algorithmic frameworks, data architectures, and model designs. Physicians play an indispensable role in analysis of medical images, identification of relevant diagnostic variables and interpretation of AI-generated output. Their domain expertise is important for training systems monitoring training and to evaluate whether algorithm decisions are aligned with current medical standards and pathophysiological realities.

However, cooperation should only proceed using physicians as an annotator. A more integrated approach includes co-design AI systems with physicians from the early stages of development. This involves defining the performance metrics that reflect clinical utility (e.g., sensitivity to the initial phase detection, or time-by-time for emergency triage tools), ensures user-centered interface design that fits into the existing clinical workflows, and identifies opportunities where AI can obstruct human decisions. For example, radiologists can help reduce functions where AI Excel (eg, identifying micro microcalcifications) requires a relevant argument (e.g., synthesizing imaging conclusions with the history of the patient). This promotes the paradigm of promoted intelligence, where it is not to replace AI but is designed to enhance the capabilities of physicians through collective interactions.

Equally important is the contribution of computer scientists, data scientists and AI engineers, who specialize in model architecture, algorithm adaptation, machine vision and statistical learning. His role includes tolerating models capable of constructing raw medical data into structures, learning formats, developing models capable of generalization in diverse population and imaging devices, and technical challenges such as overfitting, domain shifts and adverse strength. These experts should also ensure the fertility, scalability and computational efficiency of the AI system intended for clinical purposes. Importantly, they should be trained not only in technical skills but also in the principles of biomedical mortality and clinical context, which often disappear from the traditional computer science course.

The need for biomedical engineers and health information adds another layer of complexity, which serves as interoperability systems integrate and intermediaries between AI tools and existing healthcare infrastructure [41]. These professionals have been tasked to implement AI solutions within the Picture Archiving and Communication Systems (PACS), Radiology Information Systems (RIS), Electronic Health Records (EHR), and hospital IT environment. They ensure compliance with medical imaging standards such as DICOM, HL7, and FHIR, and work to optimize delays, data throughput and image quality in AI-Enhanced pipelines. Their expertise is particularly important in real-time clinical settings, where delay or system incompatibility can compromise patient safety.

Data privacy officers, cyber security experts, and bioethicists also play a growing role in interdisciplinary collaboration, especially given the sensitivity of health data and the moral implications of algorithm decision making. Their contribution includes confidentiality machine learning techniques such as federated learning and differential secrecy, algorithm bias and AI system for the AI system and the creation of guidelines for informed patient consent. When AI is used in diagnosis, the development of secrecy-conscience machine is developed. Ethical outlines should also be designed to address complex issues such as complex issues such as algorithm accountability, transparency in AI-driven decisions, and similar access to AI AI-enabled diagnosis in various population and geographical fields.

In addition, regulatory scientists, health economists and public health experts provide significant insights into scalability, cost-efficiency and social implications of AI deployment. They evaluate the long -term impact of AI on health system efficiency, resource allocation and health inequalities. For example, a cost-effectiveness analysis can suggest that an AI system for automatic mammography interpretation reduces double-reading costs while maintaining cancer detection rates-one insight that informs the policy recommendations and payment reimbursement models. These approaches are necessary to avoid adopting the AI system prematurely without adequate verification, or misuse of resources towards technologies that do not significantly improve the patient's consequences.

The importance of education and capacity building in this context cannot be eliminated. The medical course must be adapted to include AI literacy, ensuring that future physicians understand the principles, strength and limits of AI devices. Similarly, AI researchers and engineers should receive training in clinical logic, medical imaging methods and patient-focused care. Interdisciplinary training programs, joint degrees (e.g., MD-PHD in biomedical AI), and associate research environment-like AI research units are important to promote a new generation of hybrid professionals capable of navigating academic medical center-two domains with embedded AI research units.

Beyond the institutional level, international cooperation is also paramount. Global partnership between educational institutions, industry, government bodies and non-governmental organizations can speed up cross-border data, harmonize regulatory standards, and ensure that the AI systems are strong in geographical and demographic variations. Multinational consortia such as Global Alliance for Genomics and Health (GA4GH), The Radiological Society of North America AI challenges, and the European Commission's AI4HEALTH initiative is an example of how to promote collective intelligence while addressing global health challenges.

6 Navigating the Challenges Ahead

AI-Despite the impressive strides made in medical image analysis, the path ahead is neither linear nor without significant obstacles [42]. To fulfill its promise as a transformational force in healthcare for AI, it must cross a wide range of challenges spreading technical, clinical, moral, regulatory and socio-political domains. These challenges are not only casual, but are fundamental, as they directly affect the reliability, security, generality and equity of AI applications in therapy. Navigating them demands a coordinated, multi-disciplinary approach that emphasizes not only innovation, but also reflection, responsibility and flexibility.

6.1 Data Quality, Heterogeneity, and Annotation Limitations

A fundamental barrier to strengthening AI development in medical imaging is the issue of data quality and inequality. Medical images are produced using a wide range (e.g., CT, MRI, PET, ultrasound) and acquisition parameters that differ in institutions, equipment vendors, geographical areas and patient demographics. This diversity shows high level variance in training data, which can normally compromise the model if not addressed properly.

Furthermore, real-world datasets often contain noise, artifacts, missing metadata, and inconsistent labeling practices. Ground truth annotations—especially in tasks requiring fine-grained segmentation—are time-consuming to generate and subject to inter- and intra-observer variability. For example, delineating tumor boundaries in MRIs can vary significantly between radiologists, creating ambiguity in supervised training. The scarcity of well-annotated, high-fidelity datasets thus poses a critical bottleneck in model performance and validation.

Addressing this issue requires multi-pronged strategies such as:

- Data standardization protocols, including harmonization of imaging parameters and metadata fields.
- Federated learning, where models are trained on decentralized datasets from multiple institutions without transferring raw data, thereby preserving privacy while enhancing diversity.
- Semi-supervised and weakly supervised learning approaches reduce reliance on fully annotated datasets by leveraging unlabeled or partially labeled data.
- Consensus labeling frameworks using multiple expert annotators with adjudication, enhancing the reliability of ground truths.

6.2 Generalizability and Domain Shift

Even well-performing AI models frequently suffer from domain shifts when deployed outside the environment in which they were trained. This phenomenon occurs when a model trained on one dataset (e.g., a specific hospital's CT scan protocol) fails to generalize to other datasets with different imaging characteristics. Domain shift can arise from variations in patient populations, imaging modalities, disease prevalence, or even scanner calibration settings.

Mitigating domain shift involves:

- Domain adaptation techniques, such as adversarial training, style transfer, and normalization methods that align source and target feature distributions.
- External validation on independent, multi-institutional datasets prior to deployment.
- Continual learning frameworks that allow AI models to update incrementally without catastrophic forgetting of prior knowledge.
- Ensemble modeling and Bayesian approaches to quantify and mitigate predictive uncertainty in unfamiliar data contexts.

6.3 *Interpretability, Explainability, and Trust*

Another core challenge lies in the black-box nature of deep learning models, particularly CNNs and transformer architecture. These models often produce highly accurate predictions but lack transparency in their decision-making processes, which limits clinician trust and acceptance, especially in high-stakes diagnostic applications.

The push for explainable AI (XAI) is thus central to clinical adoption. Effective explainability involves:

- Visual tools such as saliency maps, Grad-CAM, and Layer-wise Relevance Propagation that highlight which regions of an image contributed most to the AI's decision.
- Counterfactual reasoning systems that generate "what-if" scenarios to illustrate how slight input changes would affect outcomes.
- Rule-based surrogate models or decision trees that approximate the behavior of complex models in an interpretable form.

However, a trade-off often exists between model accuracy and interpretability. Highly explainable models (e.g., linear classifiers) are easier to interpret but typically underperform compared to black-box models. Thus, balancing interpretability with performance remains a key unresolved issue, especially when deploying AI systems in regulatory-sensitive and medicolegal contexts.

6.4 *Bias, Fairness, and Health Equity*

AI systems are only as fair and unbiased as the data they are trained on. A growing body of evidence has demonstrated that AI models can perpetuate—and even exacerbate—existing healthcare disparities if trained on non-representative datasets. For example, models trained predominantly on data from high-income, urban hospitals may perform poorly on populations from rural areas, underrepresented ethnic groups, or low-resource settings.

Algorithmic bias can manifest at various stages, including:

- Data selection bias: Under-representation of specific demographic groups or clinical presentations.
- Measurement bias: Differences in imaging acquisition techniques or equipment across populations.
- Labeling bias: Subjectivity or systemic bias in human annotations, especially for complex or ambiguous cases.

Strategies to mitigate bias include:

- Diverse data sourcing through international collaborations and public-private data sharing partnerships.

- Bias detection and auditing tools that assess model performance stratified by age, sex, ethnicity, and socioeconomic status.
- Fairness-aware algorithms that incorporate fairness constraints during training (e.g., adversarial debiasing or reweighting methods).
- Community engagement and participatory design approaches that involve patients and marginalized communities in model development and validation.

6.5 Ethical and Regulatory Complexity

The ethical implications of deploying AI in healthcare are profound and multifaceted. Questions arise about responsibility and liability when AI-driven decisions result in adverse outcomes. The delegation of diagnostic authority to an algorithm raises normative concerns about autonomy, informed consent, and professional accountability.

Regulatory agencies such as the FDA, EMA, and MHRA are still evolving frameworks for the approval, surveillance, and governance of AI systems, particularly those that continue to learn post-deployment (adaptive AI). Key challenges include:

- Defining performance thresholds and clinical endpoints appropriate for different applications (screening, triage, diagnosis).
- Establishing explainability standards for clinical validation and approval.
- Creating post-market surveillance systems that continuously monitor AI performance and facilitate recall or update protocols when safety thresholds are breached.

Ethical frameworks must also address:

- The implications of AI replacing or overshadowing clinician judgment.
- The psychological effects on patients are informed by AI-generated diagnoses or risk scores.
- The commodification of patient data and the ethical boundaries of data monetization by commercial AI developers.

6.6 Integration into Clinical Practice and Workflow Alignment

Even the most technically advanced AI system may fail if it is poorly integrated into the clinical workflow. Clinicians are often overwhelmed by the sheer number of technologies vying for their attention. If AI systems disrupt workflows, increase documentation burden, or provide ambiguous outputs, they are likely to be underutilized or misused.

Table 3 Challenges and mitigation strategies for AI in medical imaging

Challenge	Mitigation strategy
Data Quality	Implement data standardization protocols
Bias and Fairness	Use diverse datasets and fairness-aware algorithms
Interpretability	Develop explainable AI models
Integration into Workflows	Ensure user-centered design

Effective clinical integration requires:

- User-centered design, involving clinicians in the UI/UX development process to ensure intuitive interfaces.
- Seamless integration with PACS, RIS, and EHR systems, avoiding fragmentation of data access.
- Real-time performance to support intraoperative and emergency care contexts.
- Clinical validation studies that assess not just accuracy but also usability, interpretability, and time-to-diagnosis improvements.

6.7 Sustainability and Environmental Impact

An emerging challenge often overlooked is the environmental sustainability of AI, particularly large-scale deep learning systems. Training complex models such as vision transformers or foundation models on medical imaging datasets can require massive computational resources, contributing to significant energy consumption and carbon emissions.

Future AI development must include:

- Model efficiency optimizations such as pruning, quantization, and knowledge distillation.
- Use of low-power hardware accelerators optimized for inference in clinical settings.
- Commitment to green AI principles, emphasizing accuracy-per-computation trade-offs and transparent reporting of energy usage during model training.

Table 3 outlines challenges and mitigation strategies, summarizing key findings that relate to the research hypothesis about the effectiveness of AI in medical imaging.

7 Vision for a Sustainable Future in AI-Driven Healthcare

As we enter a new era in medical diagnostics, the stability of AI- driven Healthcare is playing an important role. To pursue such technology, we must be guided not only by technical credit but also by moral -drew -wide, inclusion and long -term viability.

In this context, stability begins with responsible development. The AI algorithm must be built on a strong, representative dataset that reflects the diversity of the global population. This is not just a technical requirement; This is a moral imperative. Datasets used to train the AI system are the foundations on which these devices operate, and if the foundation is flawed - represents representation in gender, ethnicity, geography, or socio -economic background - then the outputs will reflect and strengthen those prejudices. In medical imaging, it can mean wrong diagnosis, delayed diagnosis, or even certain conditions. Such results not only compromise clinical effectiveness, but also existing health care inequalities. The AI's goal should raise care standards for all, not only for those who are already privileged by data availability.

To achieve this, healthcare AI developers and researchers must prefer diversity at every level of the data pipeline. This includes incorporating medical images from a wide range of institutions, demographics and geography and persistent auditing models for performance inequalities. Fairness -ware learning models-which are designed to detect and correct for prejudice-should become standard exercises, not alternative features. In addition, domain can help identify blind spots quickly in cooperation development with experts, moralists and affected communities. By embedding fairness in the very architecture of the AI system, we ensure that they become equipment for equity, promote a future where advanced diagnosis and care are accessible to all, regardless of the background or situation.

When trained on narrow or biased data, the AI system not only fails to serve all patients equally, but also actively deteriorates existing inequalities in healthcare. For example, assuming an AI model to detect skin cancer is mainly trained on mild skin tone images. In that case, it may diagnose or completely miss in patients with dark skin. This discrepancy may cause delayed treatment, wrong forecast, and finally, loss of confidence in medical AI technologies. Such prejudices are not always visible immediately, but their results are far-reaching, especially for marginalized people who already face systemic obstacles for quality care.

These risks highlight a deeper issue: blind spots in data collection reflect broad social inequalities. The undertaking in the dataset often reflects healthcare access, research participation and even digital record cycles. When the AI systems inherit these intervals, they can end a cycle of neglect, where some groups remain invisible in the development and deployment of state-of-the-art medical technologies. To prevent this, data diversity must be enhanced deliberately, and in the results the AI tool for equity should be constantly tested. Addressing prejudice is not just a matter of improving accuracy; It is about maintaining moral responsibility that there is no harm and ensures that the benefits of innovation reach everyone. Thus, curating the inclusive dataset and implementing the fairness-comprehensive learning model is just important steps towards healthcare solutions.

Deployment and governance also play an important role. AI tools should not act as opaque black boxes; Rather, they should be transparent, explanatory and accountable. Physicians need to rely on these systems, and patients should feel safe that artificial intelligence increases, not compromise, their care. By that end, regulatory bodies, policy makers and developers should collaborate to create guidelines that ensure safe and effective integration of AI in clinical settings.

Finally, a permanent vision includes continuous monitoring, reaction and recurrence. The AI system should be developed with medical knowledge, adapting to discoveries, changing the needs of the patient and developing with emerging diseases. In this way, AI becomes a dynamic partner in the future of healthcare, not a stable solution.

8 Final Thoughts: The Promise of AI in Revolutionizing Healthcare

Despite the challenges, the promise of AI's revolution in healthcare is very positive, inspired by the ability to increase the expertise of medical professionals. In medical image analysis, AI serves as a powerful tool that increases human intelligence by rapidly processing visual data, identifies patterns, and highlights the anomalies that may be subtle or easily ignored. For radiologists and pathologists, it means that the second set of eyes that can work tirelessly, can continuously analyze, and provide results in a fraction of time. Such capabilities are particularly important in a high-deserving environment, where time-sensitive diagnosis can significantly affect patient results.

Importantly, the integration of AI does not reduce the role of physicians, it elevates it. By automatic and streamlining the workflows, AI allows health professionals to focus on more complex decisions, patient interaction and treatment plans. In short, AI gives physicians the right to operate on top of their license, combining the speed and accuracy of machines with sympathy and significant thinking that only humans can provide. From the detection of the initial signs of cancer in the medical scan to predicting the progression of the disease using imaging biomarkers, AI is opening new frontiers in diagnosis and care that were once limited by human ability.

From the initial identity of life-drank diseases to enable real-time images to explain during surgery, AI is actively changing the landscape of modern health care distribution. Taking advantage of advanced algorithms, AI can detect abnormalities in medical images such as tumors, fractures, or internal bleeding compared to traditional methods. Long ago, symptoms also often emerged. This allows for timely intervention that can significantly improve the patient's survival rate and treatment results. Additionally, in surgical settings, A-in-operated imaging equipment helps doctors to support physicians in navigating complex procedures with real-time insights, increasing accuracy, reducing complexities and taking better decisions under pressure.

Beyond the Settings of Advanced Hospital, one of the most powerful contributions of AI lies in expanding access to care in the remote areas. In many parts of the world, the lack of radiologists and imaging experts leads to delayed diagnosis of deteriorating health inequalities or default. The AI frontline healthcare can help workers to operate this gap to conduct image-based screening and get immediate, AI-related assessment in areas without local experts. This democratization of clinical abilities not only brings high quality care closer to those who are most needed, but also helps to create more flexible, inclusive health systems capable of responding to the needs of diverse populations.

In addition, as AI becomes more individual, it paves the way for a new era of accurate therapy-where treatment is not a size-fit-everyone, but each patient's unique genetic, physical and careful to corresponding to the profile. By analyzing large datasets, which include genomic sequences, medical pictures, lifestyle factors and electronic health records, AI can identify patterns and correlations that would be almost impossible for humans to understand alone. This capacity allows physicians to predict the risk of the disease with greater accuracy, recommend highly individual treatment schemes and monitor the patient's reactions in real time, which reduces better results and adverse effects.

The fusion of AI with genomics, imaging and clinical data represents a transformative change of how we understand and treat the disease by our root cause. For example, in oncology, AI can help classify tumor subtypes based on molecular and imaging characteristics, enabling more targeted treatments. In cardiology, the AI can integrate imaging data with the wearable sensor output to estimate the heart condition before it becomes intense. This convergence of technologies not only enhances clinical accuracy but also leads to true prevention and welfare from disease management rather than reactive, healthcare. As AI continues to develop, its role in allocations of accurate therapy is not only promising but is unavoidable. Ultimately, AI's story in medical imaging is one of the empowerments - how intensive rehabilitation is provided, experienced and developed.

For healthcare professionals, AI offers an unprecedented set of devices that increase their clinical abilities, reduce cognitive charge, and allow them to focus more on patient-focused care. By automating regular tasks and providing data-powered insights, AI frees physicians to engage in deep clinical arguments and more meaningful interactions with patients. It acts not as a replacement, but as a reliable assistant that increases medical decision-making speed, accuracy and stability.

For patients, this empowerment comes through earlier detection, individual treatment plans and better access to care, especially in the areas of underestimated or remote. AI's ability to process and analyze complex data ensures that patients receive timely intervention, often before the symptoms increase, which improves the quality of life. In addition, for health systems under increasing demand, lack of staff and lack of resources, AI introduces new abilities that help to customize workflows, reduce errors and allocate resources more strategically. In every aspect, AI is a symbol of a vision of healthcare in medical imaging that is clever, sharp and more kind, offering a future where innovation supports human dignity and welfare.

9 Call to Action

The change of medical image analysis through AI is not unavoidable; It is deliberately directed by options, values and efforts that shape the future of healthcare. It is easy to see AI as an invincible force of progress, but each algorithm was developed, each dataset created, and each clinical equipment depicts human decisions show what is the priority, who to include, and how to measure success. For AI really to bring revolution in medical imaging that benefits everyone, it should be made with a conscious commitment for inclusion, transparency and patient-focused care. This means looking beyond the attraction of efficiency and accuracy to ask intensive questions: Are we solving the right problems? Are we all considering all patient population? Are we moral and accountable in our perspective?

True changes require a visionary effort of a visionary that can imagine bold possibilities, innovators who bring those vision into life through technology, moralists who maintain moral and social values, and physicians who ensure real -world's purpose and effects. It is at the intersection of these subjects that can thrive responsible and effective AI. In addition, global approaches should be welcomed - what works in one healthcare system may not be suitable for another. Especially from communities, attaching a wide range of sounds ensures that AI does not repeat or increase the existing inequalities, but becomes a force for equity and empowerment. As we stand in the tails of this new frontier, the forward route should be carved by a deepest root dedication to purpose, cooperation, and a better, fair healthcare future for the future, not with coincidence or convenience.

We call the researchers to continue the discovery of new algorithms and expand the scientific boundaries of medical imaging and beyond the scientific boundaries. As the area develops, researchers must advance innovation envelopes, develop more accurate, efficient and adaptable AI models that can address the complexity and diversity of human health. State-of-the-art technologies, such as deep learning and integration of nerve network have already achieved impressive results but still have a huge unused capacity. Researchers should continue to advance new functioning, fine-tune existing models, and identify new applications that can actually change how diseases are detected, diagnosed and treated. Their work is fundamental to increasing the continuous growth of AI in healthcare and ensure that AI is developed to meet the ever-causing challenges of therapy.

We urge physicians to be actively engaged with these techniques, providing significant reactions based on their first experiences and real -world needs, which they encounter daily. Physicians are those who understand the nuances of the patient's care, and their input is important to ensure that AI devices are not only scientifically sound, but also practically useful. By providing feedback, identifying boundaries and cooperating with AI developers, physicians can help shape the development of medical imaging technologies that actually increase their ability to diagnose and treat patients more effectively. In addition, their response may direct reforms that are responsible for the unpredictory and complexity of human health, ensuring that both AI-operated systems are accurate and optimal in the dynamic healthcare environment.

We also appeal to policy makers and regulators to prepare further -thinking structures that protect patient welfare by encouraging innovation. Since the AI continues to move forward, regulations should be coordinated with technological progress to ensure safety, privacy and moral standards. Policy makers should create rules that create a delicate balance, which protect the patient's rights and data privacy, while promoting an environment where innovation can flourish. This means developing flexible, adaptive regulatory approaches that estimate future challenges and support AI's responsible deployment in various healthcare settings. By establishing clear, well-considering guidelines, policy makers can ensure that AI in medical imaging contributes to a more efficient, accessible and equitable healthcare system while maintaining public belief in these transforming technologies.

In addition, we issue this call to all stakeholders - whether AI serves the best interests of humanity where technologists, teachers, entrepreneurs, or students are curious, important and committed to the future. AI's capacity in medical imaging is huge, but to feel this promise requires continuous engagement of all involved in this process. The technologist should contact his work with a mentality of moral responsibility, constantly questioning how his innovations worked to increase the patient results while protecting against misuse. Teachers have the responsibility to equip the next generation with knowledge and moral ideas to be necessary to carry AI forward in ways benefiting the society. Entrepreneurs should focus on the manufacture of businesses that not only produce benefits but also ensure alignment of their solutions along with the good of patients and communities. Students and learners in the field should maintain an important perspective, understanding that the future is exciting, it also comes with important moral and social challenges that require thoughtful ideas. In this collective effort, curiosity should be combined with significant thinking, and ambition should be matched with responsibility.

In addition, we issue this call to all stakeholders - whether AI serves the best interests of humanity where technologists, teachers, entrepreneurs, or students are curious, important and committed to the future. AI's capacity in medical imaging is huge, but to feel this promise requires continuous engagement of all involved in this process. The technologist should contact his work with a mentality of moral responsibility, constantly questioning how his innovations worked to increase the patient results while protecting against misuse. Teachers have the responsibility to equip the next generation with knowledge and moral ideas to be necessary to carry AI forward in ways benefiting the society. Entrepreneurs should focus on the manufacture of businesses that not only produce benefits but also ensure alignment of their solutions along with the good of patients and communities. Students and learners in the field should maintain an important perspective, understanding that the future is exciting, it also comes with important moral and social challenges that require thoughtful ideas. In this collective effort, curiosity should be combined with significant thinking, and ambition should be matched with responsibility.

AI's promise in medical imaging is real, but its feeling is in our collective hands. Each of us plays an important role in ensuring that AI has been developed and deployed in ways that we prefer human welfare and promote equity. This is a responsibility that cannot be taken lightly, as the decisions made today will shape the healthcare system for generations to come. Let us go ahead with not only hope, but also with resolve and responsibility-for the creation of an AI-operated healthcare system which is not only clever and more efficient, but also fair, more inclusive and really transformative. By embracing innovation with care and foresight, we can unlock AI's full capacity to improve health results, reduce inequalities and create more kind healthcare systems working for all.

10 Conclusion

As we attract this broad exploration closely, it is clear that artificial intelligence has not only entered the scope of medical image analysis, but it is actively shaping it again. This change appears in the clinical spectrum, ranging from increasing clinical accuracy to streamlining workflows and expanding clinical capabilities to the underserved areas. Algorithmic started once as curiosity, now mature in clinical utility, performing performance with the AI model that often crosses similarities or human expertise.

However, AI's journey in medical imaging is completely away. Future lies in promoting transparency, ensuring moral deployment and embracing interdisciplinary cooperation. Responsible innovation should prioritize fairness, interpretation and strengthening - such values that are particularly important in medicine where decisions have human results. Additionally, the capacity of multi-modal data integration and federated learning opens new frontiers for patient-specific, globally scalable solutions.

In short, this chapter has underlined a major proposal: AI is no longer an accessory tool, but a developed partner in healthcare. It brings the same access, quick diagnosis and data-operated clinical insight. The next stages require policy, practice and committed alignment of technology with human values. If thinking is done thoroughly, then the future of AI in medical imaging will not only be technically advanced but will also be deeply human.

References

1. Hammad M, Bakrey M, Bakhiet A, Tadeusiewicz R, Abd El-Latif AA, Pławiak P (2022) A novel end-to-end deep learning approach for cancer detection based on microscopic medical images. Biocybern Biomed Eng 42(3):737–748
2. Sakr AS, Pławiak P, Tadeusiewicz R, Pławiak J, Sakr M, Hammad M (2023) ECG-COVID: An end-to-end deep model based on electrocardiogram for COVID-19 detection. Inform Sci 619:324–339
3. Hammad M, ElAffendi M, Ateya AA, Abd El-Latif AA (2023) Efficient brain tumor detection with lightweight end-to-end deep learning model. Cancer 15(10):2837

4. Hammad M, ElAffendi M, Abd El-Latif AA (2025) CardioECGNet: A novel deep learning architecture for accurate and automated ECG signal classification across diverse cardiac conditions. Biomed Signal Process Control 106:107720
5. Hammad M, ElAffendi M, El-Latif AAA, Ateya AA, Ali G, Plawiak P (2025) Explainable AI for lung cancer detection via a custom CNN on CT images. Sci Rep 15(1):12707
6. Hammad M, ElAffendi M, Asim M, Abd El-Latif AA, Hashiesh R (2024) Automated lung cancer detection using novel genetic TPOT feature optimization with deep learning techniques. Results Eng 24:103448
7. Najjar R (2023) Redefining radiology: a review of artificial intelligence integration in medical imaging. Diagnostics 13(17):2760
8. Obuchowicz R, Strzelecki M, Piórkowski A (2024) Clinical applications of artificial intelligence in medical imaging and image processing—A review. Cancer 16(10):1870
9. Bulut MG, Unal S, Hammad M, Pławiak P (2025) Deep CNN-based detection of cardiac rhythm disorders using PPG signals from wearable devices. PLoS One 20(2):e0314154
10. Wang G, Badal A, Jia X, Maltz JS, Mueller K, Myers KJ et al (2022) Development of metaverse for intelligent healthcare. Nat Mach Intell 4(11):922–929
11. Suman A, Suman P, Padhy S, Kumar N, Singh A (2025) Healthcare revolution: Advances in AI-driven medical imaging and diagnosis. In: Responsible and explainable artificial intelligence in healthcare. Academic, pp 155–182
12. Ravera F, Gilardi N, Ballestrero A, Zoppoli G (2025) Applications, challenges and future directions of artificial intelligence in cardio-oncology. Eur J Clin Invest 55:e14370
13. Rashid Z, Ahmed H, Nadeem N, Zafar SB, Yousaf MZ (2025) The paradigm of digital health: AI applications and transformative trends. Neural Comput Applic 37:1–32
14. Okunlola FO, Adetuyi TG, Olajide PA, Okunlola AR, Adetuyi BO, Adeyemo-Eleyode VO et al (2025) Biomedical image characterization and radio genomics using machine learning techniques. In: Mining biomedical text, images and visual features for information retrieval. Academic, pp 397–421
15. Xiao X, Zhang J, Shao Y, Liu J, Shi K, He C, Kong D (2025) Deep learning-based medical ultrasound image and video segmentation methods: overview, frontiers, and challenges. Sensors 25(8):2361
16. Jaiswal AK, Tiwari P, Kumar S, Gupta D, Khanna A, Rodrigues JJ (2019) Identifying pneumonia in chest X-rays: A deep learning approach. Measurement 145:511–518
17. Armato SG, Giger ML, Moran CJ, Blackburn JT, Doi K, MacMahon H (1999) Computerized detection of pulmonary nodules on CT scans. Radiographics 19(5):1303–1311
18. Hou C, Yin H, Gong G, Wang L, Su Y, Lu J, Yin Y (2022) A novel approach for dose painting radiotherapy of brain metastases guided by mr perfusion images. Front Oncol 12:828312
19. Mohsen F, Ali H, El Hajj N, Shah Z (2022) Artificial intelligence-based methods for fusion of electronic health records and imaging data. Sci Rep 12(1):17981
20. Ugliotti FM, Osello A (eds) (2022) Handbook of research on implementing digital reality and interactive technologies to achieve society 5.0. IGI Global
21. Cazenave M, Cunha E, de Beer F (2024) Bakeng se Afrika: Digital skeletal repository: Advancing biological anthropology and medical. In: How to use 3D printing innovations and digital storage to democratize anatomy education, vol 6, p 63
22. Kasban H, El-Bendary MAM, Salama DH (2015) A comparative study of medical imaging techniques. Int J Inf Sci Intell Syst 4(2):37–58
23. Preston K (ed) (2012) Medical imaging techniques: A comparison. Springer Science & Business Media
24. Pesapane F, Codari M, Sardanelli F (2018) Artificial intelligence in medical imaging: threat or opportunity? Radiologists again at the forefront of innovation in medicine. Eur Radiol Exp 2:1–10
25. Aminizadeh S, Heidari A, Dehghan M, Toumaj S, Rezaei M, Navimipour NJ et al (2024) Opportunities and challenges of artificial intelligence and distributed systems to improve the quality of healthcare service. Artif Intell Med 149:102779

26. Nawrat, Z. (2013). Handbook of polymer applications in medicine and medical devices: 8. Review of research in cardiovascular devices
27. Giri A, Din FU (2025) Role of data as an interface between primary, secondary and tertiary care: Evidence from literature. Inform Health 2(1):63–72
28. Rudnicka Z, Szczepanski J, Pregowska A (2024) Artificial intelligence-based algorithms in medical image scan segmentation and intelligent visual content generation—A concise overview. Electronics 13(4):746
29. Kiziloluk S, Sert E, Hammad M, Tadeusiewicz R, Pławiak P (2024) EO-CNN: Equilibrium optimization-based hyperparameter tuning for enhanced pneumonia and COVID-19 detection using AlexNet and DarkNet19. Biocybern Biomed Eng 44(3):635–650
30. Patro KK, Allam JP, Neelapu BC, Tadeusiewicz R, Acharya UR, Hammad M et al (2023) Application of Kronecker convolutions in deep learning technique for automated detection of kidney stones with coronal CT images. Inform Sci 640:119005
31. Biswas N, Chakrabarti S (2020) Artificial intelligence (AI)-based systems biology approaches in multi-omics data analysis of cancer. Front Oncol 10:588221
32. Shukla T (2024) Beyond diagnosis: AI's role in preventive healthcare and early detection. Iconic Res Eng J 8:53–63
33. Liu Y, Chen Y, Han L (2023) Bioinformatics: Advancing biomedical discovery and innovation in the era of big data and artificial intelligence. Innov Med 1(1):100012
34. Showrov AA, Aziz MT, Nabil HR, Jim JR, Kabir MM, Mridha MF et al (2024) Generative adversarial networks (GANs) in medical imaging: advancements, applications and challenges. IEEE Access 12:35728–35753
35. Semary NA, Ahmed W, Amin K, Pławiak P, Hammad M (2023) Improving sentiment classification using a RoBERTa-based hybrid model. Front Hum Neurosci 17:1292010
36. Noura AS, Ahmed W, Amin K, Pławiak P, Hammad M (2024) Enhancing machine learning-based sentiment analysis through feature extraction techniques. PLoS One 19(2):e0294968
37. Soni N, Ora M, Agarwal A, Yang T, Bathla G (2024) A review of the opportunities and challenges with large language models in radiology: The road ahead. ANJR Am J Neuroradiol 46(7):1292–1299
38. Hammad M, Ahmed W (2025) Natural language processing techniques for social media sentiment analysis. In: Navigating challenges of object detection through cognitive computing. IGI Global Scientific Publishing, pp 33–62
39. Panayides AS, Amini A, Filipovic ND, Sharma A, Tsaftaris SA, Young A et al (2020) AI in medical imaging informatics: current challenges and future directions. IEEE J Biomed Health Inform 24(7):1837–1857
40. Ahmed Z, Mohamed K, Zeeshan S, Dong X (2020) Artificial intelligence with multi-functional machine learning platform development for better healthcare and precision medicine. Database 2020:baaa010
41. Hashemi Fotemi SG, Mannuru NR, Kumar Bevara RV, Mannuru A (2024) A systematic review of the integration of information science, artificial intelligence, and medical engineering in healthcare: Current trends and future directions. InfoSci Trends 1(2):29–42
42. Gholap AD, Uddin MJ, Faiyazuddin M, Omri A, Gowri S, Khalid M (2024) Advances in artificial intelligence in drug delivery and development: A comprehensive review. Comput Biol Med 178:108702

Index

N. Ben Aoun et al. (eds.), *AI for Medical Image Analysis*,
https://doi.org/10.1007/978-3-032-02963-8

MIX
Papier aus verantwortungsvollen Quellen
Paper from responsible sources
FSC® C105338

If you have any concerns about our products,
you can contact us on
ProductSafety@springernature.com

In case Publisher is established outside the EU,
the EU authorized representative is:
Springer Nature Customer Service Center GmbH
Europaplatz 3, 69115 Heidelberg, Germany

Printed by Libri Plureos GmbH
in Hamburg, Germany